FOGSI Focus
Imaging in Obstetrics and Gynecology

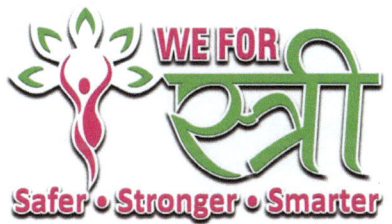

Video Content

Chapter 8: Ultrasound of Ectopic Pregnancy

Video Legend: Right Sided Ectopic Pregnancy

Description: Uterus is empty and on right side gestational sac is seen with yolk sac within it. Considerable amount of blood present in pouch of Douglas (POD) and anterior to uterus. Although patient was hemodynamically stable, presence of significant amount of blood requires urgent intervention. We did laparoscopic salpingectomy for this patient and it was incomplete tubal abortion.

FOGSI Focus
Imaging in Obstetrics and Gynecology

Editor-in-Chief

Nandita Palshetkar
MD FCPS FICOG FRCOG (UK)
Professor
Department of Obstetrics and Gynecology
Dr DY Patil Medical College, Hospital and
Research Centre
Navi Mumbai, Maharashtra, India
Past President, FOGSI, 2019
Scientific Director, Bloom IVF

Editor

Meenu Agarwal
DNB DGO FICOG
Trained in Endoscopy and IVF at Germany
Bachelor in Reproductive Surgery (European Board Certified)
Gynecological Endoscopic Surgeon and
Reproductive Medicine Specialist
National Director
Clinical Board, Morpheus IVF
Executive Board Member
International Society of Gynecological Endoscopy
Chairperson, Imaging Science Committee, FOGSI (2018–2021)
Course Director, International Training Courses in UAE

Co-Editors

Rohan Palshetkar
MS (Obs & Gyn) FRM
ART Consultant and Endoscopic Surgeon
Associate Professor
Unit Head
Dr DY Patil Medical College, Hospital and
Research Centre
Navi Mumbai, Maharashtra, India

Chinmay Umarji
MBBS DGO MRCOG (London UK) MRCP (Ireland)
Research Fellowship in Fetal Med
Consultant (Maternal and Fetal Medicine)
Visiting Expert (Maternal and Fetal Medicine)
Sassoon General Hospital, Pune
Consultant (Fetal and Maternal Medicine), Sahyadri Hospital
Deccan Umarji Hospital, Pune
Member, Antenatal Screening Committee
Government of Maharashtra
National Coordinator for Imaging Sciences Committee, FOGSI
Life Member, ISGE; Member, SLS
Editor, International Journal of Gynecological Endoscopy

Foreword

Hrishikesh D Pai

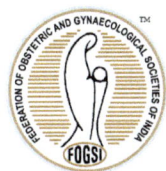

Federation of Obstetric and Gynaecological Societies of India (FOGSI)

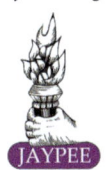

JAYPEE BROTHERS MEDICAL PUBLISHERS
The Health Sciences Publisher
New Delhi | London

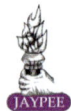 **Jaypee Brothers Medical Publishers (P) Ltd**

Headquarters

Jaypee Brothers Medical Publishers (P) Ltd
EMCA House, 23/23-B
Ansari Road, Daryaganj
New Delhi 110 002, India
Landline: +91-11-23272143, +91-11-23272703
+91-11-23282021, +91-11-23245672
Email: jaypee@jaypeebrothers.com

Corporate Office

Jaypee Brothers Medical Publishers (P) Ltd
4838/24, Ansari Road, Daryaganj
New Delhi 110 002, India
Phone: +91-11-43574357
Fax: +91-11-43574314
Email: jaypee@jaypeebrothers.com

Overseas Office

JP Medical Ltd
83 Victoria Street, London
SW1H 0HW (UK)
Phone: +44 20 3170 8910
Fax: +44 (0)20 3008 6180
Email: info@jpmedpub.com

Website: www.jaypeebrothers.com
Website: www.jaypeedigital.com

© 2021, Jaypee Brothers Medical Publishers

The views and opinions expressed in this book are solely those of the original contributor(s)/author(s) and do not necessarily represent those of editor(s) of the book.

All rights reserved. No part of this publication may be reproduced, stored or transmitted in any form or by any means, electronic, mechanical, photocopying, recording or otherwise, without the prior permission in writing of the publishers.

All brand names and product names used in this book are trade names, service marks, trademarks or registered trademarks of their respective owners. The publisher is not associated with any product or vendor mentioned in this book.

Medical knowledge and practice change constantly. This book is designed to provide accurate, authoritative information about the subject matter in question. However, readers are advised to check the most current information available on procedures included and check information from the manufacturer of each product to be administered, to verify the recommended dose, formula, method and duration of administration, adverse effects and contraindications. It is the responsibility of the practitioner to take all appropriate safety precautions. Neither the publisher nor the author(s)/editor(s) assume any liability for any injury and/or damage to persons or property arising from or related to use of material in this book.

This book is sold on the understanding that the publisher is not engaged in providing professional medical services. If such advice or services are required, the services of a competent medical professional should be sought.

Every effort has been made where necessary to contact holders of copyright to obtain permission to reproduce copyright material. If any have been inadvertently overlooked, the publisher will be pleased to make the necessary arrangements at the first opportunity. The **CD/DVD-ROM** (if any) provided in the sealed envelope with this book is complimentary and free of cost. **Not meant for sale.**

Inquiries for bulk sales may be solicited at: jaypee@jaypeebrothers.com

FOGSI Focus Imaging in Obstetrics and Gynecology

First Edition: **2021**

ISBN: 978-93-89776-35-5

Printed at Repro India Limited

Contributors

Aarti Deenadayal Tolani MD FICOG
Clinical Director
Mamata Fertility Hospital
Secunderabad, Telangana
Associate Editor, Minerva Ginecologica
Secunderabad, Telangana, India

Aashita Shrivastava MBBS MS
Consultant
Nishant Hospital
Patna, Bihar, India

Amogh Chimote MBBS MD
Gynecologist and Medical Director
Vaunshdhara Fertility Centre Pvt Ltd
Nagpur, Maharashtra, India

Anshu Baser MBBS 3rd Year
Resident
MGM Medical College and Hospital
Navi Mumbai, Maharashtra, India
Member, Mumbai Obstetrics and
Gynecological Society (MOGS)

Archana Baser MS DNB FRCOG FICOG
Director
Akash Hospital
Indore, Madhya Pradesh, India
Vice President, FOGSI, 2020
Organising Secretary, AICOG 2021, Indore
Managing Committee Member
ISAR (2018–2020)

Ashok Khurana
MBBS MD (Radiodiagnosis and Imaging)
Chairman and Consultant
(Reproductive Ultrasound)
The Ultrasound Lab
New Delhi, India

Chaitanya Nagori MD DGO
Director
Dr Nagori's Institute for Infertility and IVF
Ahmedabad, Gujarat, India

Chinmay Umarji
MBBS DGO MRCOG (London UK) MRCP
(Irelnd) Research Fellowship in Fetal Med
Consultant (Maternal and Fetal Medicine)
Visiting Expert (Maternal and Fetal Medicine)
Sassoon General Hospital, Pune
Consultant (Fetal and Maternal
Medicine), Sahyadri Hospital
Deccan Umarji Hospital, Pune
Member, Antenatal Screening Committee
Government of Maharashtra
National Coordinator for Imaging
Sciences, FOGSI
Life Member, ISGE; Member, SLS
Editor, International Journal of
Gynecological Endoscopy

Chinmayee Ratha MBBS MS (Obs & Gyn)
MRCOG (UK) FICOG FIMSA
Director
Resolution Fetal Medicine Centre
Hyderabad
Senior Consultant (Fetal Medicine)
Yashoda Hospital
Hyderabad, Telangana, India

Girija Wagh MD FICOG DIP ENDO FICS
Gynecologist, Obstetrician and
IVF Specialist
Cloudnine Hospital, Pune
Bharati Hospital
Pune, Maharashtra, India

Glossy Sabharwal MBBS MD Radiology
Director and Consultant
Department of Radiology
Jeewan Mala Hospital and WISH Clinic
New Delhi, India

Hema Desai MD
Obstetrician and Gynecologist
Mamata Fertility Hospital
Secunderabad, Telangana, India

Hitesh J Bhatt MBBS MD PGDMLS LLB
Advocate
B & S Medicolegal Consultancies
Mumbai, Maharashtra, India
Medicolegal Consultant
Past Chairperson (2014–2016)
Ethics and Medicolegal Committee, FOGSI

Indrani Suresh MD DCH
Director, MediScan Systems
Head, Fetal Medicine Unit, MediScan
Chennai, Tamil Nadu, India

Jayprakash Shah MD FICOG
Consultant and Fetal Medicine Expert
Rajni Hospital for Women
Ahmedabad, Gujarat, India

Jhillmill Kumari MBBS MD
Assistant professor
Anugrah Narayan Magadh
Medical College and Hospital
Gaya, Bihar, India

Kanchan Mukherjee MBBS CCT FRCOG
Consultant (Fetal Medicine)
Apollo Gleneagles Hospitals
Kolkata, West Bengal, India

Keshav Pai MBBS MS (Obs & Gyn) DGO
DNB (Obs & Gyn) Fellowship in Laparoscopy
Gynecologist
Ashvini Hospital
Navi Mumbai, Maharashtra, India

Liselotte Mettler PhD MD
Patroness
Kiel School of Gynaecological Endoscopy
Emeritus Professor
Department of Obstetrics and Gynecology
University Hospitals Schleswig-Holstein
Kiel, Germany
Lecturer and Visiting Professor
German Medical Center
Dubai Healthcare City, UAE

Mahima Arya MBBS 2nd Year
Junior Resident
Bharati Vidyapeeth University
Medical College and Hospital
Pune, Maharashtra, India

Mamata Deenadayal MD DGO
Founder and Medical Director
Mamata Fertility Hospital
Secunderabad, Telangana, India
President
Telangana Chapter of ISAR

Mandakini Pradhan
MBBS MD (Obs & Gyn) DNB
DM (Medical Genetics)
Professor and Head
Department of Maternal and
Reproductive Health
Sanjay Gandhi Postgraduate
Institute of Medical Sciences
Lucknow, Uttar Pradesh, India

Meenu Agarwal DNB DGO FICOG
Trained in Endoscopy and IVF at Germany
Bachelor in Reproductive Surgery (European
Board Certified)
Gynecological Endoscopic Surgeon and
Reproductive Medicine Specialist
National Director
Clinical Board, Morpheus IVF
Executive Board Member
International Society of
Gynecological Endoscopy
Chairperson
Imaging Science Committee (2018–2021)
Course Director
International Training Courses in UAE

Mumtaz P MBBS MD
Professor and Unit Chief
Department of Obstetrics and
Gynecology
MES Medical College, Kerala
Director
Mumtaz Clinic and Maternity Home
Perinthalmanna, Kerala, India

Contributors

Narendra Malhotra MD FICMCH
FICOG FRCOG FICS FMAS FIAP
President, INSARG
Past President
FOGSI/IFUMB/ISPAT/ISAR
Vice President, WAPM/SAFOG
Managing Director
Global Rainbow Health Care and
MNMH (P) Ltd
Agra, Uttar Pradesh, India
Professor, Sarajevo School of
Science and Technology, Croatia

Neeta Singh MBBS MS (Obs & Gyn)
Additional Professor
Department of Maternal and
Reproductive Health
Sanjay Gandhi Postgraduate Institute of
Medical Sciences
Lucknow, Uttar Pradesh, India

Neha Singh MS (Obs & Gyn) DNB
Fellowship in Fetal Med
Clinical fellow (Fetal Medicine)
Nowrosjee Wadia Maternity Hospital
Mumbai, Maharashtra, India

Neharika Malhotra MD (Gold Medalist)
DRM (Germany) FICMCH Fellow ICOG
(Rep Med) ICOG (USG)
Joint Secretary, FOGSI
Chair, YTP Committee, FOGSI
Director and Consultant
Global Rainbow IVF and MNMH (P) Ltd
Agra, Uttar Pradesh, India

Parth Shah MD DGO
Consultant (Fetal Medicine)
Rajni Hospital
Reshambai Hospital
Ahmedabad, Gujarat, India

Parul Choudhary Vali DGO ICOG
Consultant (Fetal Medicine)
Lara Hospital
Sara Mother and Child Hospital
Godhra, Gujarat, India

PK Shah MD
Emeritus Professor
Gynecologist and Obstetrician
Department of Obstetrics and Gynecology
KEM Hospital
Mumbai, Maharashtra, India

Pragya Nichite
MBBS DGO DNB (Obs & Gyn)
Gynecologist
Treetop Fetal Medicine and
Diagnostic Center
Navi Mumbai, Maharashtra, India

Pramod Vasantrao Patil MBBS DGO
DNB Fellowship in Fetal Medicine
Director
Fetus Day Clinic
Nashik, Maharashtra, India

Punam Dixit
MBBS (Hon) MS FRCOG (London)
Director
Punam Surgical and Maternity Clinic
Patna, Bihar, India
Member, Advisory Committee, ISUOG

Rohan Wagh MBBS
Medical Officer
Bharati Vidyapeeth Deemed University
Medical College and Hospital
Pune, Maharashtra, India

Rujul Jhaveri MS (Obs & Gyn)
Clinical Associate
Department of Fetal Medicine
Surya Mother and Child Care Hospital
Mumbai, Maharashtra, India

S Suresh MBBS FRCOG (Hon) DSc (Hon)
Director
MediScan Systems, Chennai
Visiting Professor in Perinatology
Sri Ramachandra Institute of Higher
Education and Research
PSG Hospital, Coimbatore, Tamil Nadu
Honorary Secretary
Voluntary Health Services (VHS) Hospital
Chennai, Tamil Nadu, India

Sachin Nichite MBBS DGO DNB
Fellowship in Fetal Med
Consultant (Fetal Medicine)
Treetop Fetal Medicine and
Sonography Centre
Navi Mumbai, Maharashtra, India

Seetha Ramamurthy Pal
MBBS DGO MD FRCOG FICOG RCOG/RCR
Diploma in Advanced Obstetric Ultrasound
Senior Consultant
(Fetal Medicine and Obstetrics)
Apollo Gleneagles Hospitals
Kolkata, West Bengal, India

Shreyasi Sharma
MBBS MD (Obs & Gyn) DNB
Fellowship in Fetal Med
Senior Consultant (Fetal Medicine)
Cloudnine Hospital
Gurugram, Haryana, India

Sonal Panchal MD
Ultrasound Consultant
Dr Nagori's Institute for
Infertility and IVF
Ahmedabad, Gujarat, India

Vandana Bansal MD DGO DNB MNAMS
MRCOG (Obs & Gyn) FICOG FNB (High Risk
Pregnancy and Perinatology)
Associate Professor
Nowrosjee Wadia Maternity Hospital
Mumbai, Maharashtra
Director and Head
Fetal Medicine Centre
Surya Mother and Child Care Hospital
Mumbai, Maharashtra, India

Varsha Mahajan MBBS DGO
Consultant Gynecologist
Akash Hospital
Indore, Madhya Pradesh, India

Foreword

It gives me immense pleasure to present this book to you. *FOGSI Focus Imaging in Obstetrics and Gynecology* should serve as a first reference to the reader for all day-to-day scanning queries in Obstetrics and Gynecology.

From the machine settings and room infrastructure to report writing, medicolegal tips and softwares, this book will hold the hand of the reader and walk them through.

With eminent national experts giving stepwise protocols on the relevant topics, we have made it simple, precise, and concise for your convenience.

Hrishikesh D Pai
MD FCPS FICOG MSc (USA) FRCOG
Gynecologist and Head of IVF Unit
Lilavati Hospital
Mumbai, Maharashtra, India
President Elect, FOGSI 2022
Scientific Director, Bloom IVF
Chief Administrator, FOGSI Manyata Project
Director, Corporate Affairs, IFFS
Secretary General, FOGSI (2015–2017)

Preface

There has been huge progress in the field of imaging due to advancement in technology, the availability of it across the section of society and most importantly the interest and huge efforts being taken by the emerging fetal medicine specialists. Imaging in obstetrics has become an extended arm of an obstetrician for optimizing the perinatal outcome as well as an inseparable tool for endoscopic surgeons, fertility specialists, and even for urogynecologists.

The writing of this book is driven by the enthusiasm and support of our very dear FOGSI's Past President, Dr Nandita Palshetkar.

FOGSI Focus Imaging in Obstetrics and Gynecology addresses from basic to advanced, from gynecology, infertility to obstetrics, covers all the topics with good quality images for the readers to understand and enjoy reading.

Simple language and presentation enable this as a handbook guide in the office of the consultant as a reference book for day-to-day challenges as well as for primary care obstetricians, postgraduate students, and internists.

This mammoth task was possible only with the efforts of contributing authors, who took out time to write such valuable chapters. Our heartfelt gratitude to all the contributors.

Happy reading!

Nandita Palshetkar
Meenu Agarwal
Rohan Palshetkar
Chinmay Umarji

Acknowledgments

We are extremely thankful to Shri Jitendar P Vij (Group Chairman), Mr Ankit Vij (Managing Director), Mr MS Mani (Group President), Ms Chetna Malhotra Vohra (Associate Director—Content Strategy), Ms Pooja Bhandari (Production Head), and Ms Kritika Dua (Senior Development Editor) of M/s Jaypee Brothers Medical Publishers (P) Ltd, New Delhi, India, for giving the go-ahead at the very beginning and helping us in every way possible to bring out this book.

Contents

1. Basic Principles of Ultrasound Machine 1
Sonal Panchal, Chaitanya Nagori
- Optimizing B-mode Image *1*
- Optimizing Doppler Image *3*
- Understanding the Artifacts *10*
- Safety of Doppler *11*
- Apart from this a Few Practical Tips on Planning your Setup *11*

2. Stepwise Standardized Approach to Ultrasound Examination of Female Pelvis 13
Sonal Panchal, Chaitanya Nagori
- Method *14*
- Adnexa *17*

3. Three-dimensional/Four-dimensional Ultrasound in Obstetrics: An Entertainment or an Empowerment 19
Sachin Nichite, Pragya Nichite
- Advantages of Three-dimensional/Four-dimensional or Volume Imaging *19*
- Various Modes and Tools Used in Three-dimensional/Four-dimensional Imaging *19*
- Practical Steps for Three-dimensional/Four-dimensional Ultrasound *21*
- Clinical Applications of Three-dimensional/Four-dimensional Ultrasound *22*
- Limitations of Three-dimensional/Four-dimensional Ultrasound *23*

4. Role of Color Flow and Doppler in Gynecology and Infertility 25
Amogh Chimote, Neharika Malhotra, Narendra Malhotra
- What is Color Doppler? *25*
- Variables in Doppler *25*
- Calculations in Doppler *26*
- How the Color Image is Formed? *26*
- Types of Doppler *26*
- Aliasing *26*
- Use of Doppler in Gynecology *27*
- Endometrial Polyp *29*
- Adnexal Ovarian Torsion *30*
- Endometriosis *31*
- Endometrioma *32*
- Peritoneal Endometriosis *32*
- Gestational Trophoblastic Disease *32*
- Gestational Trophoblastic Tumors *33*
- Ectopic Pregnancy *33*
- Scar Ectopic Pregnancy *34*
- Pelvic Congestion Syndrome *34*
- Malignant Uterine Tumors *34*
- Endometritis and Endometrial Carcinoma *34*

ROLE OF COLOR DOPPLER IN INFERTILITY *35*
- Study of Menstrual Cycle by Color Doppler *35*
- Changes in the Ovary *35*
- Uterine Perfusion *36*
- Changes in the Endometrium *37*
- Luteal Phase Scan *37*
- Ultrasound Technique for Uterine Biophysical Profile *38*
- Conception Rates with Uterine Scoring System for Reproduction Scores *39*

5. Ultrasound in Infertility: Follicular Dynamics and Endometrium 42
Sonal Panchal, Chaitanya Nagori, Meenu Agarwal
- Baseline Scan and Deciding the Stimulation Protocol *42*
- B-mode Features of a Mature Follicle *43*
- Doppler Features of a Good Preovulatory Follicle *44*
- B-mode Features of Pretrigger Endometrium with Good Receptivity *45*
- Secretory Phase Assessment *47*

6. Imaging in Endometriosis 49
Glossy Sabharwal, Meenu Agarwal, Liselotte Mettler
- Clinical Examination *50*
- Serum Markers *50*
- Diagnostic Imaging Modalities *50*
- Ultrasound Scan *50*
- Magnetic Resonance Imaging *51*
- Computed Tomography Scan *51*
- Laparoscopy and Biopsy with Histological Examination *52*
- Diagnostic Algorithm *52*
- Recent Advanced in the Imaging Techniques for Endometriosis *52*

7. Ultrasound in Gynecology 55
Aarti Deenadayal Tolani, Hema Desai, Mamata Deenadayal
- Requirements *55*
- Techniques *55*
- Settings *56*
- Modalities of Ultrasound *56*
- Congenital Uterine Anomalies *58*
- Morphological Uterus Sonographic Assessment *59*
- International Endometrial Tumor Analysis Group *59*
- Ovaries *62*
- International Ovarian Tumor Analysis Collaboration *64*
- Endometriosis *65*
- Pregnancy *65*
- Torsion *66*
- Reporting Pelvic Ultrasound *66*

8. Ultrasound of Ectopic Pregnancy 67
Punam Dixit, Aashita Shrivastava
- Diagnosis *67*
- Assessment of Adnexa *68*
- Different Morphological Types of Ectopic Pregnancy *68*
- Criteria for Diagnosis of Scar Ectopic *68*

9. Ultrasound of Adnexa 70
Punam Dixit, Jhillmill Kumari
- Common Indications of Ultrasound of Adnexa *70*
- Common Causes of Benign Adnexal Masses *70*
- Solid Masses of Adnexa *72*
- Malignant Adnexal Masses *72*

10. Ultrasonography for Bleeding in Obstetrics 74
PK Shah, Keshav Pai
- Causes of Bleeding in Obstetrics *74*
- Bleeding in Late Pregnancy *78*

11. Ultrasound in First Trimester 82
Archana Baser, Anshu Baser, Varsha Mahajan, Mumtaz P
- Critical Conditions in Early Pregnancy Scan *85*
- Prognostication of Pregnancy *87*

12. Ultrasound and Doppler in Multiple Pregnancy 90
Parth Shah, Jayprakash Shah
- Mechanism of Multifetal Gestation *90*
- Genesis of Monozygotic Twins *91*
- Role of Prenatal Ultrasound in Multifetal Gestation *91*
- Diagnosis of Multiple Gestation *92*
- Gestational Age Assessment in Multifetal Pregnancy *92*
- Determining Chorionicity and Amnionicity in Multifetal Pregnancy *92*
- Labeling of the Fetuses *93*
- Monitoring of the Multifetal Pregnancy *93*
- Screening for Aneuploidy in Multifetal Gestation *94*
- Invasive Prenatal Diagnosis in Multifetal Gestation *94*
- Ultrasound Screening for Structural Anomalies *94*
- Management of Twin Pregnancy Discordant for Fetal Anomaly *94*
- Fetal Reduction/Selective Termination in Multifetal Gestation *95*
- Screening for Risk of Preterm Birth in Multifetal Gestation *95*
- Fetal Growth Restriction *95*
- Managing the Surviving Twin after Demise of its Co-twin *96*
- Complications Specific to Monochorionic Twin Pregnancies *97*
- Conjoined Twins *97*
- Twin Reversed Arterial Perfusion Sequence *98*
- Twin Anemia Polycythemia Sequence *99*
- Twin-Twin Transfusion Syndrome *100*
- Monochorionic Monoamniotic Twins *102*

13. Ultrasound in Second Trimester 104
Chinmayee Ratha
- Scope of the Second Trimester Scan *104*
- Fetal Biometry in the Second Trimester *104*
- Targeted Imaging for Fetal Anomalies *106*
- Placental Localization in the Second Trimester *108*
- Uterine Artery Doppler Studies in the Second Trimester *108*
- Cervical Length Assessment in the Second Trimester *109*

14. Placental Abnormalities 111
Shreyasi Sharma
- Normal Placenta *111*
- Size and Shape Abnormalities *111*
- Extrachorial Placentation *113*
- Abnormalities of Location *113*
- Placenta Accreta Spectrum/Morbidly Adherent Placenta *114*
- Circulatory Disturbances *116*
- Placental Calcification *118*
- Placental Tumors *118*
- Abnormalities of the Umbilical Cord *118*

15. Amniotic Fluid Assessment 124
Seetha Ramamurthy Pal, Kanchan Mukherjee
- Normal Amniotic Fluid Volume *125*
- Oligohydramnios *127*
- Polyhydramnios *128*

16. Ultrasound in Third Trimester 131
Vandana Bansal, Rujul Jhaveri, Neha Singh
- Current Scenario of Obstetric Imaging in India *131*
- Third Trimester Ultrasound as a Diagnostic Tool *132*
- Indications/Components of Ultrasound Examination in Third Trimester *132*
- Imaging Parameters for a Standard Examination in Third Trimester *132*
- Fetal Central Nervous System Abnormalities *139*

- Fetal Genitourinary Anomalies *140*
- Fetal Gastrointestinal Anomalies *140*
- Congenital Lung Malformations *140*
- Cardiac Anomalies *141*
- Fetal Musculoskeletal Abnormalities *142*
- Intrapartum Ultrasonography *142*

17. Fetal Intervention ... 144
Vandana Bansal
- Genetic Counseling *144*
- Invasive Prenatal Diagnosis *145*
- Indications for Amniocentesis or Chorionic Villus Sampling *145*
- Amniocentesis *146*
- Chorionic Villus Sampling *147*
- Fetal Blood Sampling *148*
- Fetal Therapy and its Principles *149*

18. Gastrointestinal Tract Anomalies ... 156
Parul Choudhary Vali, Jayprakash Shah
- Esophageal Atresia *156*
- Duodenal Atresia *158*
- Small Bowel Atresia *159*
- Meconium Ileus *160*
- Meconium Peritonitis *161*
- Anal Atresia and Anorectal Malformations *161*
- Agenesis of Ductus Venosus *162*
- Persistent Right Umbilical Vein *163*
- Enteric Duplication Cyst *163*
- Mesenteric Cyst *164*
- Meconium Pseudocyst *164*
- Hepatic Cyst *164*
- Splenic Cyst *164*
- Choledochal Cyst *164*
- Echogenic Bowel *164*

19. Imaging in Labor ... 167
Girija Wagh, Rohan Wagh, Mahima Arya
- Imaging in Morbidly Adherent Placenta and Placental Abruption *167*
- Assessment of Fetal Well-being *168*
- Assessment of the Progress of Labor *170*
- Case Scenario *173*

20. Role of MRI in Pregnancy ... 175
Neeta Singh, Mandakini Pradhan
- Indications of MRI *175*
- Safety of MRI in Pregnancy *176*
- Advantages *176*

21. Genetic Markers in Aneuploidies ... 177
Ashok Khurana
- Sonographic Markers for Down Syndrome (Trisomy 21) *178*
- Sensitivity of Marker Detection *179*
- Significance of Individual Markers *179*
- Trisomy 18 (Edwards' Syndrome) *180*
- Trisomy 13 (Patau Syndrome) *180*
- Turner Syndrome (Xo) *180*
- Triploidy *180*
- Genetic Sonography after First Trimester Screening *181*

22. Fetal Medicine Beyond Ultrasound 184
Pramod Vasantrao Patil
- Role of Fetal Medicine Specialist *184*

23. Pre-conception and Pre-natal Diagnostic Techniques: How to Comply with the Law? 186
Hitesh J Bhatt
- Do's in Pre-conception and Pre-natal Diagnostic Techniques Act *186*
- Don'ts in Pre-conception and Pre-natal Diagnostic Techniques Act *187*

24. Writing an Ultrasound Report 189
Chinmay Umarji
- Aids to the Report Writing *189*
- Attributes of the Report Writing *189*
- Clinical Content of Report Writing *190*
- Report Storage *191*

25. Training in Ultrasound in Obstetrics and Gynecology 193
S Suresh, Indrani Suresh
- Certification *194*
- Logbook *195*
- Training for Rural India *195*
- Training of Practitioners *195*

Index 197

Basic Principles of Ultrasound Machine

Sonal Panchal, Chaitanya Nagori

INTRODUCTION

Ultrasound (US) is the most essential modality for a gynecologist. A well done US may give maximum information about the anatomy and pathology of the female pelvic organs as well as the growing fetus. It is, therefore, essential that the operator is well-acquainted with the machine and can use its different functions for the best advantage of the patient. It is true that majority of us are reluctant to operate the different knobs available for obtaining the most expected image quality probably because we fear ruining the already made settings on the machine. This is well understood by the manufacturers and therefore several presets are available on the machines, with the names of the presets suggesting, what are these best for. These presets are made keeping in mind majority of the patients, but naturally would not suit to all and several adjustments are required to produce good quality images. Good quality images are essential for correct diagnosis.

This chapter will be divided under following heads:
- Optimizing B-mode image
- Optimizing Doppler image
- Artifacts
- Safety of US
- Tips to make a good setup

OPTIMIZING B-MODE IMAGE

The image can be optimized by manipulating and adjusting the knobs on the control panel of the scanner (Fig. 1). It is essential to know about the knobs, what they do, and when to use them.

The settings that need to be often done during each scan to get an optimum information out of the scans are scanning

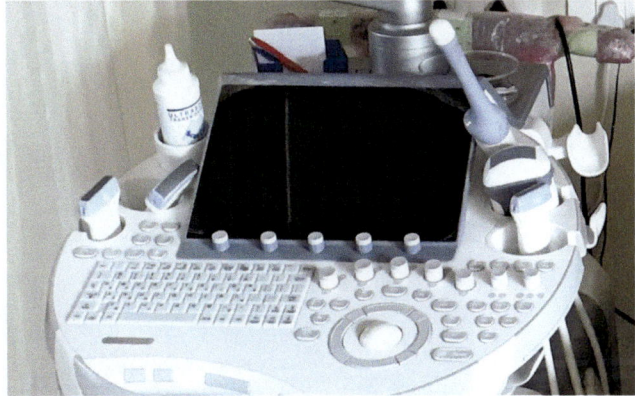

Fig. 1: Switch board of the scanner.

angle, scanning depth, probe frequency, focal zone, zoom, gains, contrast, and probe power.

- *Scanning angle*: Each probe has a maximum scanning angle. This is the maximum angle up to which the US beam can fan out. It indicates as to how far sideward can an US beam see. Maximum scanning angle for transvaginal probes usually vary from 80° to 180°. Large scanning angle is very convenient for obtaining the bird's eye view of the pelvis to see the entire uterus or first trimester fetus on a single image (Fig. 2), but it decreases the speed of scanning which is indicated by frame rate.

What is frame rate?

The real time B-mode images that we are seeing on the scanner screen are several static images seen quickly one after the other. Faster the change in frames, more real time it looks. Frame rate is the number of static images displayed in a unit time by the scanner. This means that if the frame rate is low, the image less real time.

Basic Principles of Ultrasound Machine

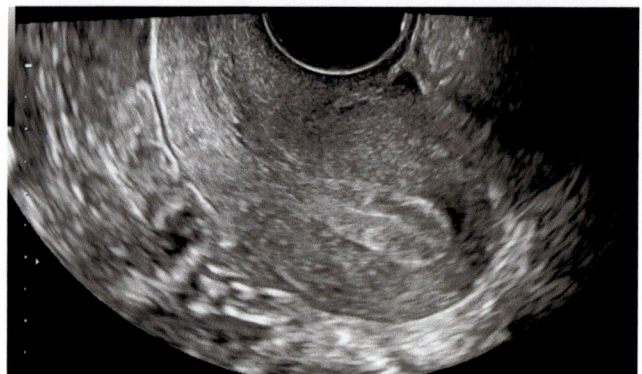

Fig. 2: B-mode image with a complete open angle.

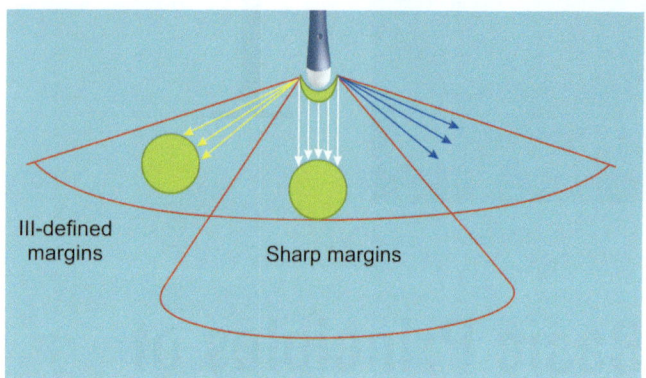

Fig. 3: Diagrammatic explanation of the sound beam direction in the central zone and in the side lobes.

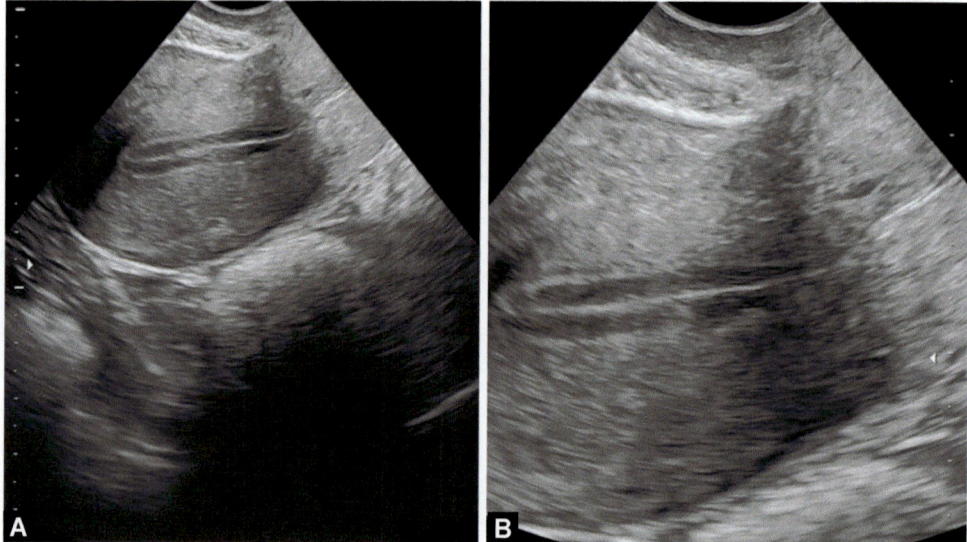

Figs. 4A and B: (A) B-mode image with more depth; and (B) B-mode image with appropriate depth.

Therefore, once the area of interest has been located, the scanning angle should be narrowed down to just a little larger than the area of interest. Narrowing the scanning angle increases frame rate. Moreover, when one decreases the scanning angle, area of interest is brought in the center. The sound beam from the transducer head then hits it at closer to right angle and gives sharper margin definition. When sound beam is emitted from the convex probe surface, the sound beam is vertical in the central part but is oblique on the sides (Fig. 3). This means that the structures that are not in the center of the image field are hit by the sound waves tangentially and lead to unsharp margins due to refraction.

- *Scanning depth*: Each probe has a limit of maximum depth up to which the US beam can penetrate. This, of course, depends on frequency of the probe. Maximum achievable depth by any probe may be used for the initial survey, but then depending on the depth at which the area of interest, the scanning depth, is to be decreased. This also increases the frame rate, and improves resolution (Figs. 4A and B). The correct depth setting is when the organ/lesion of interest fills up two-thirds of the image.
- *Setting the focal zone*: The US beam behaves like a light wave passing through the convex lens and therefore converges at a point called focal point, but since the probe (transducer) produces a series of similar sound beams the converging points of all make a plane called focal zone. Focal zone is the level at which the image is the sharpest because of the narrowest beam width. Therefore, focal zone is always set at the level of area of interest. The arrow head on right side of the image indicates the focal zone (Fig. 5). There is also an option of having more than one focal zone, when there are multiple levels at which the image needs to be sharp. But increasing the number of focal zones decreases the frame rate, and therefore usually single focal zone is selected.

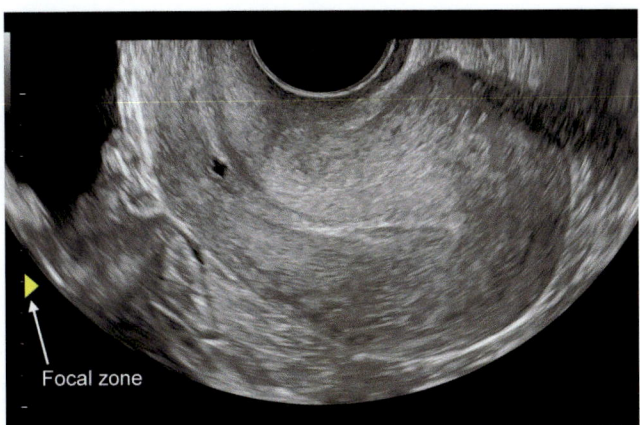

Fig. 5: B-mode image of the uterus showing yellow arrowhead on the left side indicating the focal zone.

- *Zoom*: After the overview, decreasing the scanning angle and depth and setting the focal zone, further improvement in the image quality can be achieved by zooming the image. One may zoom the whole image (panzoom) (Figs. 6A to C) or may use a zoom box to decide and define which part of the image needs to be zoomed [high-definition (HD) zoom] (Figs. 6A to C). Panzoom only enlarges the image and therefore increases the distance between the image pixels and deteriorates the image quality unless it is used after freezing the image, whereas HD zoom concentrates pixels into a smaller box and thus improves image resolution. Larger image can depict more anatomical details. Image should be zoomed large enough to fill up at least two-thirds of the screen.
- *Gains*: The US wave when travels into the body hit several tissue planes on its onward as well as return path. With each plane that it hits, the sound beam attenuates due to absorption of the energy and refraction of the sound wave. This leads to darker (hypoechoic) image of the structures that are far from the probe. Image can be made brighter by increasing the gains (Figs. 7A and B). This is potentiating of the returning beam to make the image brighter, but changing gains inadvertently may lead to erroneous diagnosis. Therefore, in all doubtful, difficult situations, the gains once set on the preset should then not be changed. If done, one must revert back to preset as soon as the scanning field is changed. Gains can be adjusted in two ways. Total gains can be increased/decreased, or gains can be adjusted layerwise, depending on the distance of the tissue plane from the probe. The latter one is known as time gain compensation (TGC) (Fig. 8). US wave returning from deeper structures takes longer time to return and is attenuated. This control compensates for the gains lost by time.
- *Probe power*: Brightness of the image can also be adjusted by increasing the power of the incident beam. Gain adjustment potentiates the returning beam, and power affects the incident beam. Probe power can be increased maximum to 100%, but usually set at between 80% and 90%. This is to control total mechanical and thermal energy transmitted to the tissues. Power may be increased only when, in spite of all adjustments, an optimum image brightness is not achieved.
- *Contrast*: Increased contrast means more black and white image with less shades of gray, and less contrast means more shades of gray in an image (Figs. 9A and B). Unoptimized contrast settings may, therefore, mask the details of soft tissues. Contrast setting may also be presented as dynamic contrast on the US machine.

OPTIMIZING DOPPLER IMAGE

What is Doppler?

Doppler effect is the change frequency of a sound wave when it hits a moving object. The difference in the emitted and the received frequency is known as Doppler shift. The shift depends on the angle at which the sound beam hits the moving object, velocity of the moving object, and the frequency of the incident beam. Looking into the equation used for calculation of the velocity from the frequency change on Doppler:

$$\text{Doppler frequency } (f_d) = \frac{2 \cdot f_t \cdot V \cdot \cos\theta}{c}$$

where,

f_d = Doppler shift
f_t = Transmitted beam
c = Speed of sound in tissue
V = Velocity of blood flow
θ = Angle of incidence between the ultrasound beam and the direction of flow

The Doppler effect can be displayed as color Doppler, power Doppler, and spectral Doppler.

Color Doppler

It displays the blood flow in two colors, and these are conventionally red and blue. The color indicates the direction of the flow. Flow toward the probe is red and away from the probe is blue (Fig. 10), but these can be interchanged by using the invert switch. When the flow is perpendicular to the sound beam, no color will be displayed in spite of presence of the flow. The arterial flow is pulsatile and the venous flow is nonpulsatile. The higher flow velocities display bright colors and the lower flow

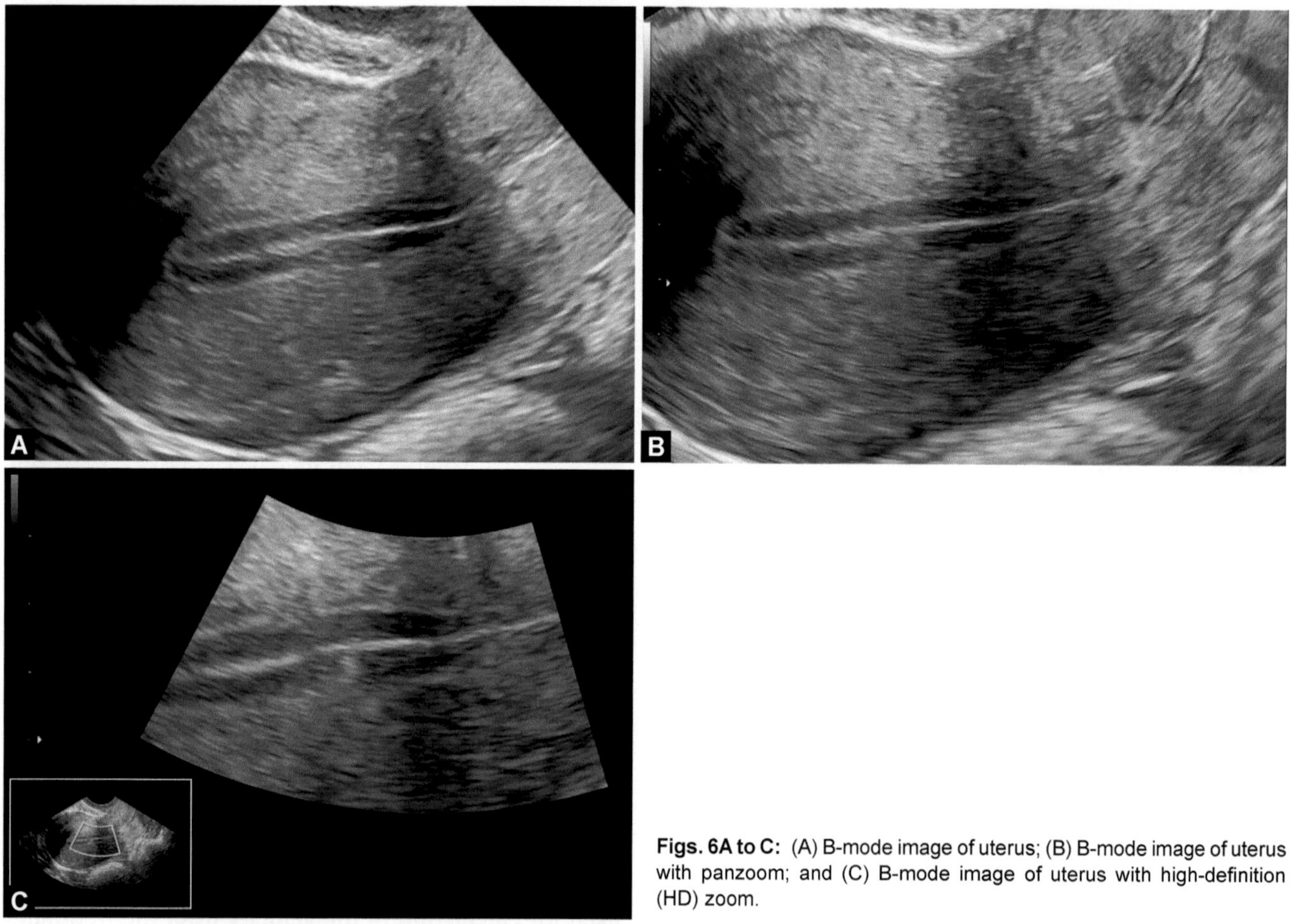

Figs. 6A to C: (A) B-mode image of uterus; (B) B-mode image of uterus with panzoom; and (C) B-mode image of uterus with high-definition (HD) zoom.

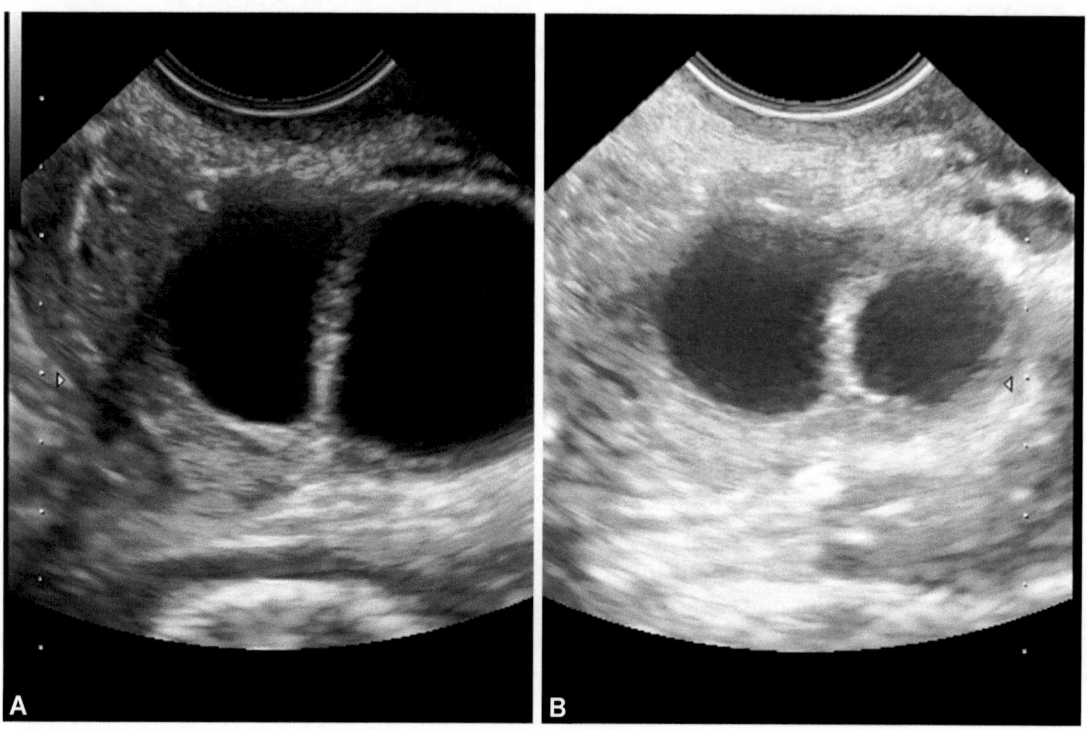

Figs. 7A and B: B-mode image of follicles with (A) Normal gains; (B) High gains.

velocities display dull colors (Fig. 11). Since color Doppler does not give exact velocity values, so it is a directional semiquantitative Doppler.

Power Doppler

Power Doppler is nonangle-dependent technology. It is known that movement of any object produces energy and this is used to depict the blood flow signals in power Doppler. This means that wherever there is a movement of blood or of body tissues, color signals will be generated. It displays color signals even in vessels that are perpendicular to the sound beam, but the disadvantage is that it is a single color display and does not show the flow direction (Fig. 12). It indigenously potentiates the signals and therefore is a useful technology for documentation of low velocity blood flows. The main application of the power Doppler, therefore, is to pick up flow in low velocity blood vessels and the blood flows in the vessels are perpendicular to the sound beam. High velocity movements show a bright color and the low velocity movements display dull color (Fig. 12).

High-definition flow is a new addition to the basic power Doppler technology. It is a directional power Doppler. Apart from high flow sensitivity, HD flow also has a color coding for the flow toward or away from the probe as in color Doppler (Fig. 13).

Spectral Doppler

Spectral Doppler is the spectral display of the blood flow/movement of a moving object. Trace above the baseline in the spectrum is the flow toward the probe and the trace below the baseline is the flow away from the probe (Fig. 14) on the spectrum. On the spectral Doppler, the arterial flow appears spiky and the venous flow appears flat. There is a scale on the side of the spectrum that calculates exact velocities of the flows can be calculated (Fig. 14).

The spectrum can be displayed for pulsed wave Doppler and the continuous wave Doppler. In pulsed wave Doppler, the sound waves are emitted in pulses and the frequency of this is called pulse repetition frequency (PRF).

To obtain the correct information about flow velocities with Doppler, certain settings and adjustments on the

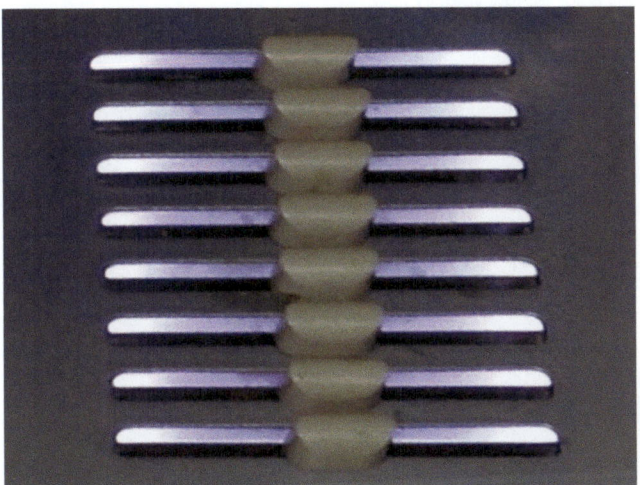

Fig. 8: Image of time gain compensation knobs.

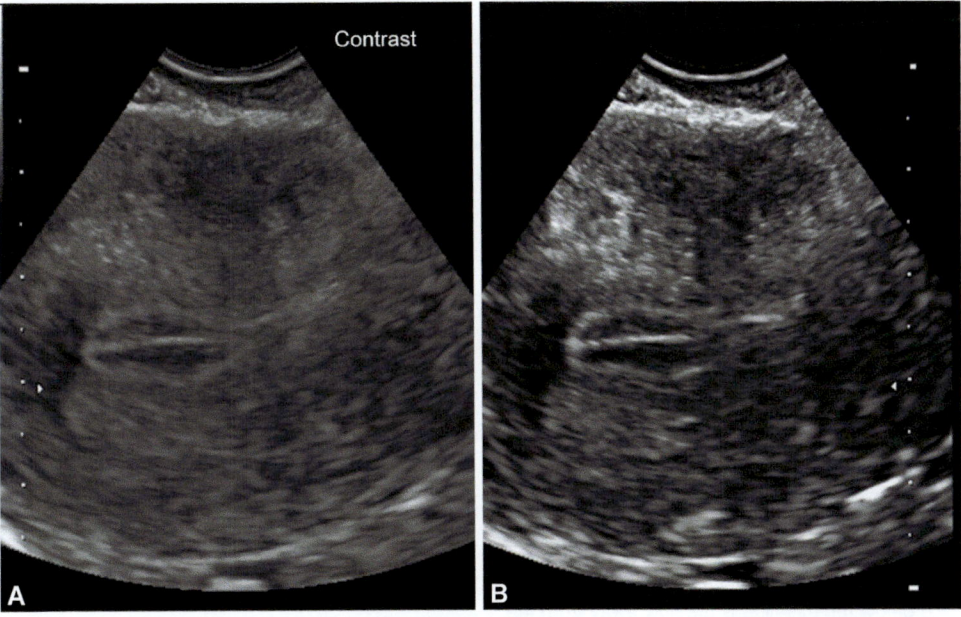

Figs. 9A and B: B-mode ultrasound image with (A) Low contrast; (B) High contrast.

Basic Principles of Ultrasound Machine

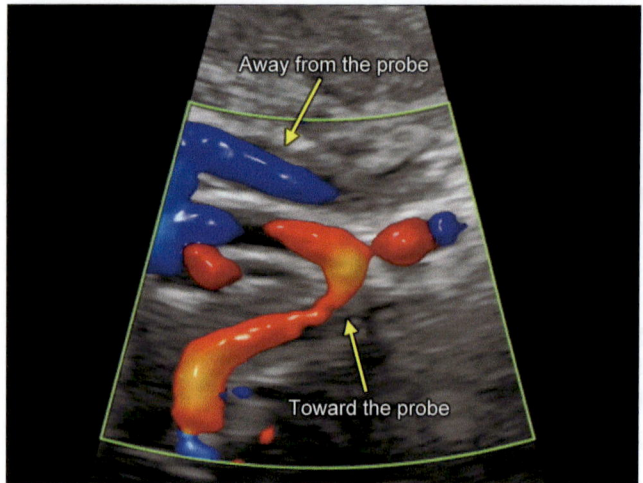

Fig. 10: Color Doppler image showing flow toward the probe in red and flow away from the probe in blue.

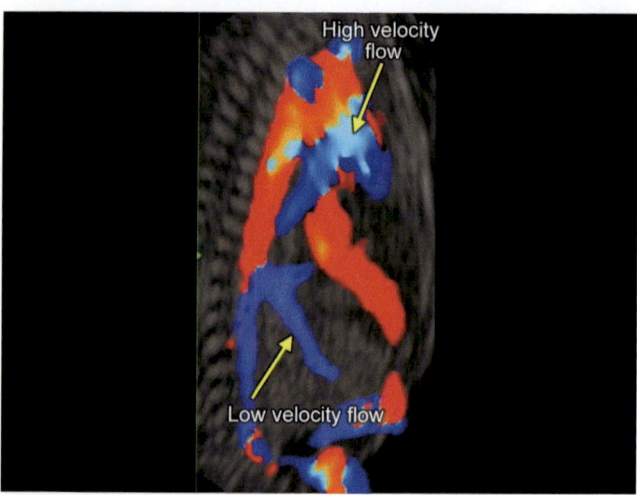

Fig. 11: Color Doppler showing bright color for high velocity flow and dull color for low velocity flow.

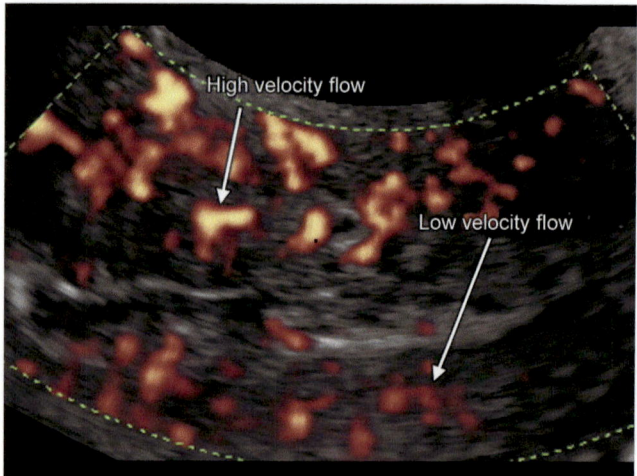

Fig. 12: Power Doppler image showing single color flow and bright color for high velocity flow and dull color for low velocity flow.

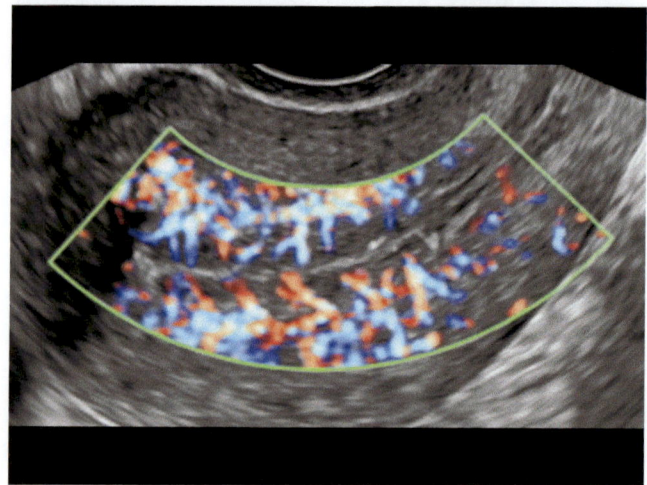

Fig. 13: High-definition (HD) flow image showing endometrial flow.

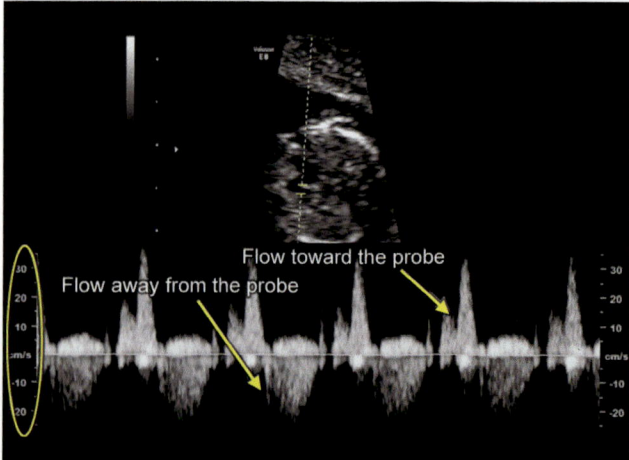

Fig. 14: Trace above the baseline in the spectrum is the flow toward the probe and the trace below the baseline is the flow away from the probe and scale on the side of the spectrum calculates the velocities.

scanner are required. Though most of these are set on the dedicated presets, it is important to understand how we can manipulate certain switches/knobs to achieve best flow information.

These are the Doppler box size, color gains, PRF, wall motion filter (WMF) and balance on color and power Doppler and sample volume, gains, PRF, WMF, and angle correction for the pulsed wave Doppler.

- *Color/power Doppler settings*:
  - *Box size*: When one switches on the color Doppler, a box appears on the screen, on the B-mode image. This box defines in which area of the B-mode image, the blood flow information will be looked for. It is important to consider here that when the Doppler is switched on, the machine has to process the B-mode information as well as the flow infor-

Basic Principles of Ultrasound Machine

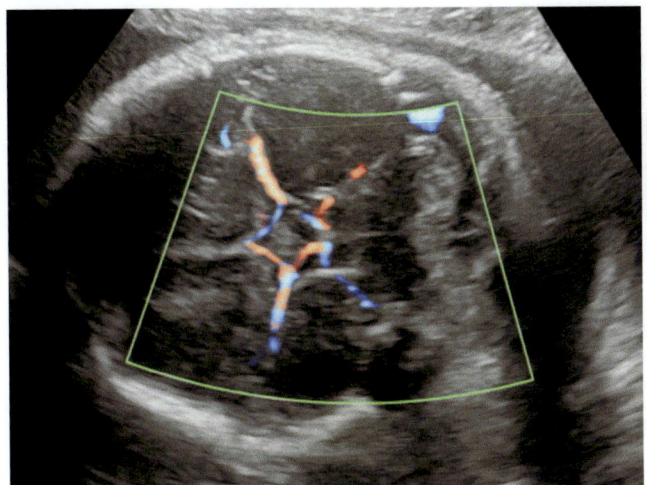

Fig. 15: Color box seen drawn by green line on the image.

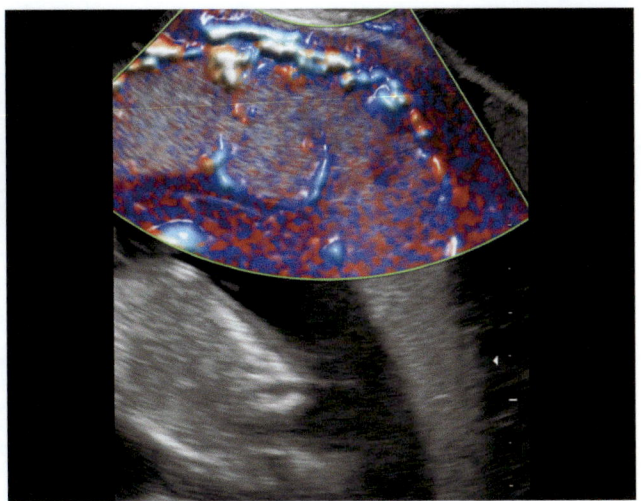

Fig. 16: High gains showing color spill outside the vessels.

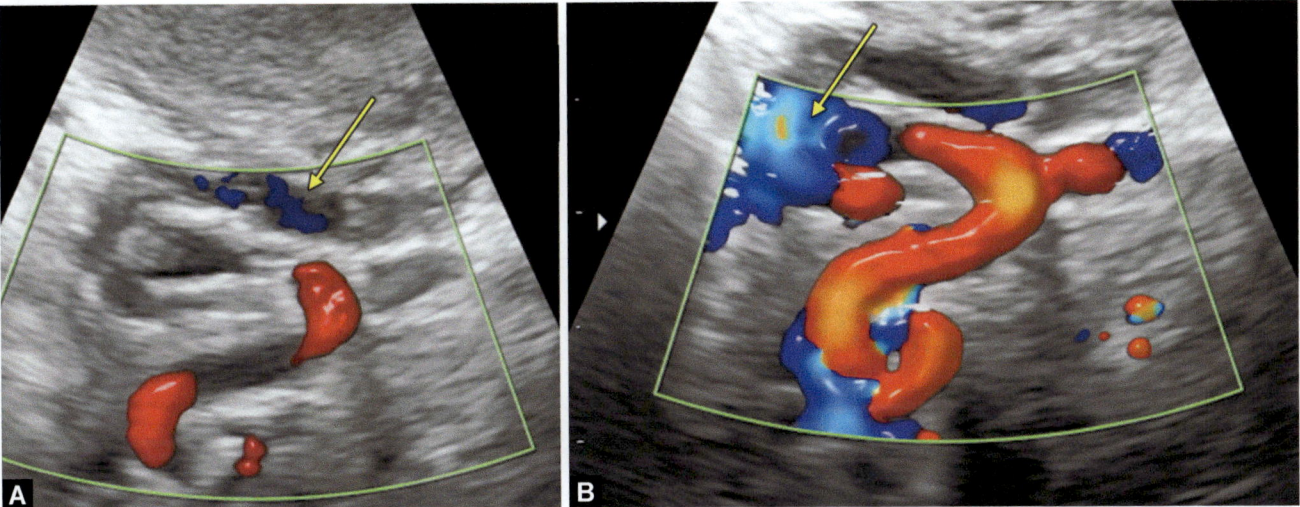

Figs. 17A and B: (A) High pulse repetition frequency (PRF) for low velocity flow shows nonfilling of the vessels (arrow); and (B) Low PRF for high velocity flow shows mixing of colors (arrow).

mation and therefore the frame rate significantly decreases. The color box size is planned just large enough to cover the area of interest. The color box can be moved all across the B-mode image and the size can be altered based on the requirement (Fig. 15).

- *Gains*: When the Doppler is switched on, it should show the blood vessels filled up with color but no color spilling out of the vessels. This is done by gain adjustment. When the gains are too high, the color will be seen spilling out of the vessels (Fig. 16). Whereas when the gains are low, the color will not completely fill up the vessel. This is because when the gains are low, the low velocity signals will not be picked up by Doppler. The correct gain, therefore, is when the entire lumen of the vessel is filled with color and there is no spill outside. Color gains can be adjusted by rotating the color knob.

- *Pulse repetition frequency*: It is important to select an optimum PRF for the velocity of the blood vessels flow studied. High PRF if used for low velocity flow, it will not be possible to pick up the color where there are flows (Fig. 17A). Instead if low PRF is used for high velocity flows, there will be aliasing mixing of red and blue colors—appears like turbulence (Fig. 17B). The PRF setting would be optimum when the color homogeneously fills the entire vessel with single color—red or blue.

- *Wall motion filter*: It is known that Doppler produces color signals wherever there is a movement and the brightness of the color depends on the velocity of the moving object. This means that the color signals

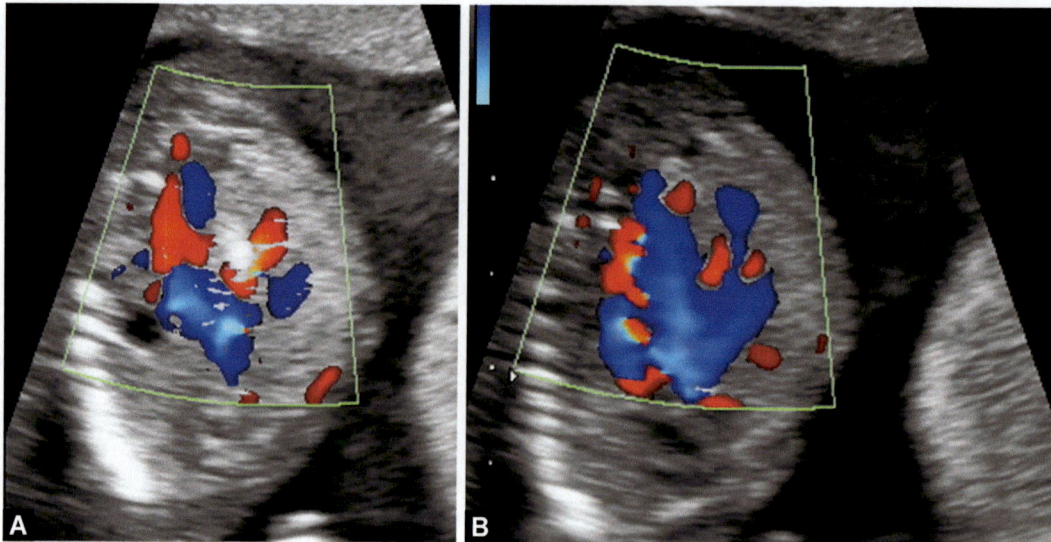

Figs. 18A and B: White patches on color Doppler due to low balance, normal color pick up with normal balance.

are produced by the red blood corpuscles in the blood, but are also produced by the wall movement of the artery and also by the pulsations transmitted to the surrounding tissues. The color signals of the blood flow are the brightest, those of wall motion are dull, and those due to transmitted pulsations from the surrounding tissues are the dullest, but these dull color signals corrupt the flow information and can be eliminated only if a low velocity filter is used. This filter is named as WMF. For larger vessels with high velocity flows, the arterial flow movement is more and higher WMF is required, whereas for small vessels with low velocity signals, the arterial wall movements are less and so low wall filters are required. Using higher wall filter for a low velocity blood, flow vessel will eliminate the slow flow information.

- *Balance*: As the name suggests, this is a balancing tool between the two modalities—the B-mode and the color Doppler. When color/power Doppler is switched on, a gray bar and a color bar appear on the left side of the screen. On the gray bar, is a green line. This line indicates the balance adjustment. When the brightness of the grayscale on the image matches the brightness below the green line on the gray bar, the color predominates and the color filling is normal, but when the brightness on the grayscale image matches the brightness above the green line on the gray bar, the B-mode predominates and therefore in these areas if the color is present to show the flows, the color will be patched up with white (Figs. 18A and B). When this happens, the correct thing to do is to change the balance to higher, or decrease the B-mode gains (Figs. 18A and B).

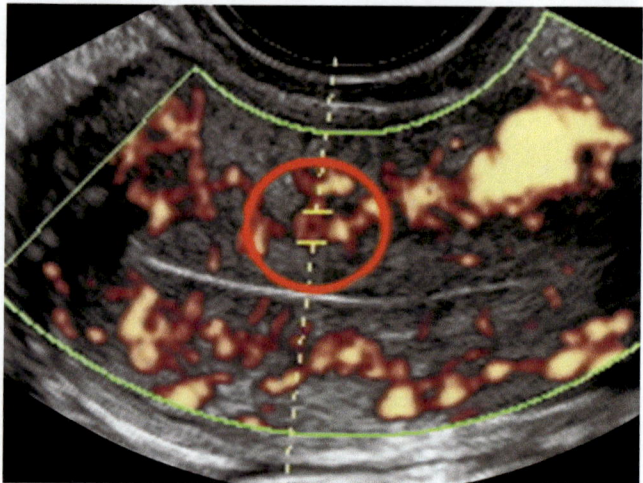

Fig. 19: Power Doppler image with pulse wave Doppler showing a dashed line with a "= line" showing the sample volume.

- *Pulsed wave Doppler*:
  - *Sample volume*: Sample volume is the selected length of the vessel to assess the flow. When pulsed wave Doppler is switched on, a dotted line appears on the screen. This line is parallel to the sound beam that can be swapped across the entire image. Two parallel short horizontal lines (=sign) appear on this line and is called sample volume/gate size (Fig. 19), this "=sign" can be moved up and down on the dotted line anywhere. This sign is to be placed on the vessel in which the flow is to be measured. The distance between the two lines decide, what length of the vessel will be evaluated for the flow assessment. If the vessel is not absolutely parallel to the sound beam (overlapping on the dotted line), the distance between the two line (sample volume)

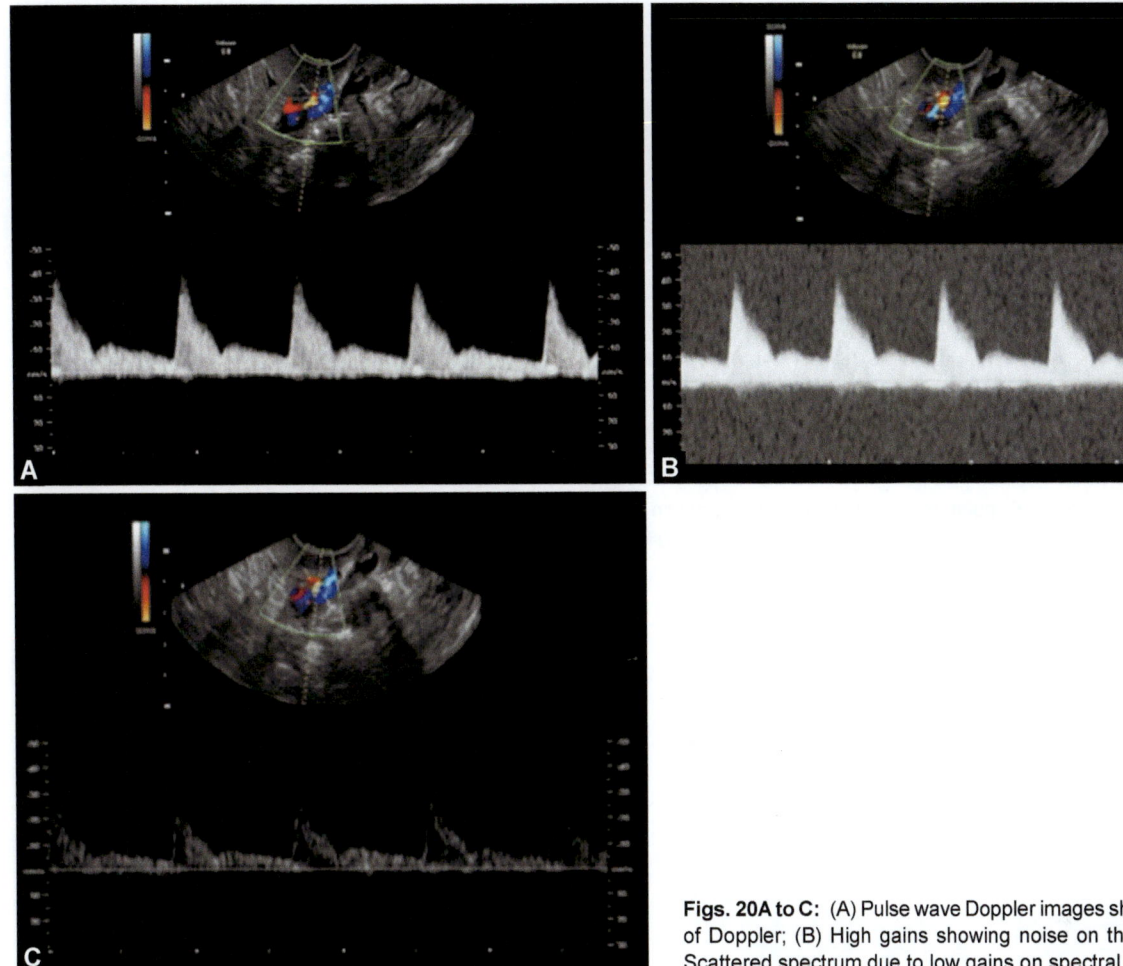

Figs. 20A to C: (A) Pulse wave Doppler images showing bold spectrum of Doppler; (B) High gains showing noise on the spectrum; and (C) Scattered spectrum due to low gains on spectral Doppler.

should be equal to the diameter of the vessel. A sample volume smaller than the diameter will lead to error in the velocity assessment.

- *Gains*: Gain settings on the pulsed wave Doppler should be such that it produces a clear well-defined bold spectrum of blood flows (Figs. 20A to C). If the gains are too high, the flow information will be corrupted by lot of noise (Figs. 20A to C). If the gains are too low, the entire spectrum will appear scarce and scattered (Figs. 20A to C).
- *Pulse repetition frequency*: PRF is adjusted according to flow velocity to be assessed, high PRF for high velocity flow and low PRF for low velocity flow. If high PRF if used for low velocity flow, it will not be possible to differentiate between the systolic and diastolic flows as the systolic flow recordings will be subdued (Figs. 21A and B). If low PRF is selected for high-velocity blood flows, there will be overlapping of systolic and diastolic signals and is known as aliasing (Figs. 21A and B).
- *Wall motion filter*: Like in color and power Doppler, the function of wall motion filter in pulsed Doppler also is to eliminate signals from low velocity movements, not to corrupt the image with wall motions. Again like color and power Doppler, the settings are low for low velocity vessels and high for high velocity vessels, but the wall filter setting in a pulsed Doppler spectrum is known to be correct only if the spectrum touches the baseline. When there is a black line or a gap between the baseline and the spectrum (Fig. 22), this trace is not to be accepted as this clearly indicates high wall filter for the case and may erroneously diagnose absence of diastolic flows. In that case if we say it eliminates low velocity information, means it interferes with the diastolic flow information and may lead to false diagnosis of absent end-diastolic flow and naturally then wrong interpretations.
- *Doppler angle*: As is discussed earlier considering the equation for calculation of the blood flow velocity from frequency of incident sound beam, frequency

Basic Principles of Ultrasound Machine

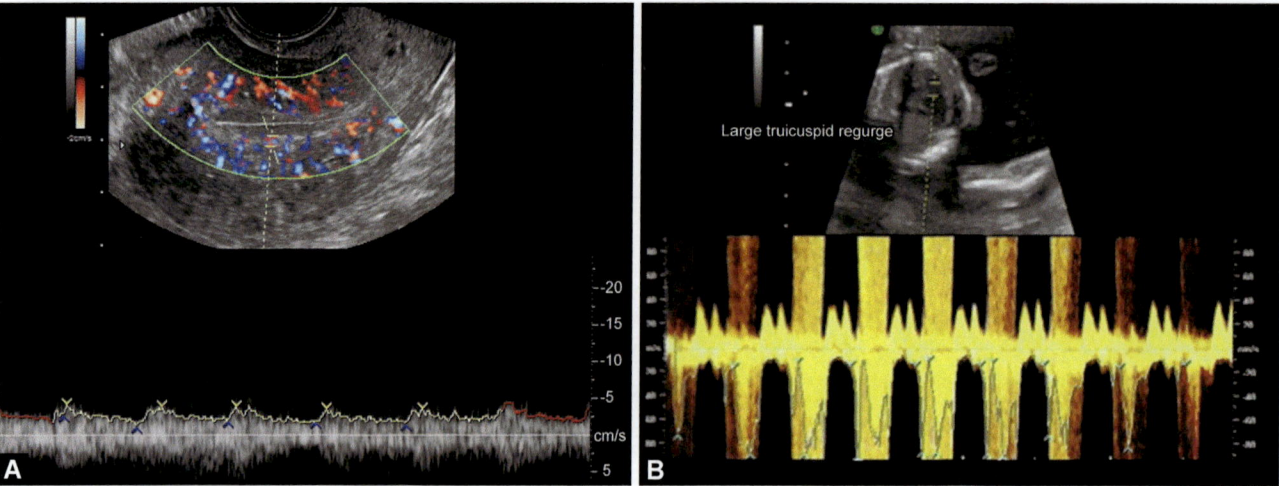

Figs. 21A and B: (A) Spectral Doppler image with high pulse repetition frequency (PRF) for low velocity flow, hardly any differentiation seen between systolic and diastolic velocities; and (B) Spectral Doppler image with low PRF for high velocity flow, showing overshooting of systolic flow on the other side of the spectrum (aliasing).

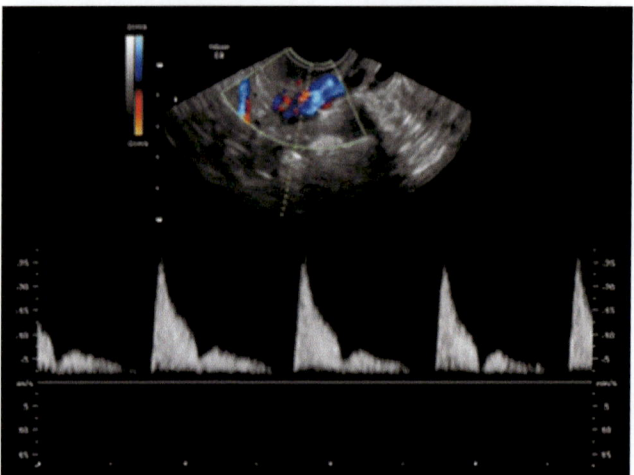

Fig. 22: High wall motion filter showing black line between the spectrum and the baseline.

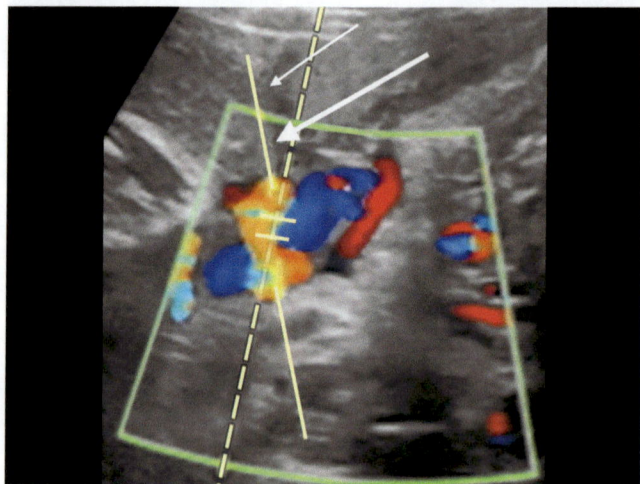

Fig. 23: Short yellow line deviating out of the dashed line when angle adjustment is done.

of received sound beam, and cos of the angle of incidence, if the angle of incidence is 90°, then the cos θ being 0, the velocity value will be 0 and also that with increasing angle from more than 60°, the percentage of error in calculation is highly significant and so the Doppler angle is always set between 0° and 60°, preferably <30°. The Doppler angle can be set at 0° when the vessel is parallel to the dotted line. This is often times possible because the dotted line can be swapped across the entire B-mode image and the probe manipulation may also help in the alignment of the two. But if it is still not possible, after achieving the smallest angle between the vessel and the dotted line, angle correction is used. This deviates out a short line from the dotted line, and is tried to align this short line to the vessel (Fig. 23).

In trying to do this, the angle between the dotted line and the short line is the Doppler angle. It is displayed on the screen or the touch pad of the scanner.
- *Setting the speed of the trace*: An ideal spectral trace is when there are four to five cardiac cycles (Fig. 24) recorded on any one spectrum image. This can be done by setting the speed of the trace. For most scans, this is possible when the speed is set as 4 or 5. Higher speed gives trace of too few cardiac cycles and lesser speed gives too many cardiac cycles traced.

UNDERSTANDING THE ARTIFACTS

In spite of all these settings used to optimize the Doppler images, certain artifacts still cannot be completely eliminated. These are aliasing, mirror image artifact, and artifacts due to electrical interferences.

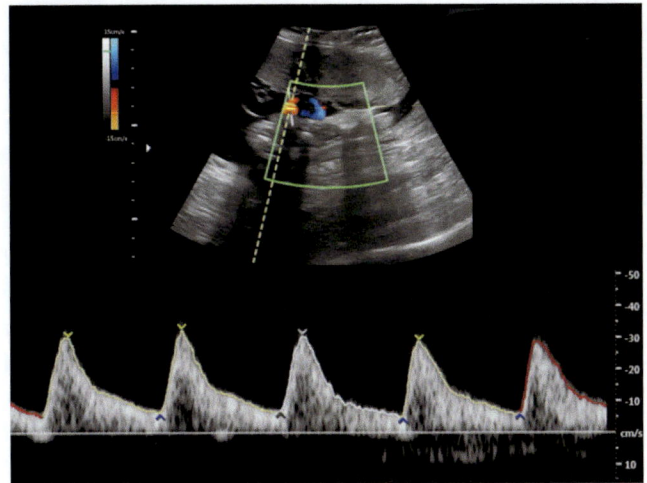

Fig. 24: Spectral Doppler showing five complete cardiac cycles on the baseline, suggesting normal speed adjustment.

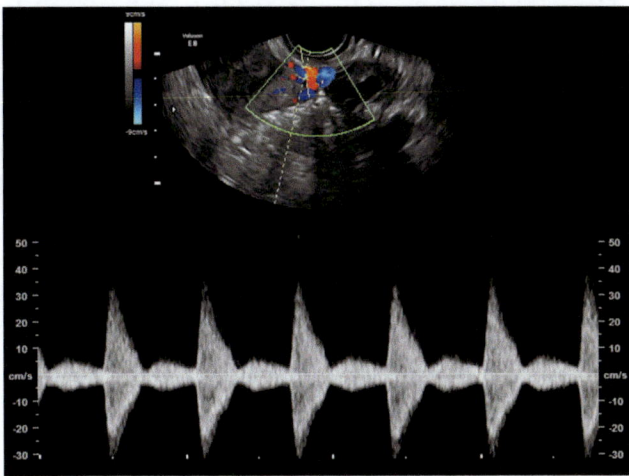

Fig. 25: Mirror image artifact seen on the spectral Doppler.

- *Aliasing*: This is overlapping effect of systolic and diastolic velocities, across the baseline on both the sides of the spectrum (*see* Figs. 21A and B). This effect is similar to what we have often observed especially in movies. The car wheels suddenly appear to start rotating in the opposite direction when the car speeds up. Adjusting the PRF can eliminate this artifact.
- *Mirror image artifact*: Mirror image artifact is when a similar spectrum is seen on both the sides of the baseline. This is especially possible when the sample volume is large and is tracing the flow in two vessels or two loops of the same vessel positioned, side by side (Fig. 25), or a large sample volume is placed on the curve of the loop, when in the proximal half of the loop the blood flow is observed away from the probe by the transducer and in the distal half of the sample volume the flow is perceived toward the probe. Decreasing the sample volume and planning to place it on one vessel only sorts out this problem.
- *Electrical interferences*: These may appear as random signals on color, power, or spectral Doppler, especially when the scanner is sharing the same electrical line as some high voltage gadget and the only way to get rid of this is to plan the electrical supply to the scanner wisely.

SAFETY OF DOPPLER

The two major effects of sound wave when it passes through the human body are:
1. *Thermal effect*: Production of heat that may damage the cells.
2. *Mechanical effect*: Due to pressure changes on the molecule.

Thermal effect: As the sound waves pass through the body tissues, there is absorption of energy and transformation of US energy into heat. The energy absorption is minimal in fluid and maximum in bones. It is also dependent on the frequency of the US waves. The absorption is higher with high frequency waves and lower with low-frequency sound waves. A temperature rise of up to 1°C is considered absolutely safe, whereas if it is >2.5°C, it can lead to significant tissue damage. This thermal effect is measured and displayed as thermal index on the screen. It is generally found that the temperature rise of 2°C is thermal index 2. The thermal index should be limited at maximum 1.

Mechanical effect: When the sound wave passes through the body tissues, it leads to oscillations of the body molecules, resulting in cavitating (low pressure) phase and a compressing (high pressure) phase. The mechanical damage caused by the sound waves is quantified as mechanical index (MI). MI is defined as "maximum estimated in situ rarefaction pressure or maximum negative pressure (in MPa) divided by the square root of the frequency (in MHz)". MI of up to 0.3 can be considered safe and more than 0.7 can lead to cavitation.[1]

APART FROM THIS A FEW PRACTICAL TIPS ON PLANNING YOUR SETUP

Ordering the Scanner

Apart from optimizing the image, it is essential to make the correct choice of the machine according to your requirements and also correctly ordering the probes and the softwares.

There is a huge choice available now in the market as there are several different brands available with a range of lower end only B-mode or portable machines to high-end 3D-4D machines loaded with lot of automations and softwares. Though the image quality, even on the B-mode, significantly improves as one moves on from lower end to the higher end scanners, 3D and 4D scanners are not essential for all. It depends on one's type of practice and the amount of work that the scanner should be selected. But as far as obstetrics and gynecology practice is concerned, in our opinion, a good quality scanner with a good quality Doppler is essential. Check for the service facilities of a particular brand around your place.

Probes must also be selected according to one's practice. It should be kept in mind always that low frequency probes are better for penetration but have a poor resolution, whereas high frequency probes have poor penetration but high resolution. Always check the B-mode and the Doppler image quality with the same probes that is to be bought during presale demonstrations. Instead of depending on the demonstration images in presentations by the company, depend on the live scans that are being done, preferably by a colleague.

When ordering the machine, confirm which softwares are optional and decide which of those are required for one's practice and specifically order for those and confirm when the written order comes to you for signature.

It is also important that in your setup, the electrical power point supplying the scanner should not be in the same line as any other equipment that consumes high power voltage. Moreover, do not fit any light-emitting diode (LED) lights in the scanning room.

CONCLUSION

Doppler is a very useful modality for assessment of circulation in the human body. Correct settings on the scanner only can give optimum results and therefore it is very important to understand the basic principles and settings of the US scanner before starting to use Doppler for interpretation of vascular flows and information of oxygenation in human fetus. US and Doppler are generally safe modalities. Their safety can be related to frequency used and the length of exposure. Therefore, Doppler should not be used for long time on a single focus and therefore as low as reasonably achievable (ALARA)[2] principle is now applied for all US scan.

REFERENCES

1. The British Medical Ultrasound Society (BMUS) (2019). Safety of ultrasound. [online] Available from www.bmus.org/public-info/pi-safety01.asp. [Last accessed November, 2019].
2. Auxier JA, Dickson HW. Guest editorial: concern over recent use of the ALARA philosophy. Health Phys. 1983;44(6):595-600.

Stepwise Standardized Approach to Ultrasound Examination of Female Pelvis

Sonal Panchal, Chaitanya Nagori

INTRODUCTION

Sonography is one of the most useful and indispensable investigations for the assessment of the female pelvis.

Pelvic organs can be scanned by:
- Transabdominal route
- Transvaginal route
- Transrectal route

The scan for pelvic organs must start as abdominal scan. Assessment of the kidneys is especially important in cases with Müllerian duct abnormalities. Moreover, an abdominal approach to the pelvic organs gives an overall idea about the pelvic organs and surrounding anatomy before the detailed study of uterus and ovaries individually. Though in those patients in whom transvaginal approach is not possible, transabdominal route may be the first option. This scan is done on full bladder.

Low ultrasound frequencies are preferred, 3–5 MHz probe, to allow visualization of the uterus and ovaries from the acoustic window of full bladder (Figs. 1 and 2). Patient is placed in supine position and is asked to relax and not to blow up her abdomen. At times, pressure with the probe may be required and probe may have to be angulated toward the pelvic cavity.

Sonography of the pelvic organs—uterus, ovaries, and adnexa is preferred by transvaginal route for better visibility and accuracy of diagnosis. This advantage is because of close placement of the probe. Because of less distance that the sound waves have to travel, these probes are high frequency (6–12 MHz) and so give better resolution. Transvaginal route cannot be used in virgins or in cases of local vaginal problems where transabdominal sonography with full bladder may be done. This route has a disadvantage of poor resolution because of the

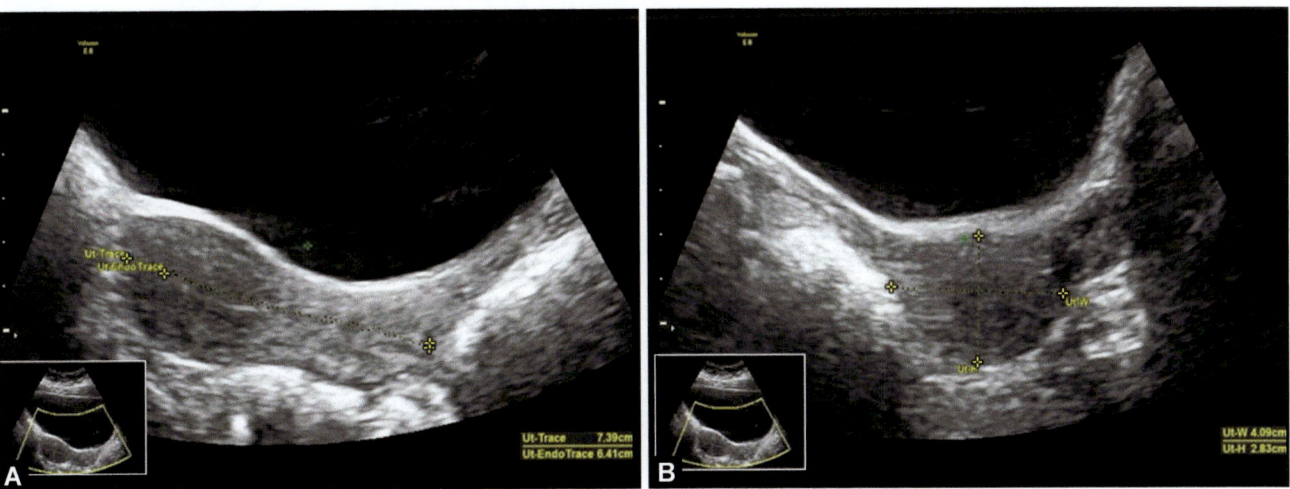

Figs. 1A and B: Uterus on longitudinal and transverse section on transabdominal scan.

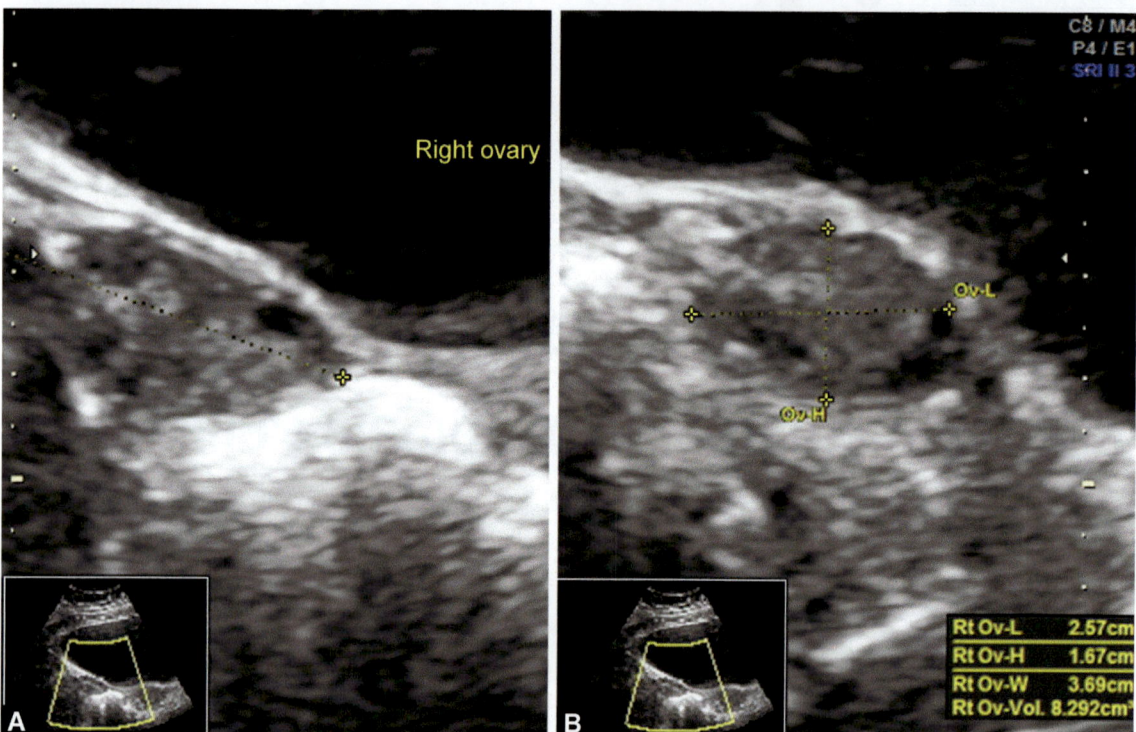

Figs. 2A and B: Right ovary in longitudinal and transverse section on transabdominal scan.

distance of the pelvic organs from the probe, maternal fat, maternal bowel loops, and the low frequency (3–5 MHz) probe which has evidently lower resolution than the high resolution, high frequency transvaginal probe.

Approximately 42% of ovarian details are missed by transabdominal scan.[1] But transrectal sonography in such cases is more preferable and informative as compared to transabdominal approach. The probe used is transvaginal probe so resolution is very similar to that of a transvaginal examination, but rectal placement is much more painful than transvaginal placement. Therefore, the approach of choice is transvaginal.

METHOD

Patient is first asked to empty the bladder. Patient is placed in lithotomy position on the gyne couch in the same way as for per speculum or per vaginal examination. Ultrasound jelly is put on the head of the transvaginal probe and then the probe is covered with the condom, not to allow any air between the probe and the condom. A small amount of jelly is then placed over the condom on the probe head and the probe is gently slided into the patient's vagina. In case of difficulty in introduction or patient's resistance to introduction, she is advised to take deep long breaths with open mouth, i.e., deep inspirations and long complete expirations. Counseling the patient before examination and explaining the whole procedure and adequate privacy

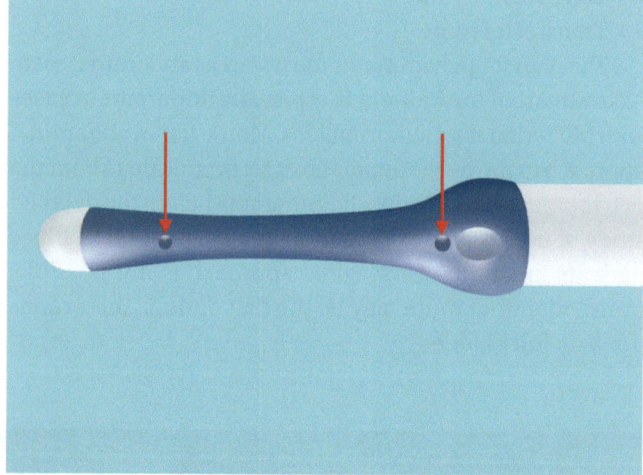

Fig. 3: The arrows showing the markers on the transvaginal probe.

help eliminate the anxiety and resistance. In spite of that if introduction of probe needs any force, the pressure should be exerted posteriorly toward the rectum which will make introduction of the probe into the vagina easier. Probe is held in the position, so that the markers on the probe face the roof of the examination room and it is introduced into patient's vagina in the same position (Fig. 3).

This indicator of the probe also matches the logo on the screen. This means that if the indicator on the screen is on the left side of the screen, the structures anteriorly placed are on the left side of the screen.

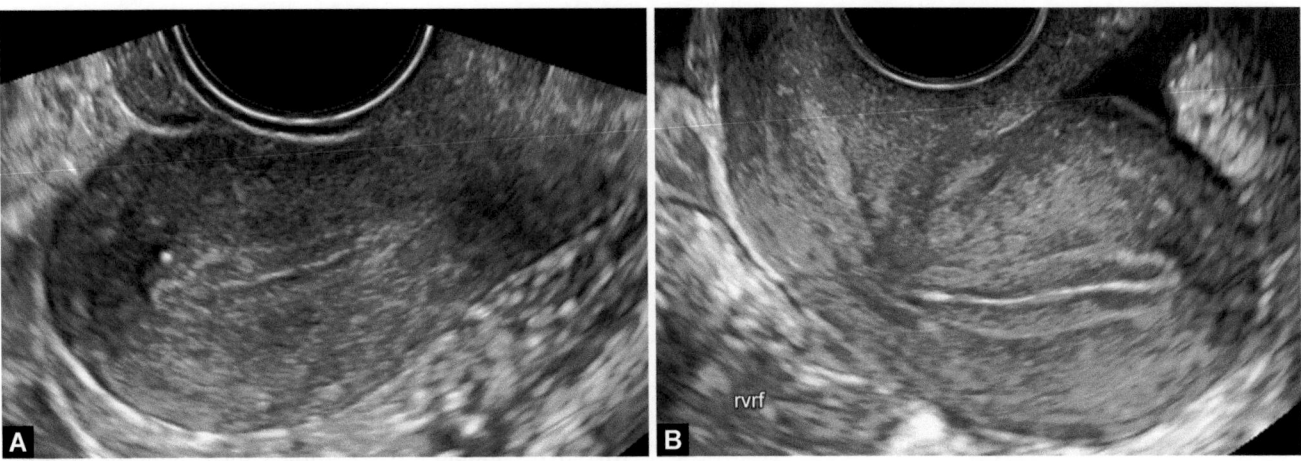

Figs. 4A and B: (A) Anteverted anteflexed uterus on B-mode ultrasound; and (B) Retroverted retroflexed (rvrf) uterus on B-mode ultrasound.

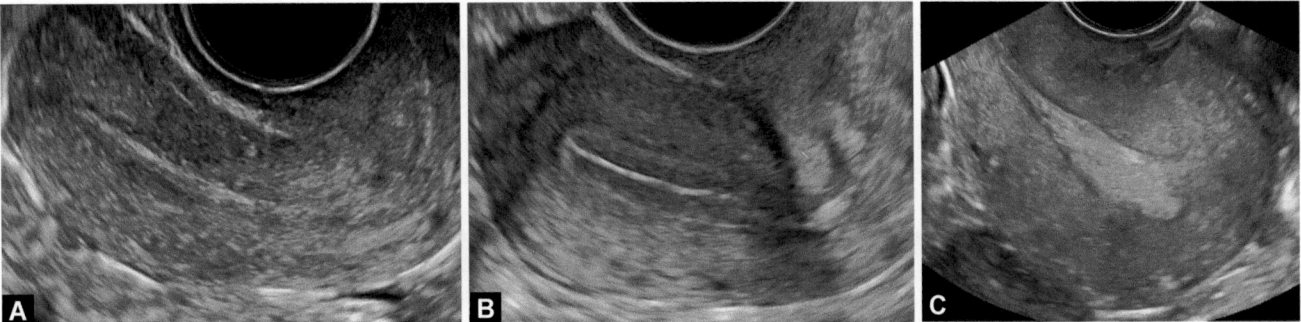

Figs. 5A to C: (A) Thin endometrium of early proliferative phase; (B) Multilayered endometrium of midcycle; and (C) Hyperechoic endometrium of secretory phase.

This longitudinal axis of the patient normally corresponds to the long axis of the uterus. That means the uterus must be seen in the long axis in this view. It may be anteverted or retroverted. When anteverted, the uterine fundus will be directed toward the indicator on the screen and urinary bladder is also seen on the same side of the screen, when retroverted fundus will be on the opposite side of the indicator and the urinary bladder (Figs. 4A and B).

If the uterus is not seen in this view, it means that the uterus is deviated toward one side. When it is deviated, it would indicate that either it is pulled on the side of the pathology like adhesions or is pushed away by the pathology which is on the opposite side say a mass. The second possibility is an abnormality of the uterus itself, most likely Müllerian duct abnormalities, such as hemiuterus or bicorporeal uterus.

Having located the uterus in the midline and decided whether it is anteverted or retroverted, its structure is evaluated as:
- *Endometrium*:
  - Corresponding with the phase of the cycle
  - Symmetry of the endometrium
  - Intraendometrial lesions such as polyp, adhesions, etc.
  - Endometrio-myometrial junction

Depending on the phase of the cycle, endometrium is expected to be thin linear in early follicular phase, triple line in preovulatory phase, and thick and echogenic in secretory phase (Figs. 5A to C). It is broadest at the fundus and narrows down smoothly toward cervix. In all the phases, there is a thin hypoechoic zone seen surrounding the echogenic outline of endometrium, which is known as endometrio-myometrial junction or junctional zone (Fig. 6). Breach in this zone is suggestive of a pathological endometrium, either infection or neoplasm. Any echogenic solid lesion in between the lines of endometrium is suggestive of pathologies such as polyps, synechiae, etc.
- *Myometrium*:
  - Homogenicity of the myometrium
  - Mass lesions
  - Scar tissues

Myometrium is homogeneously echogenic normally (Fig. 6). Any generalized heterogenicity or localized hypo-/hyperechogenicity is suggestive of pathology.
- *Serosa*:
  - Continuity
  - Smoothness of contour
  - Maintenance of tissue interface

Outer layer of uterus is covered by peritoneum and the serosal layer (Fig. 6). It defines the margins of uterus and therefore its integrity confirms that the uterus is normal. Any mass lesion in the uterus changes the contour of the uterus and therefore the smooth pear shape is distorted.

- *Cervix*:
  - *Length, mucous*: The cervical length is assessed by identifying the internal os. Internal os can be identified by two landmarks: (1) The entry of uterine vessels on transverse section, and (2) Cervical glands surrounding the cervical canal in midsagittal section (Fig. 7). Thickness of endometrio-myometrial junction is narrowest at the internal os and beyond that toward cervix, thick hypo-/hyperechoic band is seen because of cervical glands.
  - Cervical lesions, polyp, etc.
  - Serosal integrity as for the body of the uterus is also essential for the cervix.

Physiological uterocervical length also is measured in this view. It can be measured as a continuous tracing from the fundal endometrial tip to the external os, or it can be a summation of three measurements (Figs. 8A and B): (1) Fundus serosa to endometrium (myometrial length), (2) Endometrium to internal os (endometrial length), and (3) Internal os to external os (cervical length). This is uterocervical length that must be used for intrauterine insemination (IUI) and embryo transfer. The actual anatomical uterocervical length can be measured from the fundal serosa to the external os.

Now rotate the probe 90° anticlockwise. This maneuver will give transverse view of the uterus with the right side of the patient on right side of the screen (Fig. 9). In this transverse position also, the whole uterus is evaluated from the fundus to the cervix by sliding the probe up and down in the vagina. This survey should give a complete idea about the anatomy of the uterus and the exact location of any fibroids, etc.

Now deviate the probe toward right side and in transverse position at the level of uterine cornu, gradually look at the adnexal soft tissue band and follow it to the ovary. Extend the movement up to the lateral pelvic wall if ovary is not located. If the ovary is not located, the probe is moved up and down and is simultaneously moved from lateral pelvic wall to medially, to find the ovary.

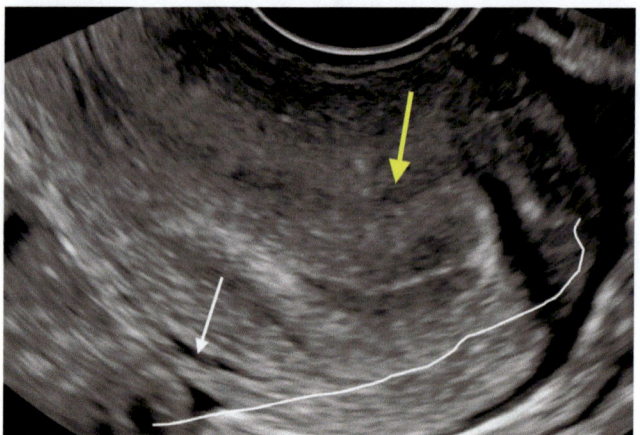

Fig. 6: Thin hypoechoic line around the endometrium is the endometrio-myometrial junctional zone (white arrow) and yellow arrow showing myometrium and the white curved line outlines the serosa.

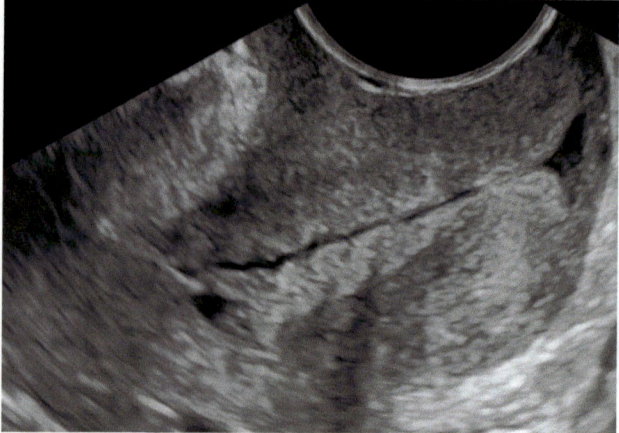

Fig. 7: Cervical glands seen on the sides of the cervical canal.

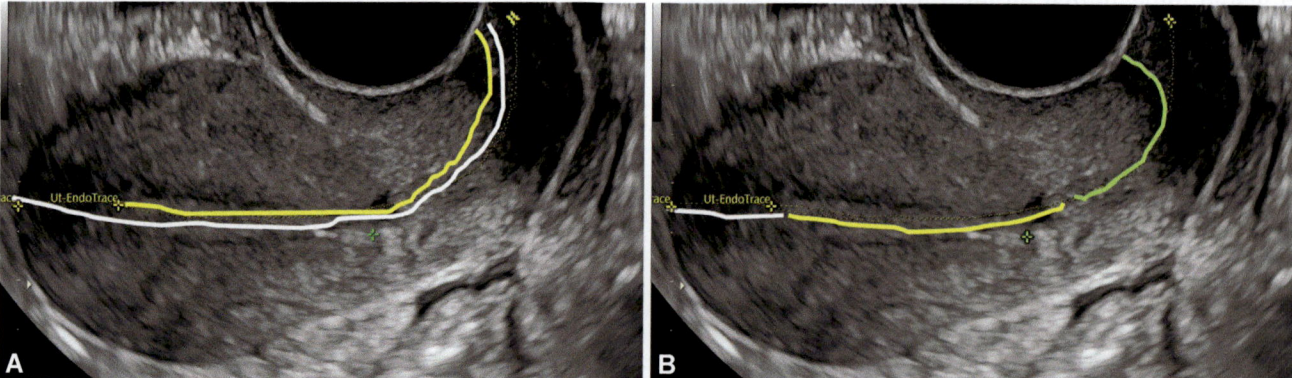

Figs. 8A and B: (A) B-mode image of the uterus, white line showing the measurement of anatomical uterocervical gland and yellow line is the physiological uterocervical length; and (B) B-mode image of the uterus, white line showing the measurement of myometrial length, yellow line is the endometrial length, and green line is the cervical length.

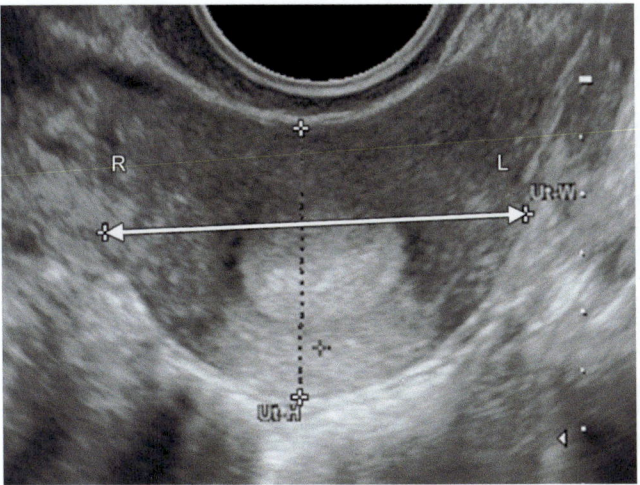

Fig. 9: Transverse section of the uterus, showing transverse diameter measurement of the uterus.

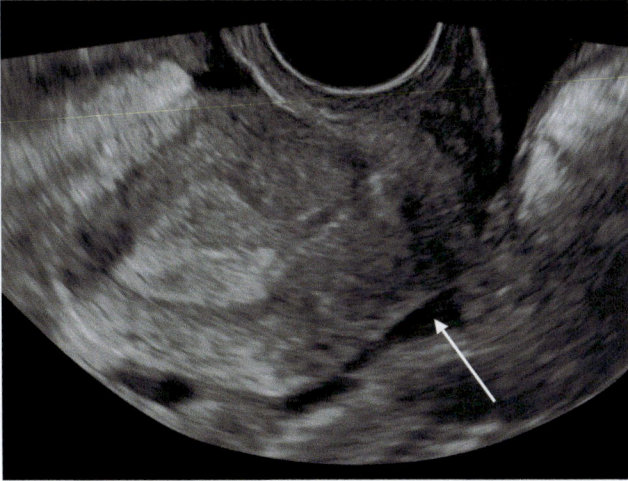

Fig. 10: B-mode image showing pouch of Douglas by white arrow.

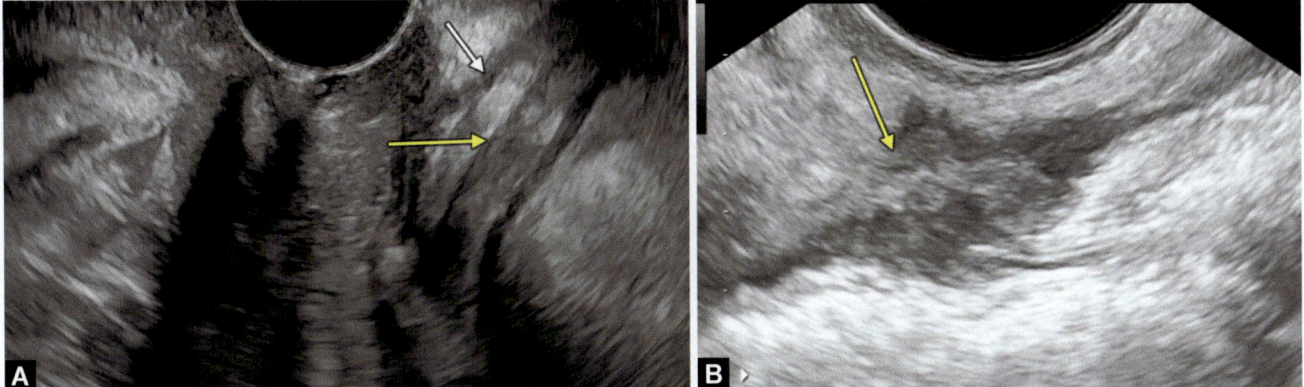

Figs. 11A and B: (A) B-mode image with probe at introitus (white arrow showing bowel muscularis and yellow arrow showing bowel lumen); and (B) Yellow arrow shows endometriotic patch in the bowel.

ADNEXA

- Look for mass lesion
- Localized fluid collection
- Thickening of the adnexa

Locate the ovary rotate probe to get a true long axis of the ovary. Scroll across on the long axis of the ovary and find the longest section and measure the longest diameter. The longest diameter perpendicular to this diameter is the anteroposterior diameter. A 90° rotation of the probe from this plane is the true transverse section and the largest side-to-side diameter is the transverse diameter (Fig. 9). These three diameters can be used to calculate the volume of the ovary. Then, move the probe to come back to the midline and follow the same procedure for the opposite adnexa.

Come back to the midline and angulate the probe head posteriorly and look for fluid in pouch of Douglas (Fig. 10).

Now before removing the probe, it is essential to check for the adhesions. Fix the probe against the uterine fundus and press over the abdomen with the hand. See if the bowel loops move against the uterine fundus. The same procedure is repeated for both the ovaries also. This is known as Timor-Tritsch test and confirms lack of adhesions. Instead of pressing on the abdomen, in and out movement of the probe can also be done to confirm the mobility of uterus and ovaries.

While removing the probe gently, have a close look at the cervical canal.

In cases where deep endometriosis is suspected, the probe is angulated slightly posteriorly toward the anal canal. This will show the bowel lumen and muscularis with interface between the vagina and the bowel (Fig. 11A). The probe is gently slided up toward the sigmoid colon. Any irregularity of the muscularis due to not very well-defined hypoechoic area suggests deep endometriosis (Fig. 11B).

This completes the two-dimensional routine transvaginal examination.

Color, pulse, or power Doppler can be added as and when required. For color Doppler of the uterine artery, the probe is brought back in the midline in longitudinal plane and then moving it laterally, serpiginous tubular structure

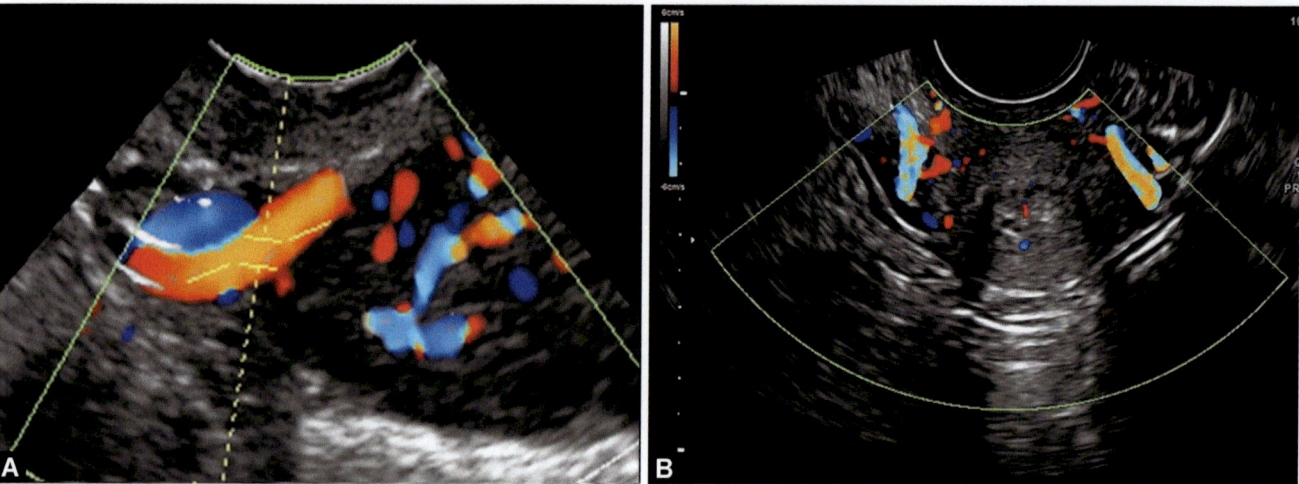

Figs. 12A and B: (A) Uterine artery seen on the sagittal section on color Doppler; and (B) Uterine arteries seen on both the sides of the internal os on color Doppler.

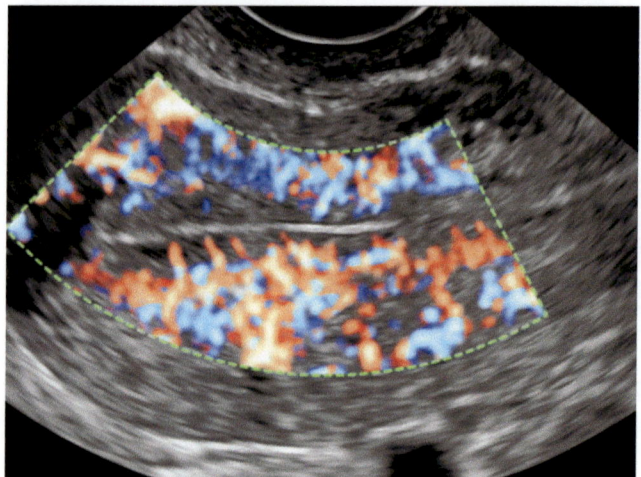

Fig. 13: Endometrial flow as seen on high-definition (HD) flow Doppler.

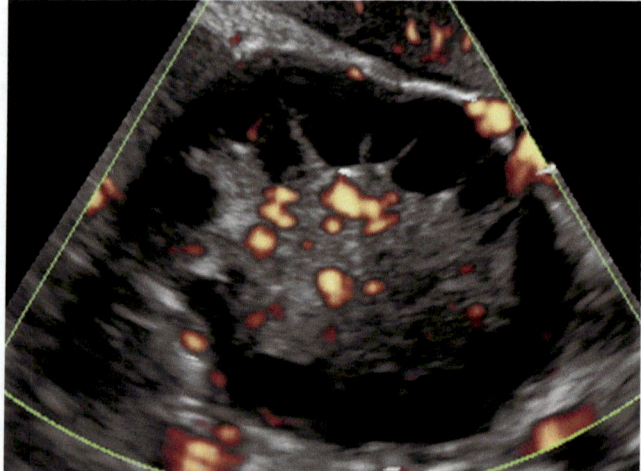

Fig. 14: Power Doppler image showing ovarian stromal flow.

is seen at the level of internal os, which is the uterine artery (Fig. 12A). It can also be traced in transverse axis of the uterus, moving the probe to the level of internal os, when arteries will be seen on both the sides (Fig. 12B).

Doppler is also used to evaluate the endometrial flow (Fig. 13). The blood vessels entering the endometrium are branches of spiral artery and are seen as vessels perpendicular to the endometrium. To document flow in the endometrial vessels, it is essential to hold the probe steadily in position on the endometrium for a few seconds to pick up this low-velocity flow. The ovarian stromal vessels are studied for baseline scan. The vessels that are seen in the ovarian stroma, not close to the follicles, are ovarian stromal vessels (Fig. 14). The main ovarian artery seen in the ovary is not the ovarian stromal vessel. Perifollicular flow is assessed in the vessels that overlap the follicular wall (Fig. 15).

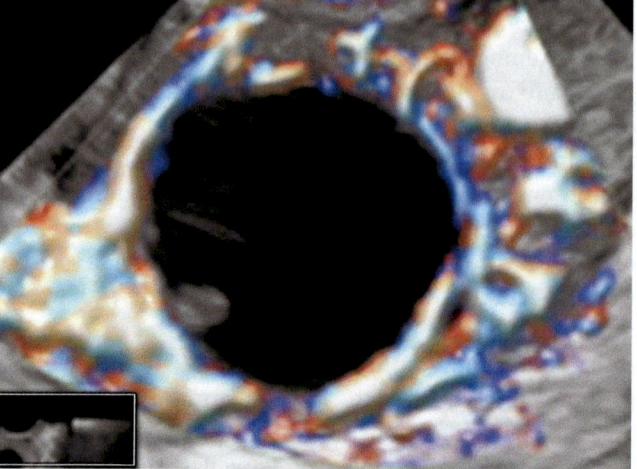

Fig. 15: High-definition (HD) flow image showing perifollicular flow.

REFERENCE

1. Hull MGR. Polycystic ovarian disease: clinical aspects and prevalence. Res Clin Forums. 1989;11:21-34.

Three-dimensional/Four-dimensional Ultrasound in Obstetrics: An Entertainment or an Empowerment

Sachin Nichite, Pragya Nichite

INTRODUCTION

Since years, two-dimensional (2D) or grayscale ultrasound has been mainstay of obstetric ultrasound. But in current era, volume imaging or three-dimensional (3D) imaging has become almost an integral part of imaging. The journey, which started from face rendering only, has now become integral part of diagnosis of fetal anomalies. So, from a source of entertainment for parents, it has moved to become empowerment for practitioners. Addition of fourth dimension, i.e., time brought to us four-dimensional (4D) ultrasound which not only made surface rendering interesting but also revolutionized the fetal cardiac imaging. In this write-up, we are going to understand the advantages, various modes and tools used, some practical aspects, clinical applications, and some limitations of this beautiful technique.

ADVANTAGES OF THREE-DIMENSIONAL/FOUR-DIMENSIONAL OR VOLUME IMAGING

- *Postprocessing*: The saved volume data of patient's sonographic 3D/4D images can be manipulated, reintegrated, and displayed in different modes.

The patient need not to be examined multiple times:[1-3]
- *Reduced operator dependency*: 3D/4D volume imaging makes it less dependent on operator's skills and eyes.[1-3]
- *Reduced dependency on fetal position*: The volume dataset can be manipulated to get desired view irrespective of position of fetus.

This also reduces the total scanning time:
- *Measurements*: Measurements can be taken that were not taken during live scanning or measurements which can only be achieved in reconstructed planes.
- *Telemedicine*: The entire dataset can be transferred to other centers for expert opinion or educational purposes.[3,4]

VARIOUS MODES AND TOOLS USED IN THREE-DIMENSIONAL/FOUR-DIMENSIONAL IMAGING (BOX 1)

- *Three-dimensional surface rendering*: This is the most common mode used and most popular among patients, often showing baby face in utero.

Box 1: Various modes and tools for 3D/4D sonography.

- 3D/4D surface rendering
- Multiplanar
- TUI/multislice
- STIC
- HDLive/realistic view
- VCI
- Inversion
- Omniview
- SonoAVC
- SonoVCAD heart
- Skeletal
- Magicut

(STIC: spatiotemporal image correlation; TUI: tomographic ultrasound imaging; VCI: volume contrast imaging; SonoAVC: sonography-based automated volume count; SonoVCAD: sonography-based volume computer-aided display)

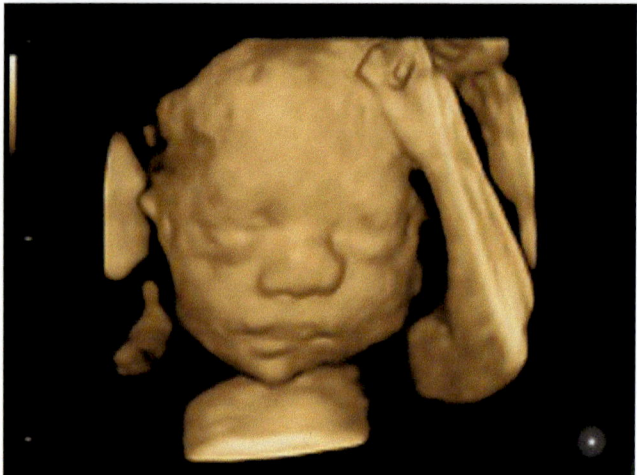

Fig. 1: Surface rendering of fetal face.

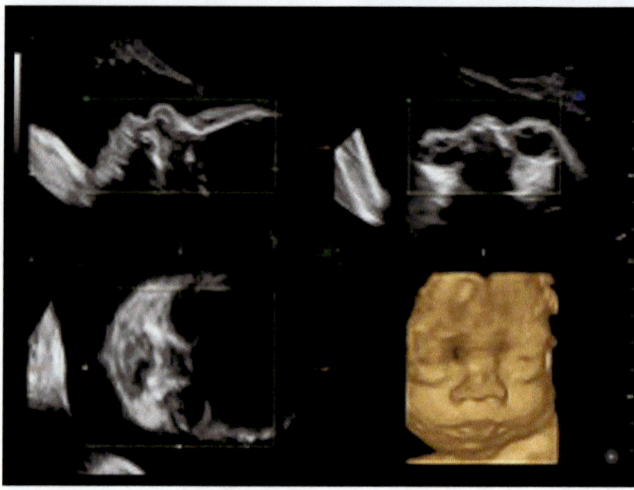

Fig. 2: Multiplanar view of fetal face.

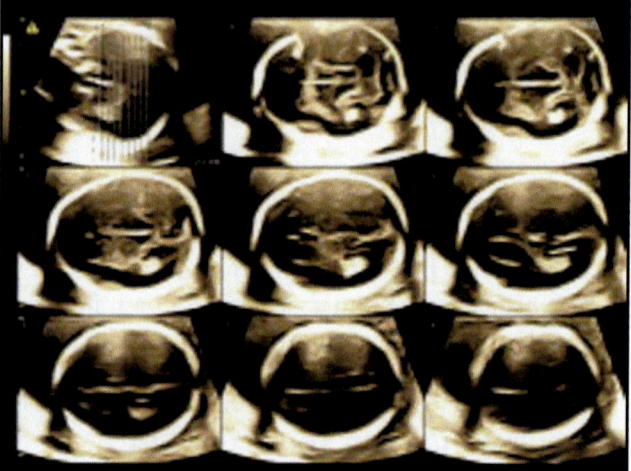

Fig. 3: Tomographic ultrasound imaging (TUI) of fetal head.

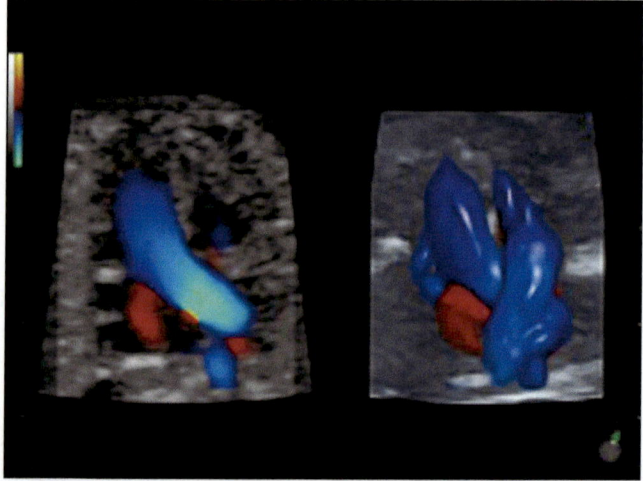

Fig. 4: Color spatiotemporal image correlation (STIC) of fetal heart.

This modality is used in evaluation of superficial parts such as face, skull, back, abdomen, and limbs (Fig. 1):[5-7]

- *Multiplanar*: This modality allows us viewing three orthogonal planes with single dot representing the point of intersection of all three planes. The volume or three planes can be manipulated by moving other dot or individual planes. Although planes A and B can be acquired from the patient using 2D ultrasound, the ability to reconstruct the C plane makes this technique unique (Fig. 2).[8-10]
- *Tomographic ultrasound imaging (TUI) or multislice*: In this technique, the volume is displayed in multiple parallel tomographic slices, similar to displays used in CT and MRI. The volume can be manipulated by changing number of slices and the distance between slices (Fig. 3).[11]
- *Spatiotemporal image correlation (STIC)*: This is a cardiac imaging technique that interrogates multiple sequential cardiac cycles and displays them as single representative volume. This volume can be manipulated using other techniques such as multiplanar, inversion, etc. (Figs. 4 and 5).[12-15]
- *High-definition (HD) live*: This method generates amazingly realistic images of human fetus. It supports shadows, a virtual light source, and advanced skin rendering techniques (Figs. 6 and 7).
- *Volume contrast imaging (VCI)*: This tool helps to improve contrast resolution and visualization of rendered anatomy within any image plane.
- *Inversion*: This is a rendering technique to suppress tissue and only show cystic/anechoic structures (Fig. 8).[16-19]
- *Omniview*: This technique allows interrogation of volume datasets and simultaneous display of up to three nonorthogonal planes by manually drawing lines from any direction or angle (Fig. 9).
- *SonoAVC (sonography-based automated volume count)*: This research tool helps visualization and measurement of hypoechoic structures within anatomy such as fetal brain, dilated kidneys, etc.

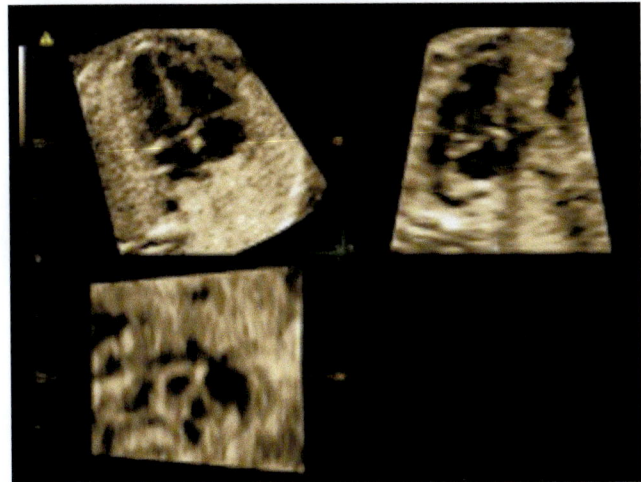

Fig. 5: Spatiotemporal image correlation (STIC) fetal heart.

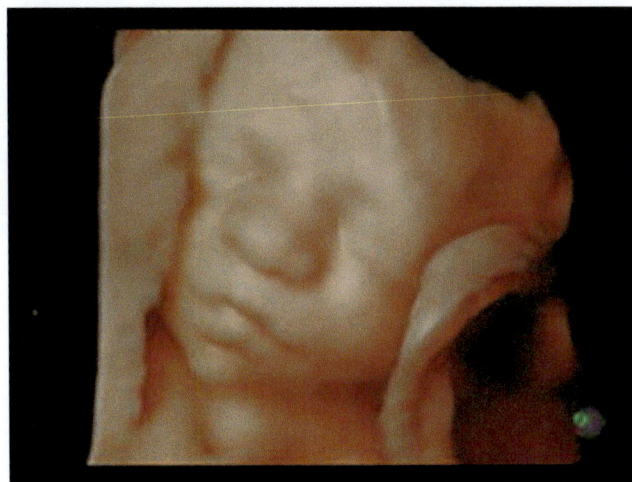

Fig. 6: HD-live mode for fetal face.

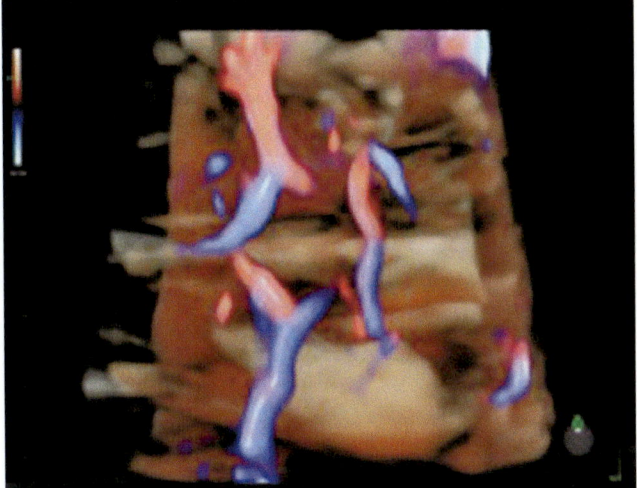

Fig. 7: HD-live flow of circle of Willis.

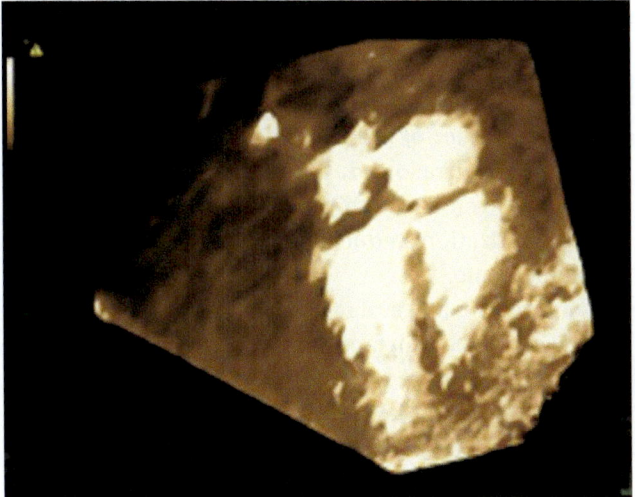

Fig. 8: Inversion mode for fetal heart.

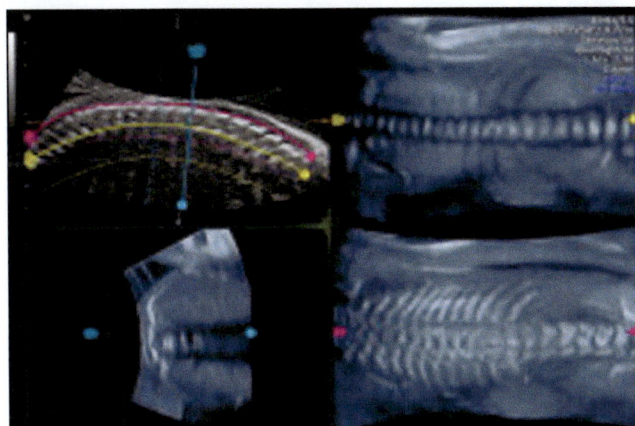

Fig. 9: Omniview of fetal spinal column.

- *SonoVCAD (sonography-based volume computer-aided display) heart:* It assists in generating standard views of fetal heart from four-chamber view.
- *Skeletal:* This mode allows us to visualize only skeletal components of volume dataset such as spine, ribs, skull, bones, hard palate, nasal bone, etc. (Fig. 10).
- *Magicut:* This is also called as electronic scalpel. This is important tool in postprocessing of 3D volumes which erases the unwanted portions.

PRACTICAL STEPS FOR THREE-DIMENSIONAL/ FOUR-DIMENSIONAL ULTRASOUND (FLOWCHART 1)

The two most important skills to learn and apply for 3D/4D imaging are placing region of interest (ROI) box and adjusting appropriate angle and speed of acquisition. It depends upon the part to be imaged, fetal movements, and amniotic fluid pocket (Figs. 11 to 13).

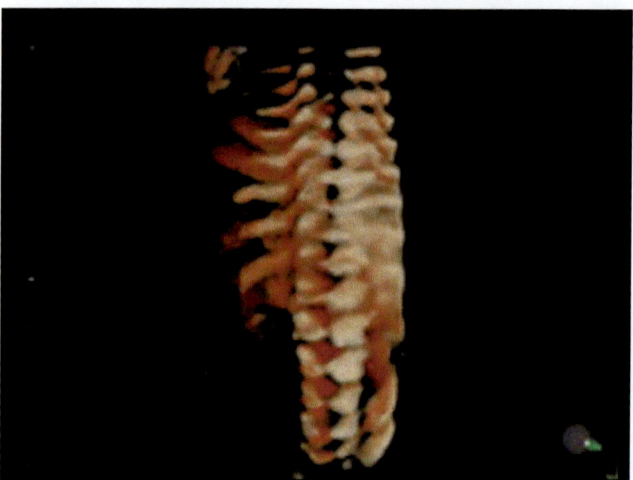

Fig. 10: Skeletal mode for spinal column.

CLINICAL APPLICATIONS OF THREE-DIMENSIONAL/FOUR-DIMENSIONAL ULTRASOUND (BOX 2)

- *Empowerment of ultrasound practice*: With the help of 3D/4D ultrasound, the ultrasound practice can be empowered due to time saving, better flexibility, standardization, reduced operator dependency, and telemedicine.
- Confirmation and evaluation of fetal abnormalities:[12-14,20]
  - *Fetal face*: Surface rendering of fetal face and multiplanar or omniview of face volumes are best for facial and palatal clefts.[21-25] A true midline sagittal plane of face can be reconstructed which is extremely helpful in diagnosis of conditions such as micrognathia,[15] Binder's syndrome, and nasal bone hypoplasia.
  - *Brain*: The diagnosis and prognostication of brain abnormalities such as absent corpus callosum, vermian agenesis, and holoprosencephaly have become easy and comprehensive due to 3D/4D modalities such as multiplanar, and omniview.
  - *Skeletal*: 3D/4D imaging has made evaluation of neural tube defects such as meningocele, encephalocele comprehensive.[26] Skeletal dysplasias can also be evaluated in details.
  - *Extremities*: Best way to demonstrate limb and finger abnormalities is by 3D reconstruction.
  - *Heart*: Invention of STIC, Doppler STIC, and inversion techniques has revolutionized cardiac and cardiac abnormalities evaluation.[11,27-31]
  - *Thoracoabdominal*: Volume imaging helps immensely in evaluation of abnormalities such as congenital diaphragmatic hernia (CDH), especially volumetric evaluation of lungs.[32-34]

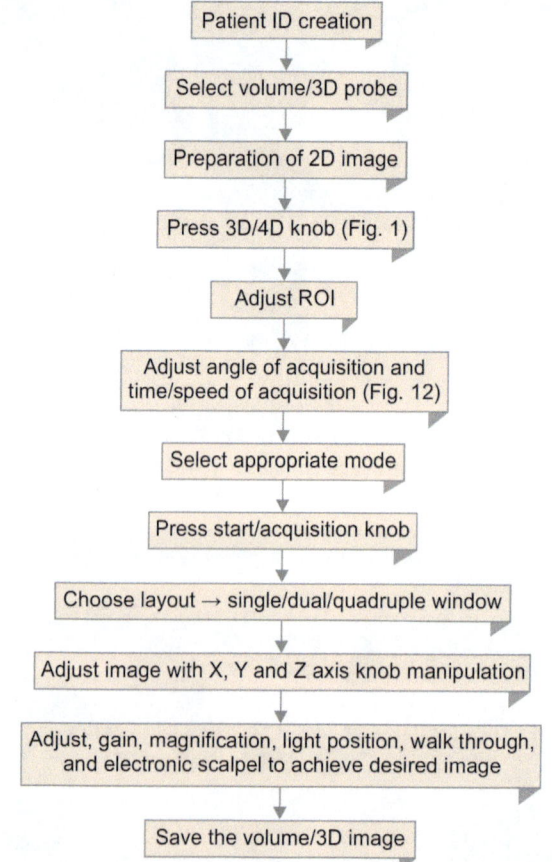

Flowchart 1: Practical steps for 3D/4D ultrasound.

(3D: three-dimensional; 4D: four-dimensional; ROI: region of interest)

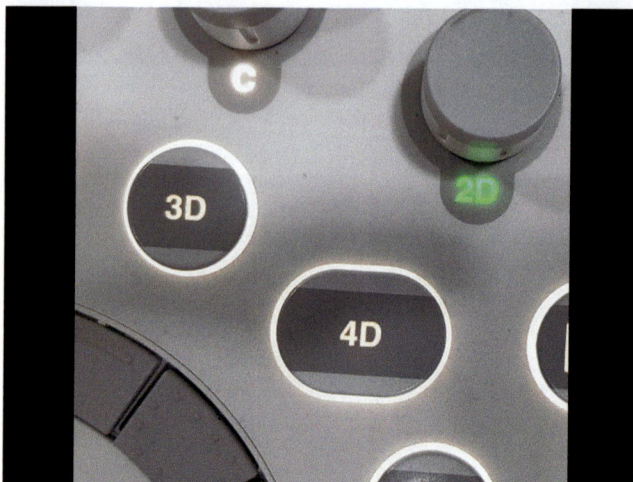

Fig. 11: 3D/4D buttons.

  - *First trimester of pregnancy*: Evaluation of normal embryo structures such as skeleton, nasal bone, vasculature, neuroanatomy, and structures such as yolk sac has improved due to volume imaging.
    Also, demonstration of first trimester abnormalities such as conjoint twins, twin reversed

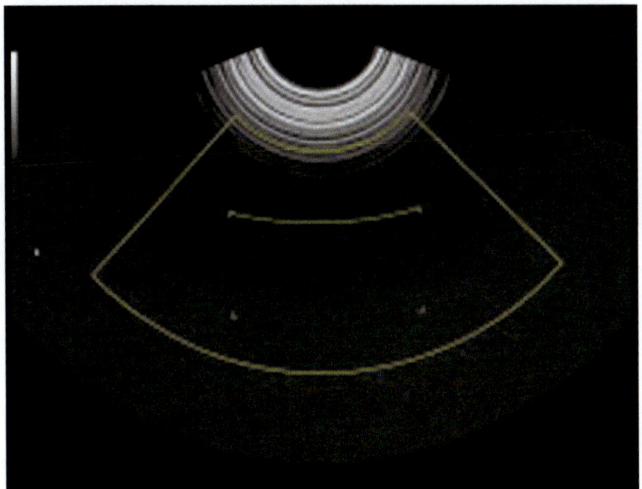

Fig. 12: Region of interest (ROI) box.

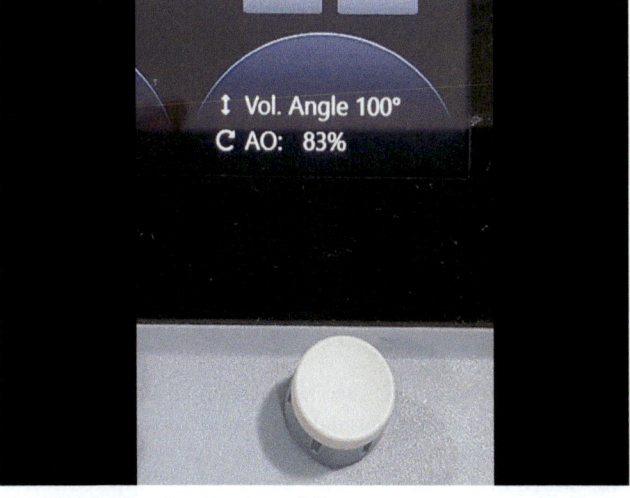

Fig. 13: Display of angle of acquisition.

Box 2: Applications of 3D/4D ultrasound.

- Empowerment of ultrasound practice
- Confirmation and evaluation of fetal abnormalities:
  - Face
  - Brain
  - Skeletal
  - Extremities
  - Heart
  - Thoracoabdominal
- First trimester evaluation and first trimester abnormalities
- Parental counseling and parent fetal bonding

arterial perfusion (TRAP) sequence, acrania, spinal defects, nasal bone hypoplasia, limb abnormalities, omphalocele, gastroschisis, bladder exstrophy, etc. has become easy and comprehensive.

- *Parental counseling and parent fetal bonding*: Direct demonstration of 3D/4D images of fetal abnormalities helps immensely in explaining and counseling to parents and relatives.

Also, watching fetal face and limbs with 3D/4D imaging is one of the most pleasurable and most sought for part of fetal scanning.

LIMITATIONS OF THREE-DIMENSIONAL/FOUR-DIMENSIONAL ULTRASOUND

- *Quality of image*: The quality of 3D/4D image depends directly on quality of 2D image. Also, the quality of orthogonal images is not as good as in plane A.
- *Dependency on patient body habitus and amniotic fluid*: The quality of rendered images is best in thin patients, first half of pregnancy, and patients with good amniotic fluid pockets near region of interest.
- *Cost*: In general, the 3D/4D ultrasound equipment is costly. Also, the maintenance and replacement cost of volume probes is very high.
- *Skills training*: Mastering 3D/4D imaging requires additional training for the operator.

So, to conclude, 3D/4D imaging is a demand of current era of imaging or era of fetal medicine. Every imaging practitioner or even obstetricians should learn this new technique and improve their clinical practice.

REFERENCES

1. Benacerraf BR, Shipp TD, Bromley B. How sonographic tomography will change the face of obstetric sonography: a pilot study. J Ultrasound Med. 2005;24:371-8.
2. Benacerraf BR, Shipp TD, Bromley B. Three-dimensional US of the fetus: volume imaging. Radiology. 2006;238:988-96.
3. Nelson TR, Pretorius DH, Lev-Toaff A, et al. Feasibility performing a virtual patient examination using three-dimensional ultrasonographic data acquired at remote locations. J Ultrasound Med. 2001;20:941-52.
4. Johnson DD, Pretorius DH, Riccabona M, et al. Three-dimensional ultrasound of the fetal spine. Obstet Gynecol. 1997;89:434-8.
5. Nelson TR, Pretorius DH. Three-dimensional ultrasound of fetal surface features. Ultrasound Obstet Gynecol. 1992;2:166-74.
6. Pretorius DH, Borok NN, Coffler MS, et al. Three-dimensional ultrasound in obstetrics and gynecology. Radiol Clin North Am. 2001;39:499-521.
7. Riccabona M, Pretorius DH, Nelson TR, et al. Three-dimensional ultrasound: display modalities in obstetrics. J Clin Ultrasound. 1997;25:157-67.
8. Benacerraf BR. Three-dimensional fetal sonography: use and misuse. J Ultrasound Med. 2002;21:1063-7.
9. Merz E, Bahlmann F, Weber G. Volume scanning in the evaluation of fetal malformations: a new dimension in prenatal diagnosis. Ultrasound Obstet Gynecol. 1995;5:222-7.

10. Pretorius DH, Nelson TR. Three-dimensional ultrasound. Ultrasound Obstet Gynecol. 1995;5:219-21.
11. Devore GR, Polanko B. Tomographic ultrasound imaging of the fetal heart: a new technique for identifying normal and abnormal cardiac anatomy. J Ultrasound Med. 2005;24:1685-96.
12. Dyson RL, Pretorius DH, Budorick NE, et al. Three-dimensional ultrasound in the evaluation of fetal anomalies. Ultrasound Obstet Gynecol. 2000;16:321-8.
13. Scharf A, Ghazwiny MF, Steinborn A, et al. Evaluation of two-dimensional versus three-dimensional ultrasound in obstetric diagnostics: a prospective study. Fetal Diagn Ther. 2001;16:333-41.
14. Merz E, Welter C. 2D and 3D Ultrasound in the evaluation of normal and abnormal fetal anatomy in the second and third trimesters in a level III center. Ultraschall Med. 2005;26:9-16.
15. Merz E, Weber G, Bahlmann F, et al. Application of transvaginal and abdominal three-dimensional ultrasound for the detection or exclusion of malformations of the fetal face. Ultrasound Obstet Gynecol. 1997;9:237-43.
16. Lee W, Gonçalves LF, Espinoza J, et al. Inversion mode: a new volume analysis tool for 3-dimensional ultrasonography. J Ultrasound Med. 2005;24:201-7.
17. Espinoza J, Gonçalves LF, Lee W, et al. A novel method to improve prenatal diagnosis of abnormal systemic venous connections using three- and four-dimensional ultrasonography and 'inversion mode'. Ultrasound Obstet Gynecol. 2005;25:428-34.
18. Benacerraf BR. Inversion mode display of 3D sonography: applications in obstetric and gynecologic imaging. Am J Roentgenol. 2006;187:965-71.
19. Timor-Tritsch IE, Monteagudo A, Tsymbal T, et al. Three-dimensional inversion rendering: a new sonographic technique and its use in gynecology. J Ultrasound Med. 2005;24:681-8.
20. Platt LD, Santulli T, Carlson DE, et al. Three-dimensional ultrasonography in obstetrics and gynecology: preliminary experience. Am J Obstet Gynecol. 1998;178:1199-206.
21. Kozuma S, Baba K, Okai T, et al. Dynamic observation of the fetal face by three-dimensional ultrasound. Ultrasound Obstet Gynecol. 1999;13:283-4.
22. Kuno A, Akiyama M, Yamashiro C, et al. Three-dimensional sonographic assessment of fetal behavior in the early second trimester of pregnancy. J Ultrasound Med. 2001;20:1271-5.
23. Pretorius DH, Nelson TR. Fetal face visualization using three-dimensional ultrasonography. J Ultrasound Med. 1995;14:349-56.
24. Lee W, Kirk JS, Shaheen KW, et al. Fetal cleft lip and palate detection by three-dimensional ultrasonography. Ultrasound Obstet Gynecol. 2000;16:314-20.
25. Chmait R, Pretorius D, Jones M, et al. Prenatal evaluation of facial clefts with two-dimensional and adjunctive three-dimensional ultrasonography: a prospective trial. Am J Obstet Gynecol. 2002;187:946-9.
26. Lee W, Chaiworapongsa T, Romero R, et al. A diagnostic approach for the evaluation of spina bifida by three-dimensional ultrasonography. J Ultrasound Med. 2002;21:619-26.
27. Viñals F, Poblete P. Giuliano A. Spatio-temporal image correlation (STIC): a new tool for the prenatal screening of congenital heart defects. Ultrasound Obstet Gynecol. 2003;22:388-94.
28. Gonçalves LF, Lee W, Chaiworapongsa T, et al. Four-dimensional ultrasonography of the fetal heart with spatiotemporal image correlation. Am J Obstet Gynceol. 2003;189:1792-802.
29. Viñals F, Mandujano L, Vargas C, et al. Prenatal diagnosis of congenital heart disease using four-dimensional spatio-temporal image correlation (STIC) telemedicine via an Internet link: a pilot study. Ultrasound Obstet Gynecol. 2005;25:25-31.
30. Gonçalves LF, Espinoza J, Romero R, et al. A systematic approach to prenatal diagnosis of transposition of the great arteries using 4-dimensional ultrasonography with spatiotemporal image correlation. J Ultrasound Med. 2004;23:1225-31.
31. Gonçalves LF, Romero R, Espinoza J, et al. Four-dimensional ultrasonography of the fetal heart using color Doppler spatiotemporal image correlation. J Ultrasound Med. 2004;23:473-81.
32. Favre R, Nisand G, Bettahar K, et al. Measurement of limb circumferences with three-dimensional ultrasound for fetal weight estimation. Ultrasound Obstet Gynecol. 1993;3:176-9.
33. Steiner H, Gregg AR, Bogner G, et al. First trimester three-dimensional ultrasound volumetry of the gestational sac. Arch Gynecol Obstet. 1994;255:165-70.
34. Hughes SW, D'Arcy TJ, Maxwell DJ, et al. Volume estimation from multiplanar 2D ultrasound images using a remote electromagnetic position and orientation sensor. Ultrasound Med Biol. 1996;22:561-72.

Role of Color Flow and Doppler in Gynecology and Infertility

Amogh Chimote, Neharika Malhotra, Narendra Malhotra

INTRODUCTION

Since the advent of ultrasound, there has been an exponential rise in its application for noninvasive diagnostic purpose especially for the pelvic region. Yet another development in this field to enhance the diagnostic capabilities of this modality was color Doppler.[1] Both these modalities have a subjective assessment and are fairly reproducible.

The role of color Doppler in obstetrics, gynecology, and infertility has been ever changing and helped us to diagnose and manage most of the complication even before they manifest.

This prediction capability of color Doppler along with ultrasound has led to its increase role and use in all these fields helping us to tackle conditions such as pre-eclampsia, intrauterine growth restriction (IUGR), benign diseases and gynecological malignancies, ovarian stimulation, infertility monitories, ovarian hyperstimulation syndrome (OHSS), and many more conditions.[2]

Doppler helps in visualizing the blood supply of almost all of the small vessels right from the endometrium, uterus, ovary, myometrium, tubes, adnexa as well as other important blood vessels of the pelvis. The sensitivity as well as the specificity of this modality is fairly high and hence has a widespread application.

WHAT IS COLOR DOPPLER?

When ultrasound energy is directed to a moving target, it is reflected back with a change in frequency. This phenomenon is what we call as Doppler shift. A waveform is constructed and this waveform is called as "Doppler velocity waveform" (Fig. 1). Studying this waveform tells us about the various changes that occur in the pelvic blood vessels which ultimately help us in formulating a diagnosis.

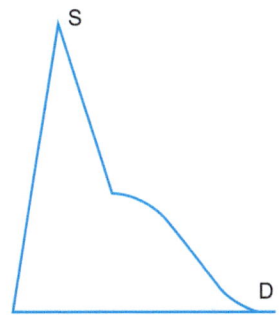

Fig. 1: A typical Doppler waveform (S: systolic wave; D: diastolic wave).

This velocity of blood flow can be determined using certain equations, if the values of the angle and of the Doppler signal are known. The processing of the Doppler signal includes sequential steps of amplification, demodulation, spectral processing, and display.

VARIABLES IN DOPPLER

- *Blood velocity*: Doppler frequency increases as the velocity of blood flow increases, i.e., high velocity blood flow will have a higher frequency depiction on the color flow.
- *Ultrasound frequency*: Doppler frequency is increased with higher ultrasound frequency. As in B-mode, lower ultrasound frequencies have better penetration. Better sensitivity to flow or better penetration depends on the choice of frequency.
- *Angle of insonation*: Angle of insonation is defined as the angle of the ultrasound beam relative to the tissue or organ of interest. The strongest echoes are produced when the angles of incidence approach the angle of reflection.

CALCULATIONS IN DOPPLER

In order to quantify the vascular resistance, various indices have been proposed.

$$\text{Pulsatility index (PI)} \atop \text{(Gosling and King, 1975)} = \frac{\text{Peak systolic velocity (PSV) - End-diastolic velocity}}{\text{Mean velocity}}$$

$$\text{Resistance index (RI)} = \frac{\text{PSV - End-diastolic velocity}}{\text{PSV}} \text{ (Bourcelot, 1974)}$$

Systolic/diastolic ratio (Stuart et al., 1980): The higher the value of these indices, more the impedance to blood flow and perfusion of the particular area. In order to understand the pathological features of different gynecological conditions, one has to know about the indices of various vessels.

HOW THE COLOR IMAGE IS FORMED?

Color images are of two types: (1) Asynchronous imaging and (2) Synchronous imaging. In asynchronous imaging, the grayscale and Doppler information are gathered at different times. In contrast, synchronous imaging information is gathered simultaneously.

Asynchronous color flow imaging: Two images are produced during scanning and are later superimposed. The grayscale comes from a real-time image. The Doppler image comes from steering another ultrasound beam at an angle to the array (0–45°). The image is composed in a digital scan converter. Two different frequencies can be used for the two image components; a system could have grayscale at 5 MHz and color at 3 MHz.

Synchronous color flow imaging: Simultaneous processing for amplitude, phase, and frequency is achieved by the same echo signal. This technology is so different that it is known as angiography. The linear array sends a dynamically focused beam, which is perpendicular to the vessels. This is good for imaging but not for Doppler. To provide the Doppler angle needed to visualize blood flow, a wedge stand off-site between the array surface and the skin surface. The image is divided into a set of sample sits, which are same in the field of view. Within this site, the system looks at the echo signal amplitude is one path, at the phase, and frequency in the other.

The machine now builds the image on a pixel basis, testing first for evidence of motion and its direction. If motion exits at a pixel, it is colored, otherwise it takes on a grayscale proportionate to the echo signal strength. Having set out the image formation, the next step is color-coding the pixels, in which motion was detected.

TYPES OF DOPPLER

There are basically two types of Doppler that are present on the ultrasound machine:
1. Continuous wave Doppler
2. Pulsed wave Doppler

Continuous Wave Doppler

As the name suggests, this type of Doppler emits continuous wave and receives them simultaneously. The beam of sound flows continuously until it is completely attenuated by the depth of the tissue and it transmits the Doppler wave from every blood vessel it encounters in its path. Owing to this property, continuous wave Doppler is unable to determine the source as well as the location of the velocities which it passes and hence there is lack of a color flow image. This type of color flow is generally more useful in cardiac scans.

Pulsed Wave Doppler (Fig. 2)

Pulsed wave, as the name suggests, emits and receives sound waves in a pulsatile manner. This small interval in pulsed wave enables it to locate the depth as well as velocity of the vessel. Additional advantage of this type of Doppler is that the range gate can be changed according to the diameter of the vessel, hence getting a more accurate flow velocity and interpretation. It allows simultaneous B-mode and color flow images to be seen together. Obstetric or gynecological ultrasound use pulsed wave Doppler as to continuous flow.

ALIASING

At a given sampling frequency when the pulses are transmitted (pulse repetition frequency), the maximum

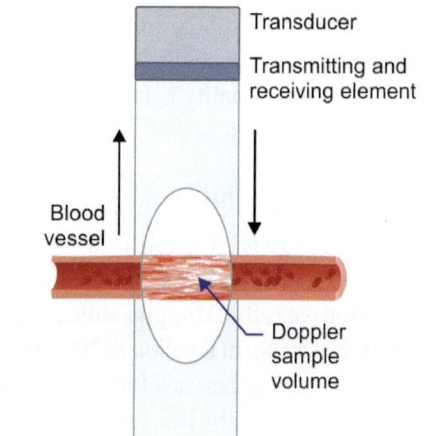

Fig. 2: Pulsed wave Doppler.

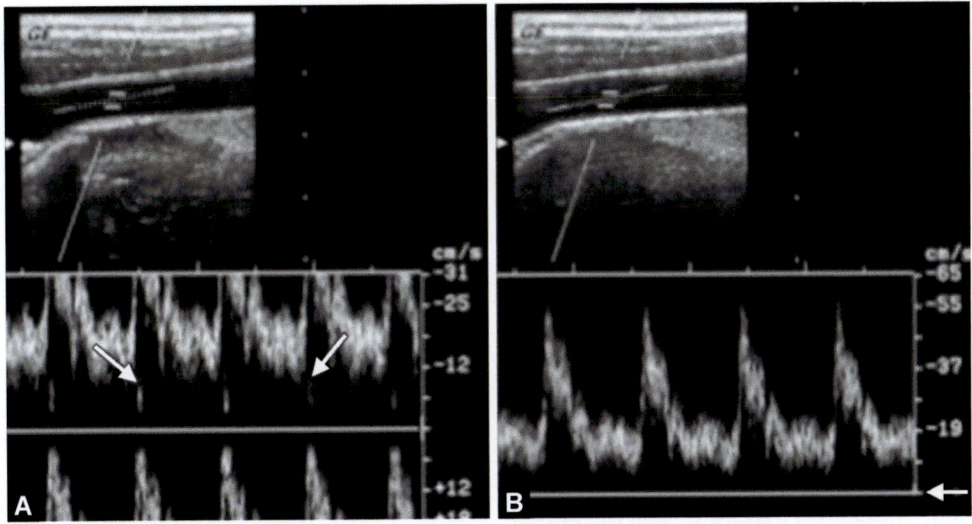

Figs. 3A and B: Aliasing and correction of aliasing by shifting the baseline (arrows).

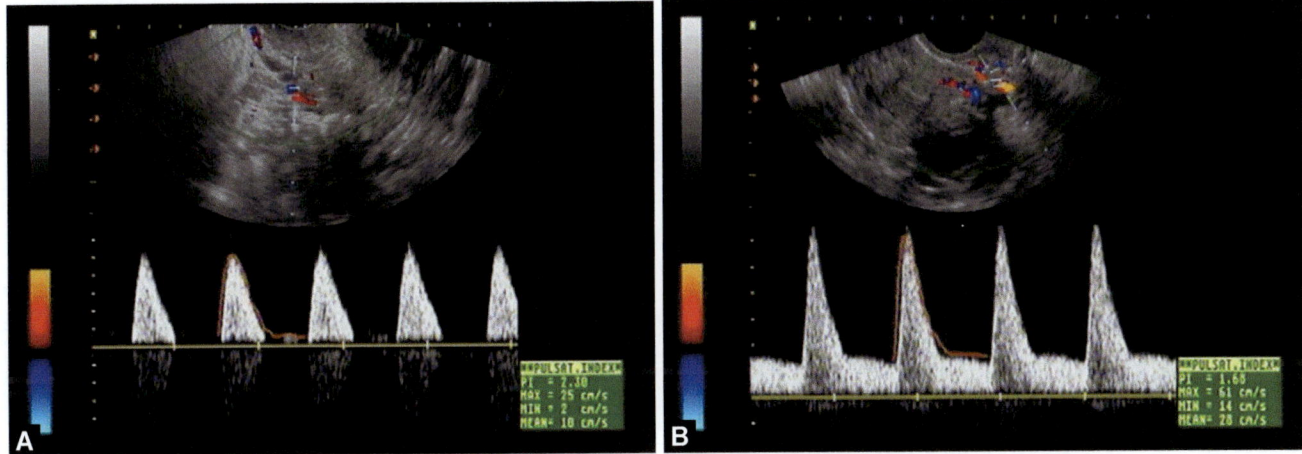

High resistance: Diastolic flow is very less, less than 10% of systole (RI around 0.9)

Resistance decreases as menstrual cycle and now the diastolic flow is about 30% (RI around 0.7)

Figs. 4A and B: (A) In early proliferative phase resistance index (RI) 0.94 ± 0.04; and (B) Day 18 (secretory phase) RI 0.74 ± 0.04.

Doppler frequency (fd) that can be measured without ambiguity is exactly the half of pulse repetition frequency. So, if the flow angle and the blood velocity combine to give an fd which is more than half of the rules of repetition frequency, the Doppler signal becomes ambiguous, this is what is called as aliasing (Figs. 3A and B).

A simple example is when we see backward rotation of a wheel on a film if the frame rate is low even when the wheel is moving forward.

USE OF DOPPLER IN GYNECOLOGY

The use of color Doppler in gynecology has opened many avenues for diagnosing and preventing various diseases which were previously ambiguous or difficult to diagnose and required invasive diagnostic techniques calculating various indices in all the pelvic vessels that gives an idea of the resistance to blood offered by that vessel.[3-10] Usually, all muscular arteries, due to the musculature, let blood go through to the organ in diastole. This blood is approximately 30% of the systolic push.

Main Uterine Vessel

The color Doppler signal from the main uterine vessels may be seen in all patients lateral to the cervix. The small branches of uterine artery can be followed by searching the corpus, ascending along the lateral wall. Waveform analysis shows high velocity and high resistance flow. The RI depends on the age, phase of menstrual cycle, and any special condition such as pregnancy or tumor (Figs. 4A and B).

Table 1: Resistance index (RI) for ovarian vessels during menstrual cycle.			
Active ovary: RI (corpus luteum)	0.44 ± 0.09	PSV	27 ± 10 cm/s
Inactive ovary: RI	0.76 ± 0.22	PSV	8.9 ± 3.8 cm/s

(PSV: peak systolic velocity)

Ovarian Vessels

It is difficult to visualize the ovarian vessels but an experienced operator using modern color Doppler unit can detect them in most patients in the lateral upper pole of the ovary.

Color flow is usually not prominent, velocity is low, and resistance varies according to the menstrual cycle. A low velocity, high impedance pattern is seen during the follicular phase. At ovulation, there is maximum increase in the velocity and *RI decreases, reaching a dip of 0.44 ± 0.09* (Table 1). 4–5 days later, it slowly increases by 0.04–0.05 before menstruation.

Iliac Flow

The common and external iliac arteries show plug flow (triphasic flow), a window under the waveform, and a reversed component during diastole. The internal iliac vessel in contrast has a parabolic flow with an even distribution of velocities within the waveform. These can be generally located near the ovary on the caudal side.

Ovarian Masses

A recent new classification and terminology for distinguishing ovarian mass is the International Ovarian Tumor Analysis (IOTA) classification. It follows certain modified terminologies which are as follows.

Classification of Adnexal Masses According to the International Ovarian Tumor Analysis (Table 2)[11,12]

- *Benign ovarian*: Polycystic ovaries, functional cysts, endometriomas, serous cystadenoma, mucinous cystadenoma, mature teratoma, fibroma (rare, can cause Meigs syndrome: ascites and pleural effusion), and thecoma (very rare, can secrete estrogen and progesterone).
- *Benign nonovarian*: Paratubal cyst, hydrosalpinges, tubo-ovarian abscess, peritoneal pseudocysts, appendiceal abscess, diverticular abscess, and pelvic kidney.
- *Primary malignant ovarian*:
  – Epithelial carcinoma
    - Borderline
    - Serious cystadenocarcinoma

Table 2: Characteristics of masses in the IOTA classification.	
Locules	Unilocular, unilocular-solid, multilocular, multilocular-solid, or solid
Cyst contents	Anechoic, low level, ground glass, and hemorrhagic or mixed—solid material or papillary structures or wall irregularity (presence and size)
Vascularity	PI and RI of the ovarian vessels
Shadows	–
Ascites	–

(IOTA: International Ovarian Tumor Analysis; PI: pulsatility index; RI: resistance index)

- Mucinous cystadenocarcinoma
- Pseudomyxoma peritonei
- Clear cell carcinoma
– Germ cell tumor
- Malignant teratoma
- Dysgerminoma
– Sex cord tumor
- Granulosa cell tumor
- *Secondary malignant ovarian*: 10% of ovarian malignancy, predominantly: breast gastrointestinal carcinoma (Krukenberg tumor).

International Ovarian Tumor Analysis Terminologies

So, color Doppler helps us in determining the vascularity score and determine if the mass is benign, borderline malignant, or malignant.

Uterine Masses

A lesion or a mass in the uterus is an alarming finding in women of any age and needs to be diagnosed further.[13-15]

Uterine fibroids are one of the most common pathologies seen in abnormal uterine bleeding (AUB) ranging from 20% to 50% of women globally.[21] An uterine fibroid needs to be differentiated from an adenomyoma or focal patch of adenomyosis as well as malignant transformation of the fibroid. This differentiation can be very well-established by the use of color Doppler and each entity has its own characteristic vascularity as well as Doppler finding.

Color flow Doppler and spectral Doppler findings are variable in uterine fibroids reflecting their natural history with growth followed by episodes of degeneration. The vascularity in fibroids is typically peripheral with very high velocities and low resistance. In contrast, the center of fibroids is often avascular and necrotic.[16,17]

A pedunculated fibroid can simulate an ovarian cancer. On endovaginal color flow, copious vascularity may be seen with perfusion characteristics identical to those in ovarian cancer. The pitfall can be avoided by demonstrating the connecting pedicle.

There is an increase in blood flow and a decrease in impedance in both uterine arteries in patients with fibroids. The degree of vascularity of a fibroid can determine how the patient should be managed, i.e., when myomectomy should be offered and by which route, whether gonadotropin-releasing hormone (GnRH) agonists should be given or when hysterectomy should be performed.[18-20]

In adenomyosis, there is an inherent increase in vascularity owing to the muscular hyperplasia and hypertrophy. The vascularity of the adenomyoma is such that there is myometrial involvement with increased tortuosity of the penetrating vessels.

Differentiation of Fibroid from Adenomyosis

The differentiation of fibroid from adenomyosis is given in Figures 5A to D.

The differentiating features of fibroids and adenomyoma are described in Table 3.

ENDOMETRIAL POLYP

Ultrasound is the most accepted investigation for evaluation of abnormal uterine bleeding.[22] In about 25% of patients, abnormal uterine bleeding is the result of a well-defined organic abnormality.[23] Endometrial polyps account for abnormal vaginal bleeding in 39% and 21–28% of pre- and postmenopausal women, respectively.[24]

The grayscale characteristics of a polyp are:
- Isoechoic uniform echotexture similar to the endometrium

Table 3: Differentiating features of fibroids and adenomyoma.

Characteristics	Fibroid	Adenomyoma
Vascularity	Peripheral/circumferential	Dispersed/diffuse
Pulsatility index (PI)	1.1 ± 0.04	1.52 ± 0.25
Resistance index (RI)	0.74 ± 0.09	0.56 ± 0.12

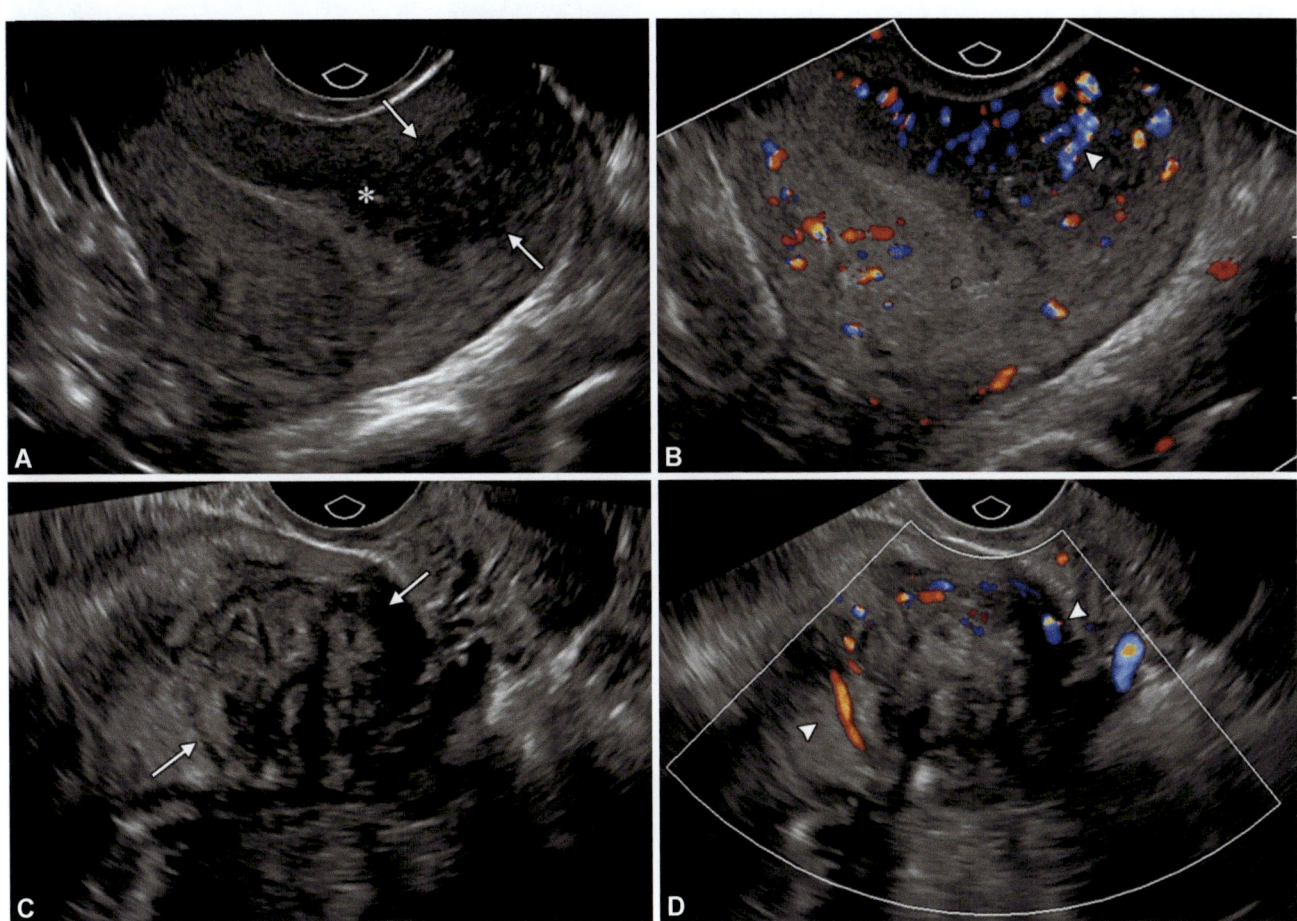

Figs. 5A to D: (A) Adenomyosis: A heterogeneous myometrium (abnormal) with small echogenic nodules and myometrial cysts (arrows) with loss of endomyometrial junction (*); (B) The color flow pattern of the adenomyosis which is diffuse with multiple tortuous penetrating vessels dispersed around the heterogeneous mass (arrowhead); (C) Sagittal view with a distinct area of differentiation between the mass and the myometrium circumferentially (arrows), a typical characteristic of fibroid; and (D) A typical circumferential vasculature pattern with minimum to no vascularity in the central part of the lesion suggestive of fibroid (arrowheads).

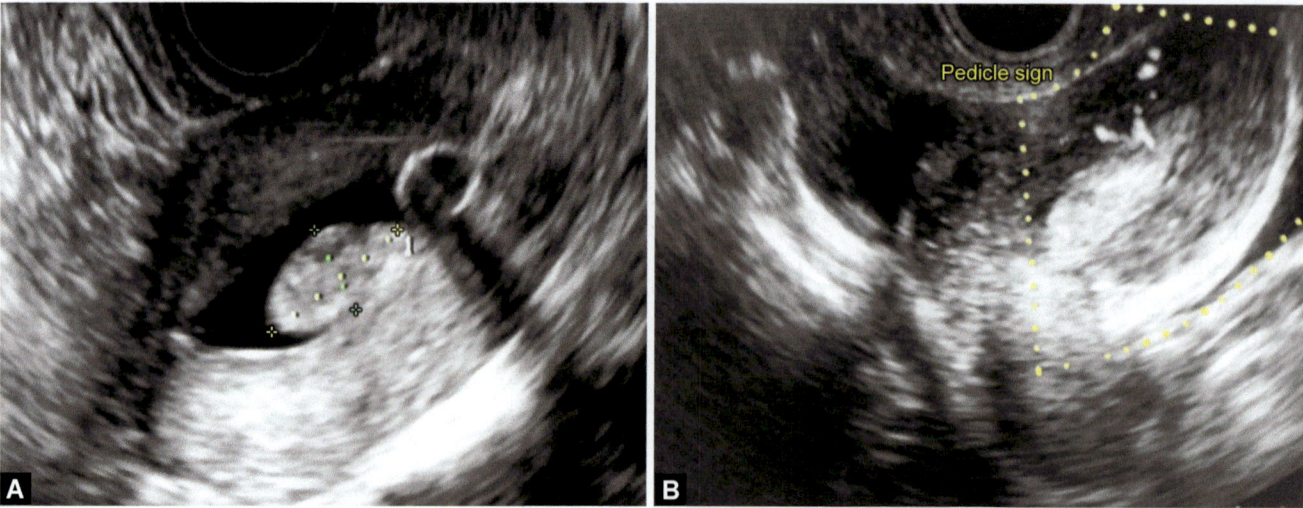

Figs. 6A and B: (A) Saline infusion sonography delineating the polyp; and (B) The pedicle artery sign seen on power Doppler.

- An acute angle to the endometrium
- The endomyometrial junction is intact with smooth margins.

A good method to diagnose a polyp is saline infusion sonography (SIS) which easily demarcates the polyp once the cavity is distended with saline. But with the use of color Doppler, there is seldom a need for SIS as putting color at a thickened endometrial lining shows the pedicle artery sign that is a single pulsating feeding vessel to the thickened endometrium. This "pedicle artery sign" was described by Timmerman et al. as visualization of the feeding blood vessel of the endometrial polyp (Figs. 6A and B).[22]

The pedicle artery sign is characteristic of the endometrial polyp whereas multiple feeding vessels can indicate endometrial hyperplasia, carcinoma, or even in submucous fibroid.

Timmerman et al. in a prospective study found sensitivity of pedicle artery sign as a marker for diagnosis of endometrial polyp to be 76.4%, specificity of 95.3%, positive predictive value (PPV) of 81.3%, and negative predictive value (NPV) of 93.8%.[22] Cil et al. also found a similar finding with sensitivity of 81.2%, specificity of 88.2%, PPV of 92.9%, and NPV of 71.4%.[25] Talat et al. in a study concluded that pedicle artery sign has 94% sensitivity and 100% specificity.[26] Cogdez et al. reported in their study a sensitivity, specificity, PPV, and NPV of single feeding vessel in diagnosing polyp to be 80%, 100%, and 69.2%, respectively.

ADNEXAL OVARIAN TORSION

Ovarian torsion can occur in females of all ages; however, women in their reproductive years have the highest prevalence with 17–20% of cases occurring in pregnant women.[27] This is a difficult diagnosis on either clinical or imaging criteria. The appearances on ultrasound are almost infinitely variable. Transvaginal sonography (TVS) is one of the best imaging techniques for diagnosing torsion as it is noninvasive, accessible, and cost-effective with reproducible and accurate results. A series of study showed that PPV of ultrasound diagnosis of ovarian torsion to be 87.5% and specificity of 93.3%, hence forming a basic yet effective tool for diagnosing torsion (Fig. 7).[28]

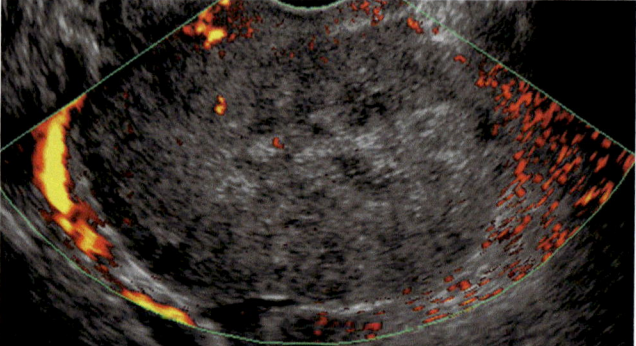

Fig. 7: Absence of color flow in the ovary suggestive of ovarian torsion, the central foci is a motion artifact.

The ovarian torsion can be broadly divided into two types depending on the compromise of the blood vessels and twist on the pedicle are as follows:
1. Complete
2. Incomplete

Color flow Doppler will not distinguish the condition from other pathologies since flow has been demonstrated both centrally and peripherally in lesion. However, it has been suggested that the absence of flow within a twisted ovary identifies one that is beyond salvage by conservative

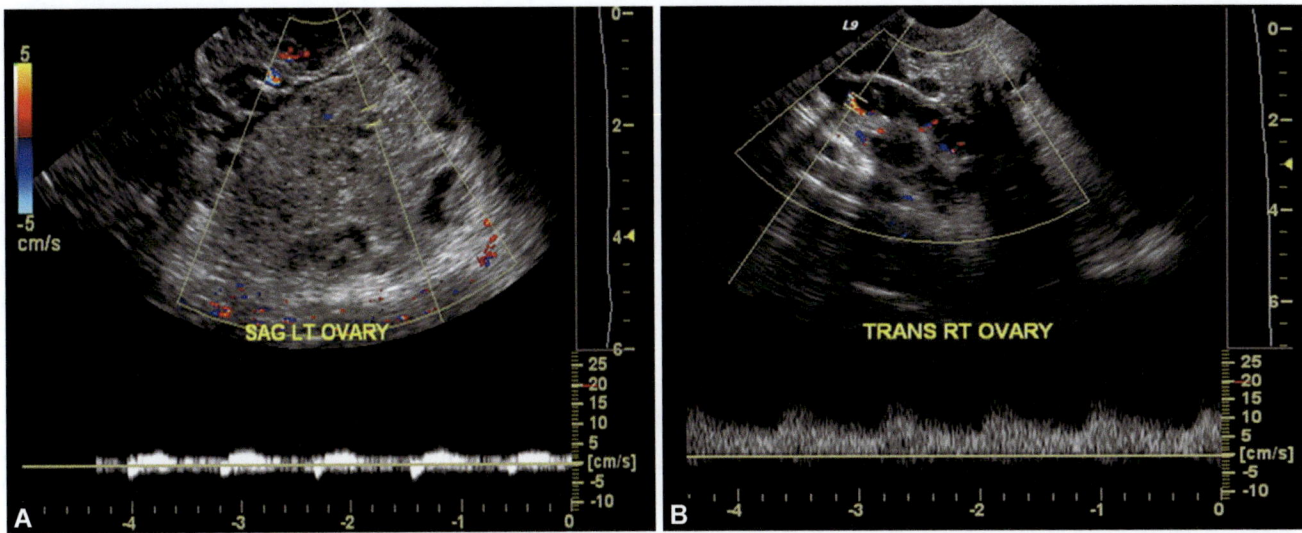

Figs. 8A and B: (A) Sagittal view of the ovary with dampened arterial color flow suggestive of partial torsion and hence the ovary can be salvaged; and (B) A relatively normal color flow of the right ovary which helps in confirming the diagnosis of torsion in the contralateral ovary.

surgery and this may help in the surgical management of this condition.

Doppler findings in ovarian torsion can be as follows (Figs. 8A and B):

- Minimum or no intravenous flow in the ovarian vessels
- Absence of flow in the arteries (poor prognosis, less commonly seen)
- Diastolic flow is reversed or absent
- Vascularity is normal (does not rule out torsion as ovaries receive dual blood supply)
- Whirlpool sign (twisted ovarian pedicle) (Fig. 9)[29]
- Probe tenderness over the ovary[30]

Ultrasound has a sensitivity of approaching 100% and specificity of 97%, if there is an enlarged ovary with an absence of arterial and venous blood flow.[31]

In an incomplete torsion (<360°), there are certain signs which can be seen. The vascular pedicle which is twisted may appear as round hyperechoic with multiple concentric hypoechoic strips called as the target sign. This sign instead of circular can also be beak shaped (concentric low echogenic strips), ellipsoid (internal heterogeneous echoes). The whirlpool sign seen as concentric low echoic intrapedicular structure. The presence of whirlpool sign can be either medial or lateral that is between the lateral pelvic wall and ovary or the ovary and the uterus.[32] The hypoechoic rings comprise of fallopian tube, the utero-ovarian ligament, broad ligament, and branches of ovarian vessels.

Depending on the size of the mass, the whirlpool sign can either be medial or lateral. Greater the volume of the ovarian mass, higher is the tendency toward lateral

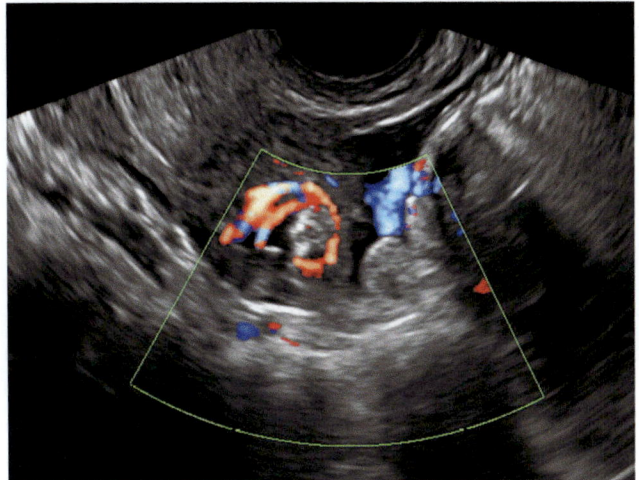

Fig. 9: Whirlpool sign on the medial aspect of the ovary suggestive of a relatively small mass.

whirlpool sign as due to the large mass the ovary is pulled downward and the components of whirlpool sign cannot fit between the ovary and the uterus hence the lateralization. In a small mass, the components of the whirlpool sign can fit between the mass and the uterus hence the medialization. This finding can further help us in determining the size of the mass.[33]

Hence, a positive whirlpool or a target sign in a twisted vascular pedicle is the most definitive sign for ovarian torsion.[34]

ENDOMETRIOSIS

The word endometriosis was introduced by Sampson in 1927[35,36] based on the description of endometrium-like tissue in the myometrium by Rokitansky[37] in the rectovaginal septum by Cullen, who called this entity an adenomyoma[38-40] and in "hemorrhagic (chocolate) cysts in the ovaries".[41] Endometriosis was defined as "endometrium-like glands and stroma outside the uterus". Therefore, stromatosis[42,43] is not considered to be endometriosis despite similarities.

Color Doppler may demonstrate flow within these apparent solid structures thereby confirming the diagnosis. The vessels at the periphery of the endometriotic cyst show relativity high vascular impedance. If inflammatory changes occur, there may be altered flow showing reduction in impedance to flow (D/D malignancy).

Though endometrioma being the most predominant finding in cases of endometriosis, deep-seated endometriosis and endometriotic nodules cause a significant hindrance to the quality of life as well as the fertility potential of the female. To diagnose these nodules and deep-seated endometriosis, the color Doppler can be used and give a better insight to the disease process. Endometriosis, especially cystic ovarian and deep endometriosis[44,45] and adenomyosis,[46,47] are associated with abnormal placentation, insufficient physiologic changes in the spiral arteries, and an increased risk of preterm birth, small for gestational age (SGA) babies, and pre-eclampsia.[45]

ENDOMETRIOMA

Transvaginal color Doppler (TVCD) is one of the best noninvasive, in-vivo modalities for assessment for ovarian endometrioma vascularization.[48-51] To the best of knowledge, no other study has evaluated the relationship between clinical symptoms and the vascularization features, as assessed by TVCD, in patients with histologi--cally proven ovarian endometrioma. There seems to be a direct correlation of increased vascularization of endometrioma with pelvic pain or dyspareunia. The correlation of low resistance flow in the pouch of Douglas (POD) as well as in the lateral fornices along with pelvic pain is an indicator of endometrioma.

These color Doppler findings should be correlated with grayscale (B-mode) features of endometrioma.

The typical hilar vascularity with low-resistance flow in the affected ovary is a good marker for an endometrioma (Fig. 10).

PERITONEAL ENDOMETRIOSIS

Peritoneal endometriosis is a rather difficult entity to diagnose only on grayscale ultrasound. But with introduction of sensitive power Doppler which can pick up the smallest vessels and lowest of velocity have made our work much simpler to diagnose pelvic endometriosis. Transvaginal probe tenderness is one of the clinical signs suggestive of an inflammatory change which may be endometriosis or pelvic inflammatory disease (PID). The differentiating factor in both is that the endometriotic lesions appear more echogenic on color Doppler and have a rather low RI ($<0.59 \pm 0.2$) (Fig. 11).

GESTATIONAL TROPHOBLASTIC DISEASE

These include molar pregnancy (both partial and complete), invasive mole, and choriocarcinoma. Patients with moles usually present in early pregnancy as a threatened abortion and serum human chorionic gonadotropin (hCG) levels are found to be greater than 100,000 U/L. Examination of the uterus by endovaginal ultrasound discloses echogenic contents, and the application of color flow shows these contents to be highly vascular with placental like flow.

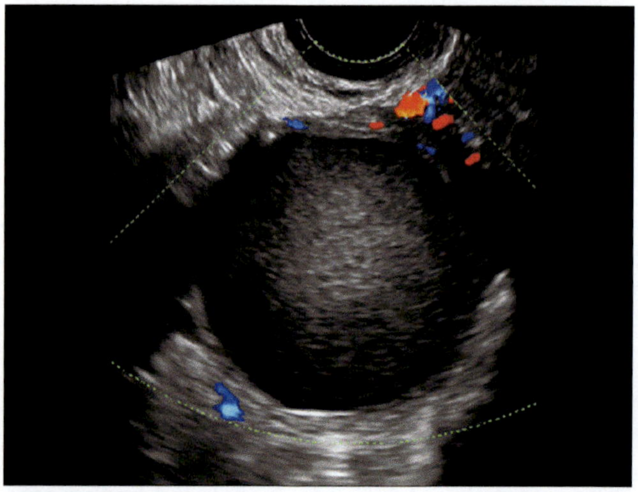

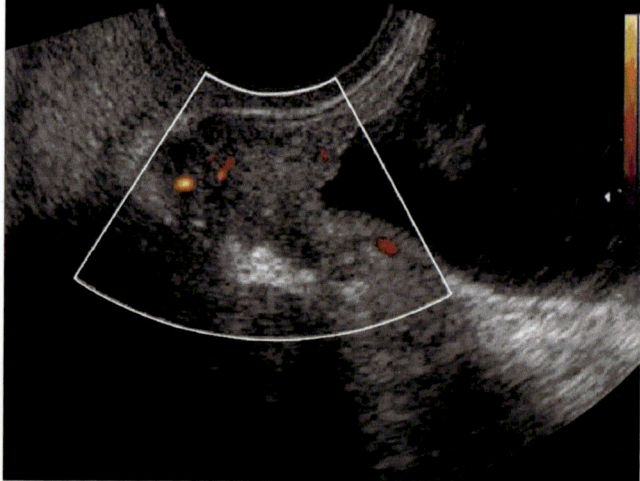

Fig. 10: No peripheral vascularity is noted in the endometrioma. Endometrioma is identified by characteristic ground-glass appearance of the mass and no jelly sign.

Fig. 11: High-velocity, low-resistance tortuous vessels at the uterovesical fold suggestive of endometriotic nodules.

If a normal gestation is seen within uterus, the serum hCG should be repeated because errors in dilutions are not uncommon and may lead to erroneously high serum levels.

Color is extremely helpful in possible recurrence. Myometrial invasion or invasion of adnexa may be seen by the application of color flow. Moles have extensive arteriovenous communications, which account for high-velocity, low-impedance flow. Choriocarcinoma displays a typical color-coded "hot" area representing pre-existing and newly formed blood vessels. All these vessels show high-velocity, low-impedance blood flow signals.

GESTATIONAL TROPHOBLASTIC TUMORS

There is reduction in the resistance indices of uterine artery Doppler spectra—this pattern correlates well with aggressive trophoblastic tumors and with prognosis. Those tumors exhibiting high RI value require massive chemotherapy and fewer treatment cycles.

There is a low uterine arterial resistance to flow with high peak systolic velocities.[52] The gestational trophoblastic neoplasia (GTN) shows a very high blood flow that is a high-diastolic flow due to decreased tone of the vessels in proliferating neoplasm in persistent GTN. These vascular tumors tend to show very high blood flow.[53] Although the myometrial vasculature has a high-velocity flow, the ambiguity of diagnosis is decreased by the presence of low-velocity flow in the uterine artery with low pulsatility along with persistently high βhCG levels (Figs. 12A to D).[54,55]

ECTOPIC PREGNANCY

The advent of color Doppler to transvaginal probe has improved the diagnostic accuracy to almost 98%. Color flow imaging shows classical fire ring with trophoblastic flow pattern. Also, color flow helps in monitoring medical treatment with methotrexate and in planning medical treatment, but this sign can also be seen as a corpus luteum or an hemorrhagic cyst (Figs. 13A and B). The

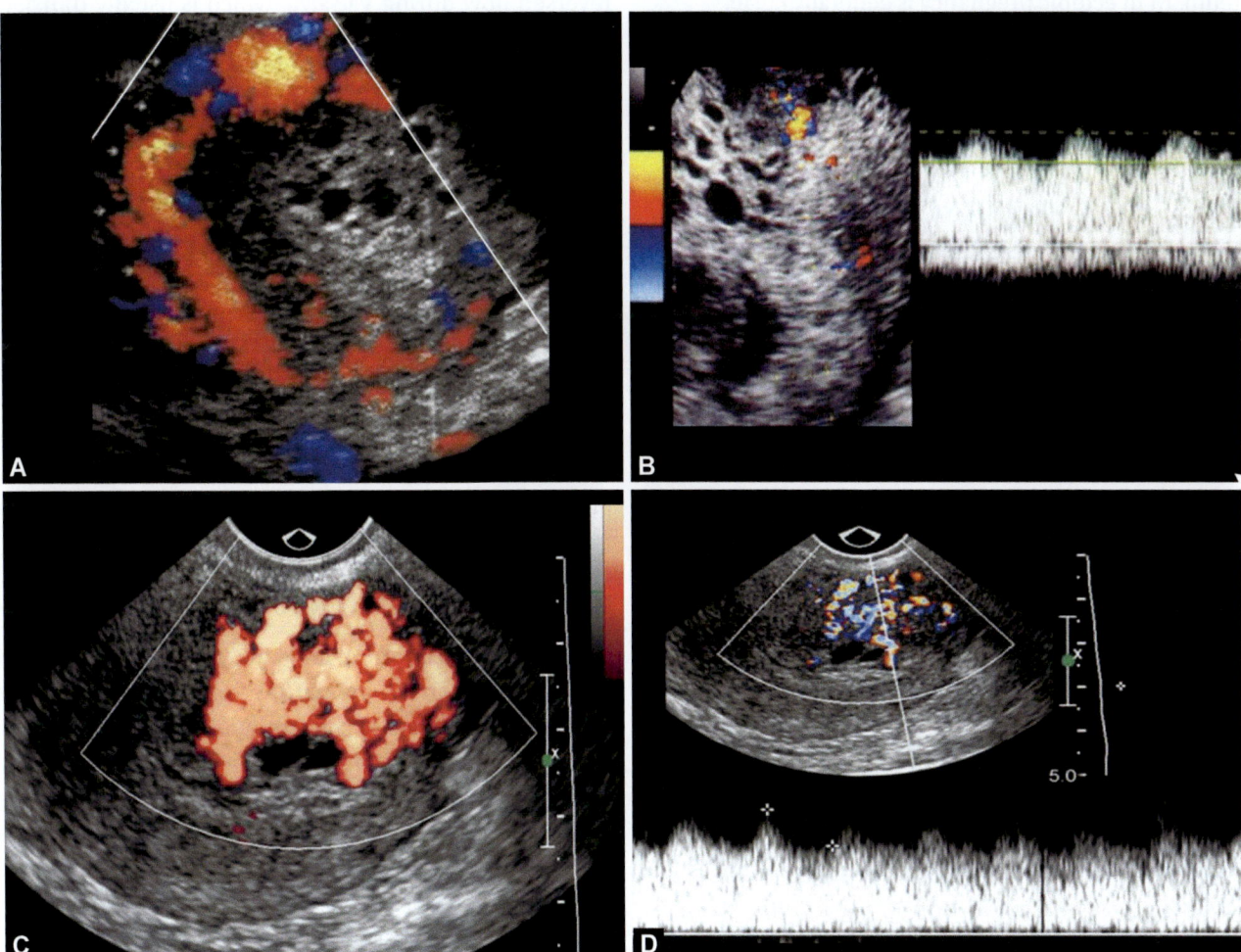

Figs. 12A to D: (A) Snowstorm appearance on TVS color Doppler in molar pregnancy; (B) Reduced vascular impedance on pulsed Doppler in molar pregnancy (RI < 0.2); (C) Power Doppler showing increased vascularity; and (D) Low vascular resistance on color Doppler (RI: resistance index; TVS: transvaginal sonography).

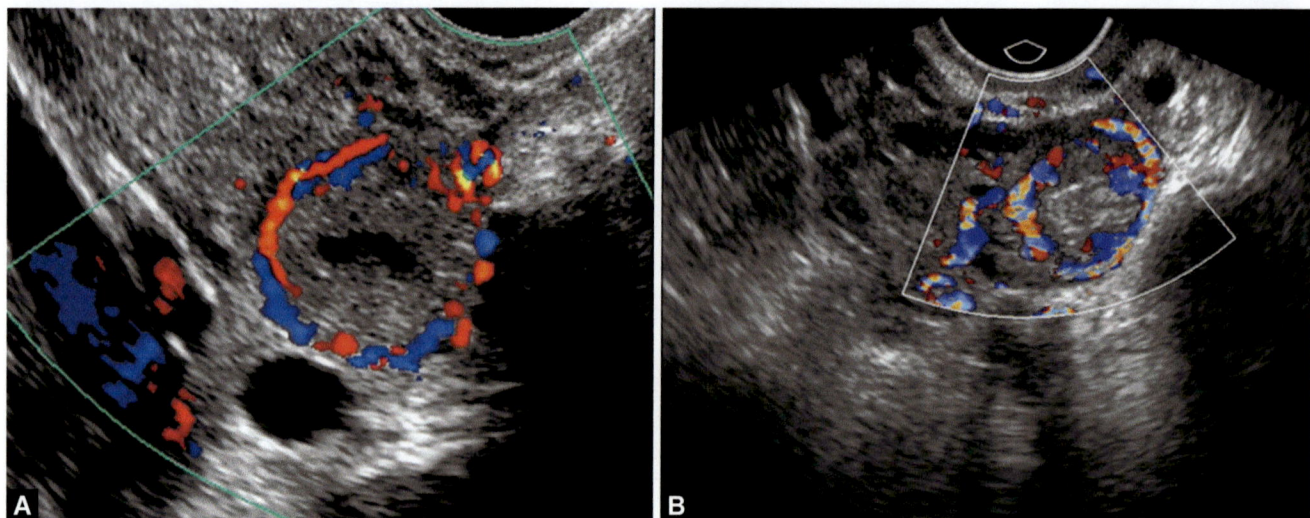

Figs. 13A and B: (A) The characteristic ring of fire sign of ectopic pregnancy in the adnexa, generally separate from the ovary; and (B) The circumferential vascularity in a hemorrhagic cyst/corpus luteum.

way to differentiate between them is the velocimetry. RI in tubal ectopic pregnancy is lower as compared to the corpus luteum. RI in ectopic pregnancy is generally <0.40.[56]

PPV and NPV calculated in this study were 97% and 89%, respectively. The RI can be used as a diagnostic marker for adnexal ectopic pregnancy with TVS when no intrauterine gestational sac is noted.[56]

SCAR ECTOPIC PREGNANCY

Color flow Doppler has been used in some studies to see the invasion of trophoblastic cells in the serosa or the bladder, but the diagnostic efficacy is not very reliable for this invasion.[57]

Diagnostic criteria for scar ectopic pregnancy included:
- Presence of trophoblast between the bladder and anterior uterine wall
- No fetal parts in the uterine cavity
- Discontinuity in the anterior uterine wall must be present on a sagittal view
- On Doppler, the vascularity should be present and invading the serosa or bladder wall (trophoblastic invasion).

PELVIC CONGESTION SYNDROME

The association between chronic pelvic pain, dyspareunia, and pelvic varices has been termed as pelvic congestion syndrome. There is dilatation of pelvic veins with congestion of the ovaries with resultant ovarian swelling and cyst formation, occasionally there may be vulvar and leg varices. Dilated pelvic veins can be seen in the absence of symptoms and not all patients with characteristic congestion exhibit the typical ultrasound appearance. Large serpiginous pelvic veins of diameter >4 mm with flow velocities <5 cm/s in association with cystic ovaries is characteristic. Similarly, reversed flow during Valsalva, which is usually transient, is maintained in this condition with reverse flow of 2 cm/s or greater.

Color Doppler sonography is excellent for the diagnosis of uterine and ovarian plexus varicosities. It differentiates arteries from veins.

MALIGNANT UTERINE TUMORS

Uterine sarcomas appear as inhomogeneous mass with increased tumor vascularity showing low impedance flow. In addition, PSV also shows a decline from normal. Abnormal blood vessels are seen in all cases with sarcoma, whereas only 30% of fibroids show abnormal vessels. Richly vascularized necrotic and large uterine myoma has to be properly evaluated for its blood flow in order to differentiate from sarcomas.

ENDOMETRITIS AND ENDOMETRIAL CARCINOMA

Endometritis results from infection, trauma such as D and C, prolonged labors, premature rupture of membranes, or retained products of conception. Endometritis may be associated with considerable hyperemia, and this may be of the low impedance pattern described in endometrial carcinoma (Taylor et al.). In patients with postmenopausal bleeding due to endometrial carcinoma, the mean PI was 0.91 with a range of 0.31–1.49 (Bourne et al.). Women with other causes for postmenopausal bleeding had a mean PI of 3.83 with a range of 1.95–6.40. Unfortunately, due to the confusion with similar flow found in both hyperplasia of endometrium and in endometritis, the value of this

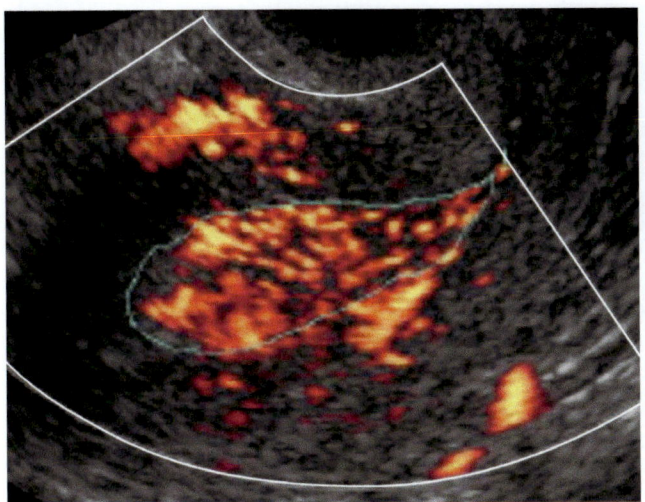

Fig. 14: Typical vascular pattern seen in endometrial carcinoma with low spiral artery resistance index (RI < 0.40) and high velocity.

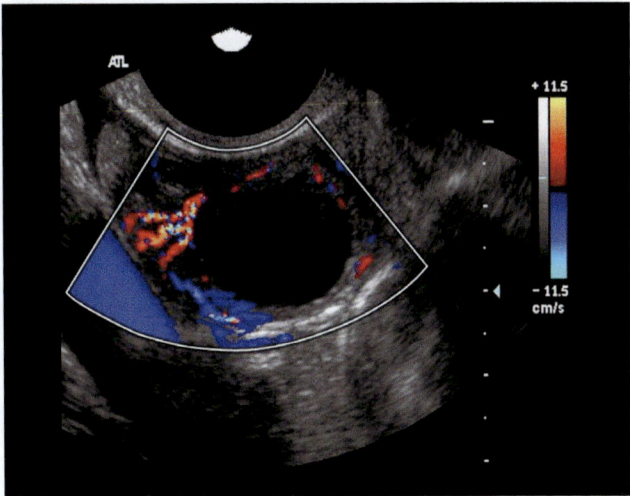

Fig. 15: The dominant follicle in the ovary is determined by ring of angiogenesis around the follicle, which becomes more marked with increased size.

ratio is not clear. In practice, any postmenopausal woman presenting with endometrial thickness of >6 mm needs to undergo biopsy (Fig. 14).

It has recently become apparent that tamoxifen may also be associated with some significant endometrial abnormalities. From the National Cancer Institute (NCI) report, it appears that the risk of endometrial cancer in patients receiving tamoxifen is approximately three times that of normal population.

The differentiating point between endometrial hyperplasia and carcinoma is presence of vascularity when the endometrial thickness is >5 mm in postmenopausal women and absence of intralesional vascularity in endometrial hyperplasia. Clinical usefulness of color Doppler ultrasound in patients with endometrial hyperplasia and carcinoma is seen.[58,59]

Carcinoma of the Cervix

Doppler appears to have little applications in the diagnosis of carcinoma of the cervix. However, cervical carcinoma can be seen on endovaginal ultrasound and neovascularity can be demonstrated.

ROLE OF COLOR DOPPLER IN INFERTILITY

INTRODUCTION

The advent of transvaginal color Doppler sonography has added a new dimension to the diagnosis and treatment of infertile female. Color Doppler innovation is a unique noninvasive technology to investigate the circulation of organs like uterus and ovaries. Dynamic changes occur almost every day of the menstrual cycle in a reproductively active female. These events are picked up very well by transvaginal color Doppler and definite conclusions can be drawn regarding the diagnosis, prognosis, and treatment of infertile patients. As the vaginal probe lies close to the organs of interest, various vessels supplying these structures can be studied in detail like the uterine artery, ovarian artery, and their branches.

STUDY OF MENSTRUAL CYCLE BY COLOR DOPPLER

It is very important to study the whole of the menstrual cycle by transvaginal color Doppler during the evaluation of infertility. It provides vital information about follicular dynamics like blood flow to the growing follicle, the vascular supply of the endometrium, and corpus luteum vascularization which are very important for a successful outcome in terms of pregnancy.[60]

CHANGES IN THE OVARY

The ovaries are situated on either side of the uterus and measure about 2.2–5.5 cm in length, 1.5–2.0 cm in width, and 1.5–3.0 cm in depth and are recognized by the presence of follicle of different sizes. The blood supply is by ovarian artery via the infundibulopelvic ligament and ovarian branch of the uterine artery. There is anastomosis between the two sources of blood supply. The primary and secondary branches of the ovarian artery grow along with the development of the follicle. Dominant follicle within the ovary can be recognized by transvaginal color Doppler by day 8th or 10th of the cycle by a ring of angiogenesis around it, when compared to the subordinate follicles which do not demonstrate this. These vessels become more abundant and prominent as the follicle grows to about 20–24 mm in size (Fig. 15).

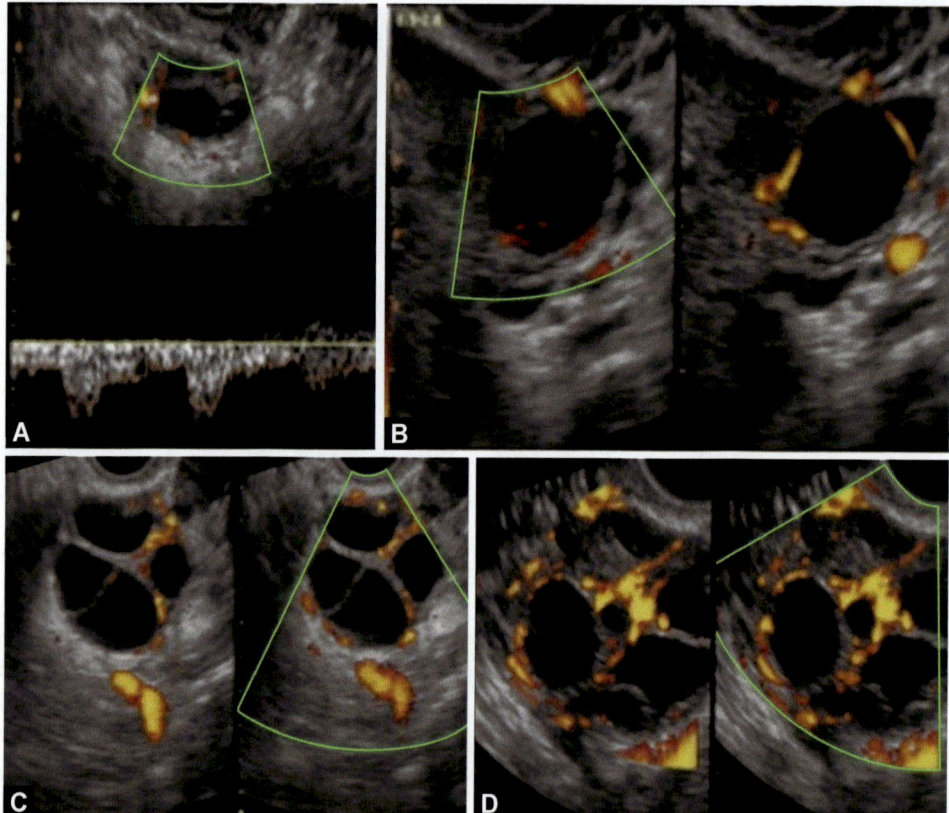

Figs. 16A to D: (A) Power Doppler image of early follicular phase follicle in which vascularity is <10%; (B) Late follicular phase follicle showing 10–25% vascularity; (C) Early luteal phase vascularity (days 14–17) shows 25–50% vascularity; and (D) Late luteal phase (days 18–24) shows 50–75% vascularity.

The phases are described as early follicular (days 5-7), late follicular (days 11-13), early luteal (days 15-17), and late luteal (days 26-28) (Figs. 16A to D). In general, the index values are high in the early part of menstrual cycle and fall as ovulation approaches. According to Kurjak et al., the RI in the early proliferative phase is 0.54 ± 0.04 and declines the day before ovulation [luteinizing hormone (LH) peak] when it is about 0.44 ± 0.04.

This is the best time for administration of surrogate hCG. The increase in PSV with a relatively constant is a particularly interesting finding that might herald impending ovulation. It is hoped that information on ovarian perfusion may be used to predict ovulation and to investigate ovulatory dysfunction. The lowest RI values were obtained during the midluteal phase (RI 0.42 ± 0.06) with a return to higher vascular resistance (0.50 ± 0.04) during the late luteal phase:
- Rising PSV (>10) and steady low RI (0.4-0.6) suggest follicle is close to rupture.
- Decreasing PSV (<10) and rising RI (>1) suggest follicle is likely to become luteinized unruptured follicle (LUF).
- Fertilization of a follicle with PSV of <10 cm/s may result in an embryo with chromosomal abnormality.

The dominant ovary corpus luteum shows a low impedance waveform with a RI of 0.39-0.49, characteristic of blood flow in early pregnancy. The contralateral ovary shows a high impedance flow with a RI of 0.69-1.00 characteristic of nondominant ovary (Kurjak et al.). If the ovary having corpus luteum shows high RI (>0.50), it is associated with nonviable outcome.

Predictors of poor ovarian response are:
- Ovarian volume < 3 cc
- Antral follicles < 3
- Ovarian RI > 0.6
- Ovarian PSV < 5 cm/s
- Stromal flow index (SFI) < 11

All these suggest poor ovarian response and higher doses of gonadotropins will be required for stimulation.

UTERINE PERFUSION

The uterine artery gives rise to the arcuate arteries which are oriented circumferentially in the outer third of the myometrium. These vessels give rise to the radial arteries, which after crossing the myometrium-endometrium border, further branch and give rise to the basal arteries and the spiral arteries.

The uterine artery RI lies around 0.88 ± 0.04 until day 13 of the 28 days menstrual cycle. After 3 days of the peak of LH levels, there is increase in the uterine artery impedance, i.e., around day 16. This can be explained by the fact that the increased contractility and compression of the uterine vessels traversing the myometrium cause decrease in their diameter and hence cause a higher resistance to the flow. The peak luteal phase records the lowest blood flow impedance (RI 0.84 ± 0.04) during which implantation is likely to occur. At this time, the RI of the radial vessels is 0.78 ± 0.10.

Blood flow velocity waveform changes in the spiral arteries during normal ovulatory cycles are characteristics of lower velocity and lower impedance to blood flow than are those observed in the uterine arteries with larger diameter. It seems that features of endometerial blood flow may be used to predict the implantation success rate and to reveal unexplained infertility problems more precisely than evaluation of the main uterine artery alone.

CHANGES IN THE ENDOMETRIUM

Michael Applebaum in his study with transvaginal color Doppler divided the endometrium and periendometrial areas into four zones. In the study conducted by him, no pregnancy was reported in in vitro fertilization (IVF) patients unless vascularity was demonstrated in zone III or within zone III or IV prior to transfer (Figs. 17 to 20).

LUTEAL PHASE SCAN

- A healthy corpus luteum shows a good vascular ring on color Doppler (Fig. 21)
- Resistance index of 0.35–0.50
- Pulsatility index of 0.70–0.80

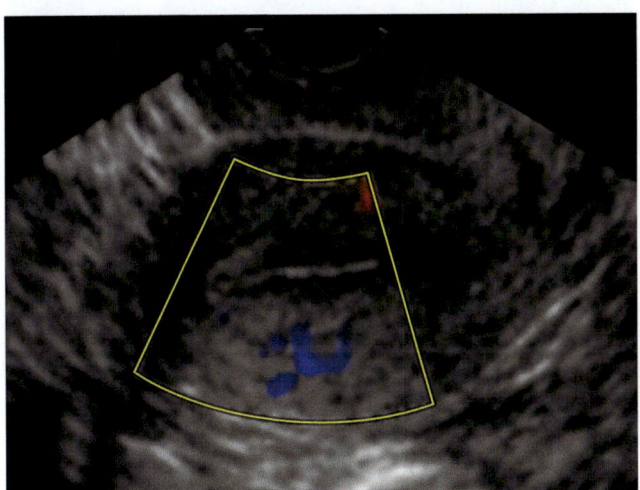

Fig. 17: *Zone 1*: 2 mm thick area surrounding the hyperechoic outer layer of the endometrium.

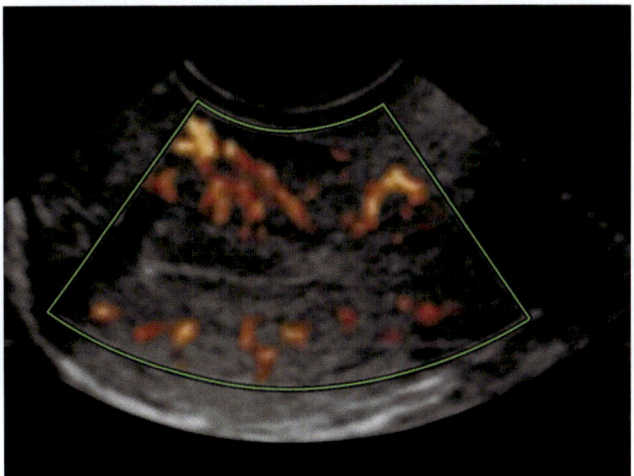

Fig. 18: *Zone 2*: The hyperechoic outer layer of the endometrium.

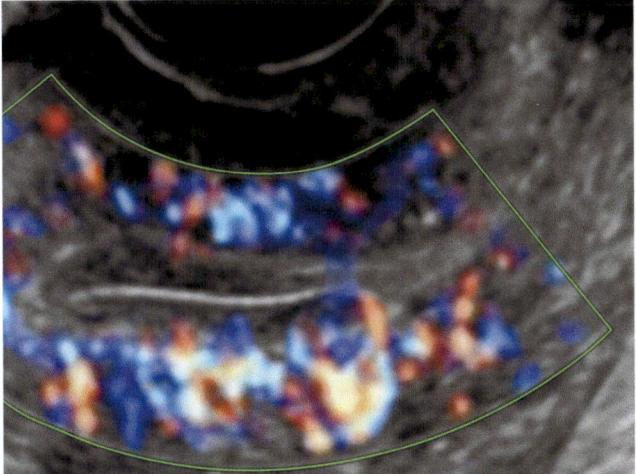

Fig. 19: *Zone 3*: The hypoechoic inner layer of the endometrium.

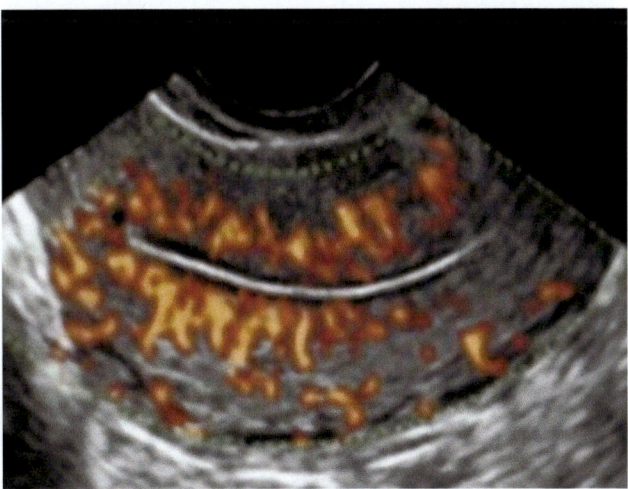

Fig. 20: *Zone 4*: The endometrial cavity.

- Peak systolic velocity of 10–15 cm/s
- Resistance index of corpus luteum correlates well with plasma progesterone level which is an index of luteal function.

ULTRASOUND TECHNIQUE FOR UTERINE BIOPHYSICAL PROFILE

To perform the uterine biophysical profile (UBP), special care should be taken. The following guidelines are recommended (Applebaum 96):
- Presence of a five-line endometrium may be demonstrated on both transabdominal and transvaginal ultrasonography (USG) as this may be present on transabdominal scan and may sometimes may not be seen on TVS due to the position of the uterus and vice versa. At the same time, the endometrial vascularity should also be seen while visualizing the five-line endometrium (Figs. 22A and B).
- The endometrial blood flow is difficult to visualize and the machine may take sometime to register this blood flow and represent it by the image. If the sweep is too fast, the flow may not be seen. The endometrial blood flow has a very erratic behavior as it may sometimes be easily visible in some areas and in some areas it may be totally absent, hence patience is required to note the vascularity in the endometrium.
- To observe and make the endometrium as specular as reflector as possible, manual manipulation of the uterus with probe pressure or counter pressure from above can be done.
- Both coronal and sagittal planes should be seen as there may be some difference in the blood flow seen in either of the planes.
- Endometrial thickness should be taken when there is contraction affecting the endometrial thickness with complete and continuous visualization of the endometrial cavity [sagittal plane, anteroposterior (AP) measurements].

Uterine Biophysical Profile

Certain noteworthy points seen in a midcycle (normal) uterus are as follows:
- Full-thickness measurement in greatest AP dimensions is 7 mm
- A distinct/hazy five layer appearance of the endometrium
- The endometrial blood flow is noted till the zone 3 on color Doppler

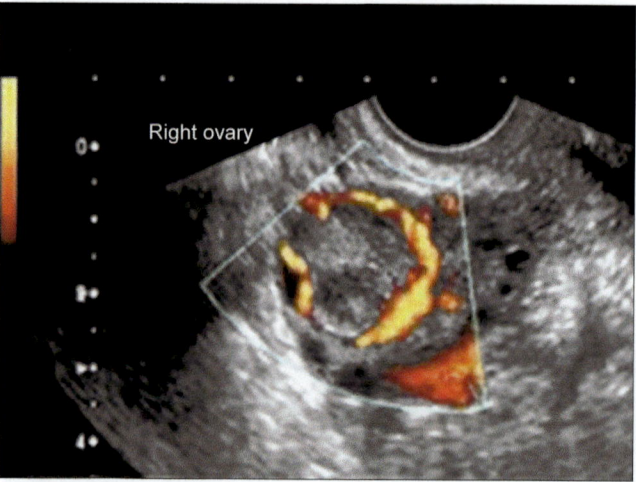

Fig. 21: Color Doppler of a corpus luteum.

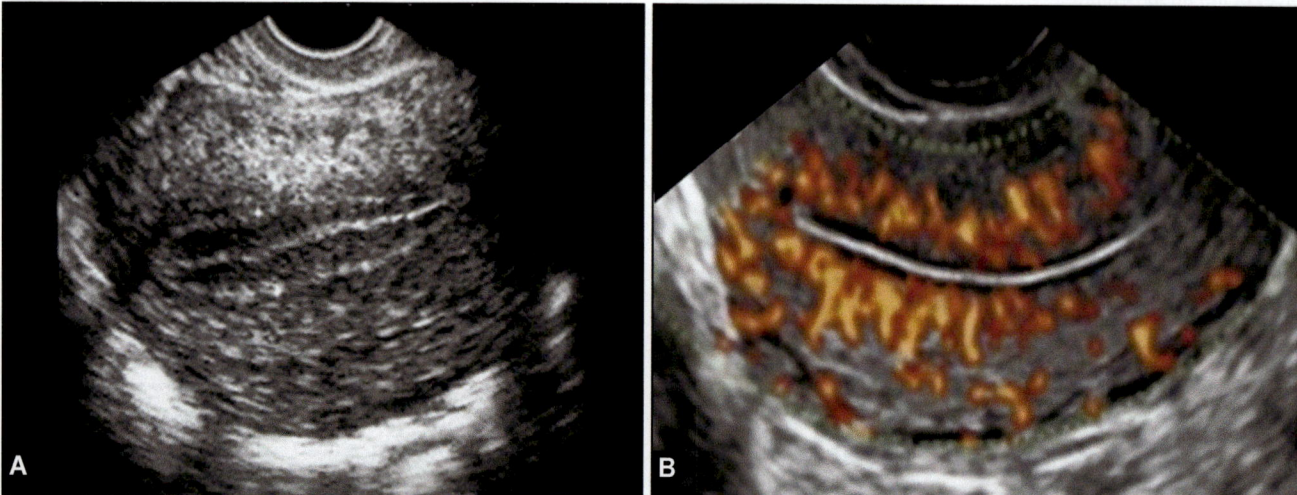

Figs. 22A and B: A distinct five-line endometrium, measuring 10–14 mm with a relatively homogeneous myometrium with presence of myometrial blood flow and zone 4 vascularity. This is an ideal endometrium for embryo transfer and will yield a good pregnancy outcome.

- Myometrial contractions are noted (wave-like motion of the endometrium)
- Uterine artery PI < 3
- Myometrial echogenicity appears to be homogeneous
- Visualization of myometrial blood flow on gray (internal to the arcuate vessels).

The uterine scoring system includes the following points that are to be evaluated before embryo transfer (ET) (Table 4).

One can safely assume a technically adequate USG which suggests no abnormalities of the uterine shape, development or gross abnormalities (significant masses) and a normal ovarian cycle (w/o evidence of dyscoordination of the ovarian-uterine cycles), and absence of male factor infertility.

According to the literature, a perfect score of 20 [uterine scoring system for reproduction (USSR)] is associated with conception rate of 100% (the number of patients on which this finding is based in the USSR study was 5). This group included two spontaneous conceptions [non-assisted reproductive technology (ART) or intrauterine insemination (IUI)], two IUI, and one IVF.

CONCEPTION RATES WITH UTERINE SCORING SYSTEM FOR REPRODUCTION SCORES (TABLE 5)

Absent endometrial flow, despite highest values for the other parameters, has always been associated with no conception.

CONCLUSION

Today the advent of color flow imaging, Doppler, and Power Angio has opened a new diagnostic horizon for understanding physiology and vascular pathology of gynecology, infertility, uteroplacental, and fetal circulation.

The diagnostic ability with use of Doppler in routine practice has increased.

"See better with sound
Use color to improve you image
Explore the 3rd and 4th dimensions
Practice better medicine with better images"

Table 4: USSR parameters of uterine scoring.

Parameter	Determination	Score
Endometrial thickness (mm)	<7	0
	7–9	2
	10–14	3
	>14	1
Endometrial layering	No layering	0
	Hazy 5 line appearance	1
	Distinct 5 line appearance	3
Myometrial echogenicity	Coarse, inhomogeneous	1
	Relative homogeneous	2
Endometrial motion (No. of myometrial contraction in 2 min) (Real time)	<3	0
	≥3	3
Uterine artery Doppler flow (PI)	2.99–3.00	0
	2.49	1
	<2	2
Endometrial blood flow	Absent	0
	Present but sparse	2
	Present multifocally	5
Myometrial blood flow (grayscale)	Absent	0
	Present	2

(PI: pulsatility index; USSR: uterine scoring system for reproduction)

Table 5: Conception rates with uterine scoring system for reproduction (USSR) scores.

USSR scores	Conception rates
20	100%
17–19	80%
14–16	60%
<13	0

REFERENCES

1. Campbell S. Ultrasound in Obstetrics and Gynecology: Recent Advances. Philadelphia: WB Saunders Company Ltd.; 1983.
2. Callen PW. Ultrasonography in Obstetrics and Gynecology, 5th edition. Philadelphia: WB Saunders Company Ltd.; 2007.
3. Kurjak A, Zalud I. Doppler and Color Flow Imaging. United States: Mosby Year Book; 1992. pp. 285-94.
4. Bourne TH. Transvaginal color Doppler in gynecology. Ultrasound Obstet Gynecol. 1991;1:359-73.
5. Kurjak A, Kupesic S. Transvaginal color Doppler and pelvic tumor vascularity: lessons learned and future challenges. Ultrasound Obstet Gynecol. 1995;6:145-59.
6. Steer CV, Campbell S, Pampiglione JS, et al. Transvaginal colour flow imaging of the uterine arteries during the ovarian and menstrual cycles. Hum Reprod. 1990;5:391-5.
7. Taylor KJ, Burns PN, Wells PN. Clinical Applications of Doppler Ultrasound, 2nd edition. New York: Raven Press; 1995.
8. Hackelöer BJ, Fleming R, Robinson HP, et al. Correlation of ultrasonic and endocrinologic assessment of human follicular development. Am J Obstet Gynecol. 1979;135:122-8.
9. Zandt-Stastny D, Thorsen MK, Middleton WD, et al. Inability of sonography to detect imminent ovulation. Am J Roentgenol. 1989;152:91-5.
10. Picker RH, Smith DH, Tucker MH, et al. Ultrasonic signs of imminent ovulation. J Clin Ultrasound. 1983;11:1-2.
11. Jaffe R, Ben-Aderet N. Ultrasonic screening in predicting the time of ovulation. Gynecol Obstet Invest. 1984;18:303-5.
12. Kerin JF, Kirby C, Morris D, et al. Incidence of the luteinized unruptured follicle phenomenon in cycling women. Fertil Steril. 1983;40:620-6.
13. Sakamoto C. Sonographic criteria of phasic changes in human endometrial tissue. Int J Gynaecol Obstet. 1985;23:7-12.
14. Sharma RP. Fallopian tube patency by ultrasound scan. Obstet Gynaecol India. 1989;39:700-1.
15. Brundin J, Dahlborn M, Ahlberg-Ahre E, et al. Radionuclide hysterosalpingography for measurement of human oviductal function. Int J Gynaecol Obstet. 1989;28:53-9.
16. Henry-Suchet J, Tesquiter L, Pez JP, et al. Prognostic value of tuboscopy vs. hysterosalpingography before tuboplasty. J Reprod Med. 1984;29:609-12.
17. Donnez J, Langerock S, Lecart C, et al. Incidence of pathological factors not revealed by hysterosalpingography but disclosed by laparoscopy in 500 infertile women. Eur J Obstet Gynecol Reprod Biol. 1982;13:369-75.
18. Brosers IA, Vasquez G. Funeral microbiopsy. J Reprod Med. 1976;16:171-8.
19. Allahbadia GN. Fallopian tubes and ultrasonography: the Sion Experience. Fertil Steril. 1992;58:901-7.
20. Malhotra N, Kumar P, Shah PK, et al. Ultrasound in Obstetrics and Gynecology, 4th edition. New Delhi: Jaypee Brothers Medical Publishers; 2000.
21. Woźniak A, Woźniak S. Ultrasonography of uterine leiomyomas. Menopause Rev. 2017;16:113-7.
22. Timmerman D, Verguts J, Konstantinovic ML, et al. The pedicle artery sign based on sonography with color Doppler imaging can replace second-stage tests in women with abnormal vaginal bleeding. Ultrasound Obstet Gynecol. 2003;22:166-71.
23. Brenner P. Differential diagnosis of abnormal uterine bleeding. Am J Obstet Gynecol. 1996;175:766-9.
24. Garza-Cavazos A, de Mola JR. Abnormal uterine bleeding: new definitions and contemporary terminology. Female Patient. 2012;37:1-9.
25. Cil AP, Tulunay G, Kose MF, et al. Power Doppler properties of endometrial polyps and submucosal fibroids: a preliminary observational study in women with known intracavitary lesions. Ultrasound Obstet Gynecol. 2010;35:233-7.
26. Talaat S, Mostafa N, Alrauof MA. Diagnostic value of ultrasound and colour Doppler in endometrial and cervical polyps. Med J Cairo Univ. 2009;77:397-403.
27. Hata K, Hata T, Senoh D, et al. Change in ovarian arterial compliance during the human menstrual cycle assessed by Doppler ultrasound. Br J Obstet Gynaecol. 1990;97:163-6.
28. Bouguizane S, Bibi H, Farhat Y, et al. Adnexal torsion: a report of 135 cases. J Gynecol Obstet Biol Reprod. 2003;32:535-40.
29. Graif M, Itzchak Y. Sonographic evaluation of ovarian torsion in childhood and adolescence. Am J Roentgenol. 1988;150:647-9.
30. Lee EJ, Kwon HC, Joo HJ, et al. Diagnosis of ovarian torsion with color Doppler sonography: depiction of twisted vascular pedicle. J Ultrasound Med. 1998;17:83-9.
31. Amirbekian S, Hooley RJ. Ultrasound evaluation of pelvic pain. Radiol Clin North Am. 2014;52:1215-35.
32. Nizar K, Deutsch M, Filmer S, et al. Doppler studies of the ovarian venous blood flow in the diagnosis of adnexal torsion. J Clin Ultrasound. 2009;37:436-9.
33. Navve D, Hershkovitz R, Zetounie E, et al. Medial or lateral location of the whirlpool sign in adnexal torsion: clinical importance. J Ultrasound Med. 2013;32:1631-4.
34. Vijayaraghavan SB. Sonographic whirlpool sign in ovarian torsion. J Ultrasound Med. 2004;23:1643-9.
35. Sampson JA. Peritoneal endometriosis due to the menstrual dissemination of endometrial tissue into the peritoneal cavity. Am J Obstet Gynecol. 1927;14:422-69.
36. Sampson JA. Metastatic or embolic endometriosis due to the menstrual dissemination of endometrial tissue into the venous circulation. Am J Pathol. 1927;3:93-110.
37. von Rokitansky KF. Ueber Uterusdrüsen-Neubildung in Uterus- und Ovarial-Sarcomen (on the neoplasm of uterus glands on uterine and ovarian sarcomas). Zeitschr Ges Aerzte Wien. 1860;16:577-81.
38. Cullen TS. Adenomyoma of the round ligament. J Hopkins Hosp Bull. 1896;7:112-4.

39. Cullen TS. Adenoma-myoma uteri diffusum benignum. J Hopkins Hosp Bull. 1896;6:133-7.
40. Cullen TS. The distribution of adenomyomata containing uterine mucosa. Am J Obstet Gynecol. 1920;1:215-83.
41. Sampson JA. Perforating hemorrhagic (chocolate) cysts of the ovary. Their importance and especially their relation to pelvic adenomas of the endometrial type. Arch Surg. 1921;3:245-323.
42. Hughesdon PE. The endometrial identity of benign stromatosis of the ovary and its relation to other forms of endometriosis. J Pathol. 1976;119:201-9.
43. Batt RE, Smith RA, Buck Louis GM, et al. Mullerianosis. Histol Histopathol. 2007;22:1161-6.
44. Pan ML, Chen LR, Tsao HM, et al. Risk of gestational hypertension-preeclampsia in women with preceding endometriosis: a nationwide population-based study. PLoS One. 2017;12:e0181261.
45. Koninckx PR, Zupi E, Martin DC. Endometriosis and pregnancy outcome. Fertil Steril. 2018;110:406-7.
46. Hasdemir PS, Farasat M, Aydin C, et al. The role of adenomyosis in the pathogenesis of preeclampsia. Geburtshilfe Frauenheilkd. 2016;76:882-7.
47. Hashimoto A, Iriyama T, Sayama S, et al. Adenomyosis and adverse perinatal outcomes: increased risk of second trimester miscarriage, preeclampsia, and placental malposition. J Matern Fetal Neonatal Med. 2018;31:364-9.
48. Alcázar JL. Transvaginal colour Doppler in patients with ovarian endometriomas and pelvic pain. Hum Reprod. 2001;16:2672-5.
49. Kurjak A, Kupesic S. Scoring system for prediction of ovarian endometriosis based on transvaginal color and pulsed Doppler sonography. Fertil Steril. 1994;62:81-8.
50. Aleem F, Pennisi J, Zeitoun K, et al. The role of color Doppler in the diagnosis of endometriomas. Ultrasound Obstet Gynecol. 1995;5:51-4.
51. Guerriero S, Ajossa S, Mais V, et al. The diagnosis of endometriomas using colour Doppler energy imaging. Hum Reprod. 1998;13:1691-5.
52. Szulman AE, Surti U. Linear relationship between gestational age and size of villi. Am J Obstet Gynecol. 1978;132:20.
53. Taylor KJ, Schwartz PE, Kohorn EI. Gestational trophoblastic neoplasia: diagnosis with Doppler ultrasound. Radiology. 1987;165:445-8.
54. Carter J, Fowler J, Carlson J, et al. Transvaginal color flow Doppler sonography in the assessment of gestational trophoblastic disease. J Ultrasound Med. 1993;12:595-9.
55. Kurjak A, Zalud I, Predanic M, et al. Transvaginal color and pulsed Doppler study of uterine blood flow in the first and second trimesters of pregnancy: normal versus abnormal. J Ultrasound Med. 1994;13:43-7.
56. Kurjak A, Zalud I, Schulman H. Ectopic pregnancy: transvaginal color Doppler of trophoblastic flow in questionable adnexa. J Ultrasound Med. 1991;10:685-9.
57. Jurkovic D, Hillaby K, Woelfer B, et al. First-trimester diagnosis and management of pregnancies implanted into the lower uterine segment cesarean section scar. Ultrasound Obstet Gynecol. 2003;21:220-7.
58. Emoto M, Tamura R, Shirota K, et al. Clinical usefulness of color Doppler ultrasound in patients with endometrial hyperplasia and carcinoma. Cancer. 2002;94:700-6.
59. Kaijser J. Towards an evidence-based approach for diagnosis and management of adnexal masses: findings of the International Ovarian Tumour Analysis (IOTA) studies. Facts Views Vis Obgyn. 2015;7:42-59.
60. Pan HA, Wu MH, Cheng YC, et al. Quantification of Doppler signal in polycystic ovary syndrome using three-dimensional power Doppler ultrasonography: a possible new marker for diagnosis. Hum Reprod. 2002;17:201-6.

5

Ultrasound in Infertility: Follicular Dynamics and Endometrium

Sonal Panchal, Chaitanya Nagori, Meenu Agarwal

INTRODUCTION

Ultrasound is a modality of choice for monitoring of ovulation induction which is inevitable for any fertility treatment. It is patient friendly, easy to use repeatedly, and is financially also viable. When used with Doppler, it gives a precise idea about morphological changes and vascular changes which represent hormonal changes.

Ultrasound during the entire treatment cycle will be divided into three phases for the ease of discussion:
1. Baseline scan and deciding the stimulation protocol
2. Preovulatory scan and decision on trigger
3. Luteal phase scan

BASELINE SCAN AND DECIDING THE STIMULATION PROTOCOL

Transvaginal scan is done on days 2–3 of the menstrual cycle. The ovaries are silent, and have no active follicle or corpus luteum at this stage.

Total number of antral follicles and ovarian stromal blood flow were the two most significant predictors of ovarian response and ovarian volume was highly significant predictor of number of follicles and oocytes retrieved.[1-3]

The parameters that we have used to calculate the dose for gonadotropins stimulation protocol for intrauterine insemination (IUI) cycles in our study are antral follicle count (AFC), ovarian volume, ovarian stromal resistance index (RI) and peak systolic velocity (PSV), age, and body mass index (BMI). Linear correlation is seen between AFC and anti-Müllerian hormone (AMH) and both help to predict the extremes of response. AFC had the highest accuracy for predicting ovarian response in patients with abnormal ovarian reserve test and was statistically significant (number of oocyte aspirated, p value < 0.001) than AMH (p value 0.06), and follicle-stimulating hormone (FSH) (p value 0.212) in predicting ovarian response. For prediction of poor ovarian response, a model including AFC + AMH was found to be almost similar to that of (p value 0.001) using AFC alone.[4] AFC can be calculated by two-dimensional (2D) ultrasound or by three-dimensional (3D) with inversion mode rendering and SonoAVC a specialized 3D ultrasound software for calculation of antral follicle number and volume of follicles. This method is more precise as there is least chance of follicles being missed or being counted twice because of color coding, but postprocessing is required for accurate calculations (Fig. 1).

It is known that smaller ovarian volume indicates lower reserve and thus larger ovarian volume raises the risk of ovarian hyperstimulation syndrome (OHSS). Volume can be calculated by taking three orthogonal diameters or by VOCAL software on 3D ultrasound (Fig. 2).

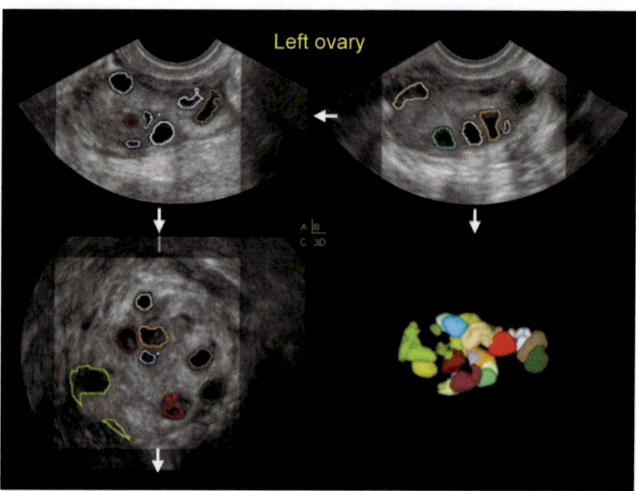

Fig. 1: Three-dimensional (3D) ultrasound image of the ovary with SonoAVC for calculating antral follicle counts.

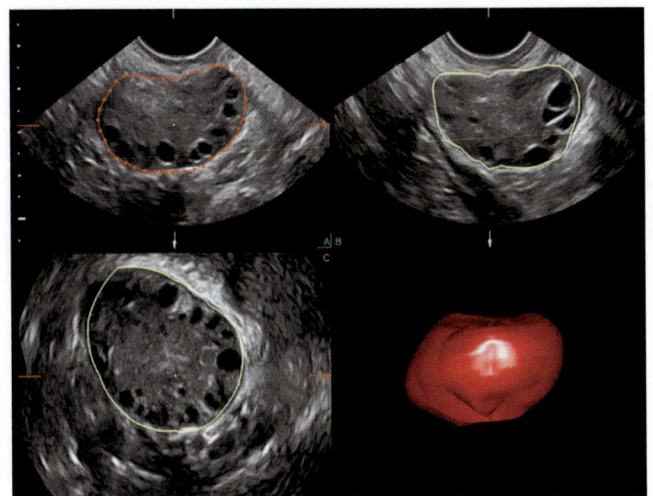

Fig. 2: Three-dimensional (3D) ultrasound calculated ovarian volume by a software called VOCAL.

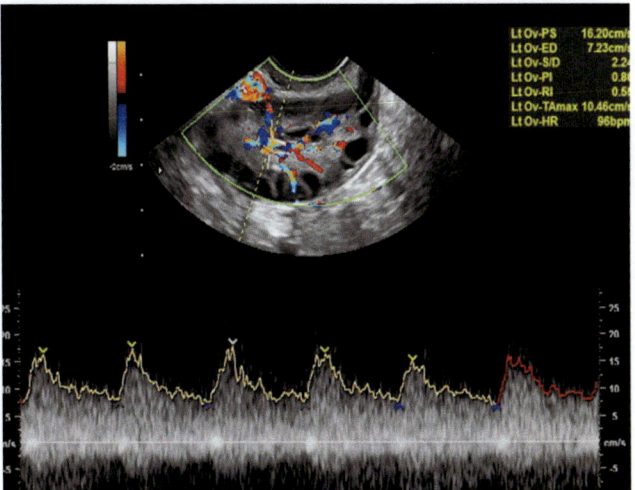

Fig. 3: Ovarian stromal flow as seen on color Doppler and pulse Doppler.

Table 1: Scoring system based on clinical and ultrasound findings.					
Score	1	2	3	4	5
Age	>40	35.1–40	30.1–35	25.1–30	<25
BMI	>30	30–28.1	28–25.1	25–22.1	<22
AFC	<5	5–10	10–15	15–20	>20
Ovarian volume	<3	3.1–5	5.1–7	7.1–10	>10
Stromal RI	>0.75	0.75–0.66	0.65–0.56	0.55–0.46	<0.45
Stromal PSV	<3	3.1–5	5.1–7	7.1–10	>10

(AFC: antral follicle count; BMI: body mass index; PSV: peak systolic velocity; RI: resistance index)

Ovarian stromal blood flows, and stromal PSV (Fig. 3) are related to subsequent ovarian response in in vitro fertilization (IVF) treatment even after down-regulation.[5,6]

Age is known to be one of the most important factors that reduce not only the ovarian reserve, but also the oocyte quality. BMI is also an important determinant of the ovarian response. This is because flow in the ovarian stroma is less in obese patients as compared to controls.[7]

A scoring system is developed based on these clinical and ultrasound findings as given in Table 1.

The starting stimulation doses according to the patient's score are as follows (for IUI cycles):
- >25: 25 IU
- 20–24: 37.5 IU
- 15–20: 75 IU
- 10–15: 112.5 IU
- 6–10: 150 IU

The doses for stimulation for IVF cycle according to the patient's score are as follows:

Score of:
- >23: 75 IU
- 20–22: 150 IU
- 16–20: 225 IU
- 11–15: 300 IU
- 6–10: 375 IU

This scoring system is highly reliable way of deciding the stimulation protocol with negligible cycle cancelation due to poor response and also negligible OHSS rate.[8,9]

A follicle, that is of >10 mm in diameter (dominant follicle), grows at a rate of 2–3 mm/day, has no internal echogenicity, and has thin (pencil line-like) walls. This follicle is likely to mature into healthy ovum.

B-MODE FEATURES OF A MATURE FOLLICLE

The follicular diameter is measured as a mean of three orthogonal diameters. A mature follicle is 16–18 mm (Fig. 4), has thin walls, regular round shape, and no echogenicity in the lumen. It shows a thin hypoechoic rim surrounding the follicle and sometimes (about 35–40%) cumulus-like shadow may be seen approximately 36 hours before rupture. A flimsy irregular line or internal low level echoes are seen inside the follicle parallel to the wall about 6–10 hours before rupture (Fig. 5).

44 *Ultrasound in Infertility: Follicular Dynamics and Endometrium*

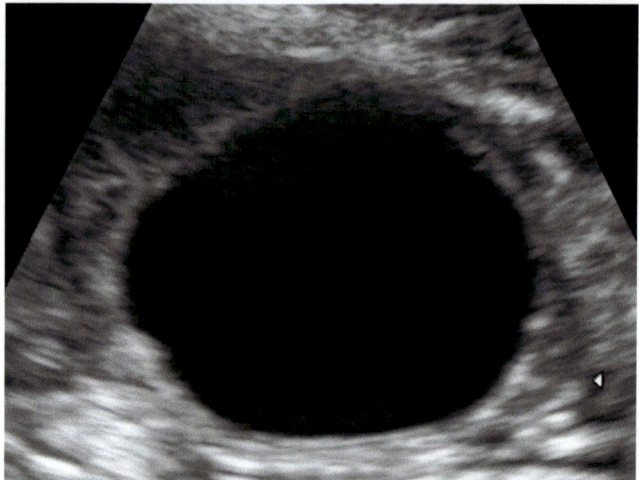

Fig. 4: B-mode ultrasound image of a mature follicle.

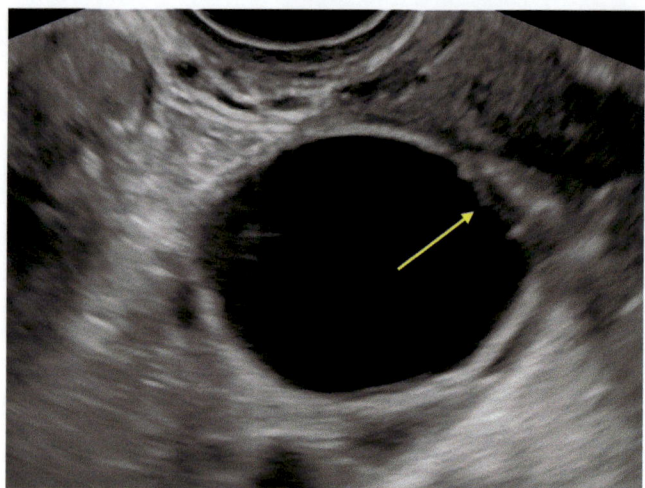

Fig. 5: B-mode ultrasound image of a follicle of which rupture is impending showing mild separation of inner wall (arrow).

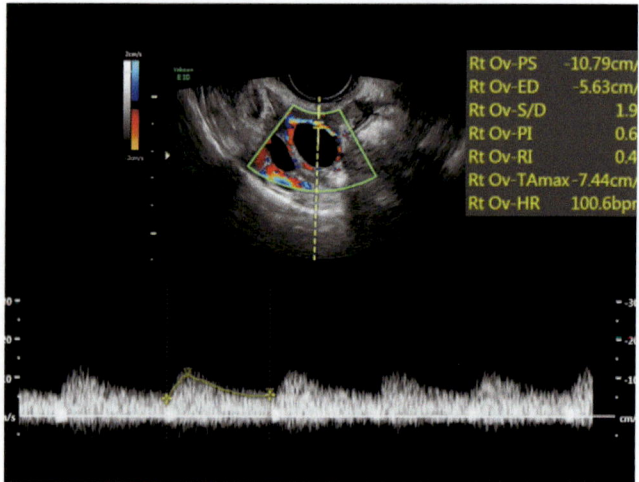

Fig. 6: Pulse Doppler image of follicle showing flow on color Doppler and the low-resistance flow as seen on spectral Doppler.

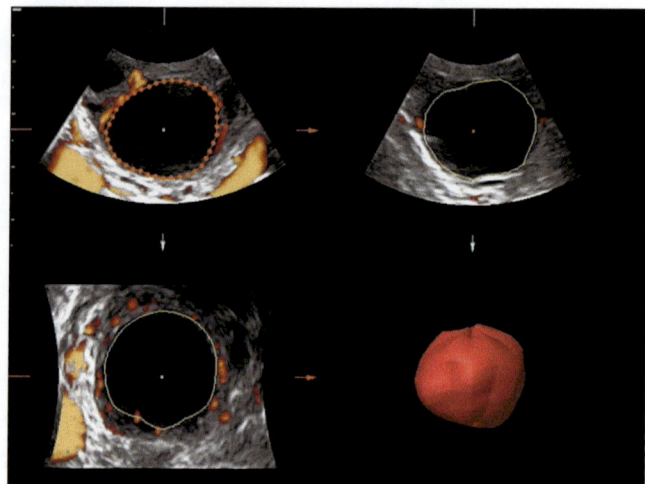

Fig. 7: 3D US acquired, VOCAL calculated volume of follicle.

DOPPLER FEATURES OF A GOOD PREOVULATORY FOLLICLE

Fall in perifollicular RI starts 2 days before ovulation, and reaches <0.5 at the start of the surge. When functionally mature, on color Doppler, the follicle shows blood vessels covering at least three-fourths of the follicular circumference (Fig. 6). On pulse Doppler, these blood vessels show RI of 0.4–0.48[10] and PSV of >10 cm/s (Fig. 6).

The pulse repetition frequency (PRF) settings for color Doppler are set at 0.3 and wall filter at the lowest. The perifollicular vessels are only those that overlap the follicular wall with color Doppler. Decision for trigger should be based on the Doppler findings as ovarian and this correlates well with oocyte recovery rates. Moreover, oocytes from severely hypoxic follicles are associated with high frequency of abnormalities of organization of chromosomes on metaphase spindle and may lead to segregation disorders and catastrophic mosaics in embryo.[10] On 3D ultrasound with VOCAL, the follicular volume of 3–7.5 cc has been found to be optimum in our study and correlated with follicular size of 18–24 mm in diameter (Fig. 7).[11]

It has also been suggested that the follicles-containing oocytes capable to produce a pregnancy have more uniform perifollicular vascular network.[12] This can also be better studied by 3D power Doppler ultrasound.

Human chorionic gonadotropin (hCG) plays a major role in inducing influx of blood within follicles. Under the effect of rising luteinizing hormone (LH), the perifollicular PSV keeps on rising constantly till an hour before rupture.[13]

Endometrium is also assessed by transvaginal 2D ultrasound and color Doppler before planning for hCG during any assisted reproductive technologies. Endometrial study for its morphology and vascularity can explain the mysteries of implantation failure.

B-MODE FEATURES OF PRETRIGGER ENDOMETRIUM WITH GOOD RECEPTIVITY

On transvaginal sonography (TVS), an endometrial thickness of minimum 6 mm is required on the day of trigger, but 8–10 mm is optimum. Morphology of the endometrium is as important as thickness of the endometrium. In all the healthy endometria, the endometrio-myometrial interface should be intact. Breach or irregularity of endometrio-myometrial junction is an indication of unhealthy endometrium and, therefore, poor receptivity.

Popularly multilayered endometrium is considered as a desired endometrial pattern. The endometrium becomes multilayered as early as days 6–7 of the cycle and then under the effect of rising estrogen levels, secreted from the dominant follicle, it grows from grade B–A and then to grade C. Grade B endometrium is multilayered with almost anechoic intervening area and is seen with one mature follicle, with two to four mature follicles grade A endometrium is expected which is multilayered with intervening area as echogenic as the anterior normal myometrium and with multifollicular development, a grade C endometrium is seen which is an isoechoic homogeneous endometrium (Figs. 8A to C).

Doppler Features of Endometrium with Good Receptivity

Segmental uterine artery perfusion demonstrates significant correlation with hormonal and histological markers of uterine receptivity, reaching the highest sensitivity for subendometrial blood flow. On color Doppler, the endometrium, which has good receptivity, shows vascularity in zones 3 and 4.

Endometrial Vascularity: Its Relation to Implantation Rates (Table 2)[14]

Zaidi et al. found that absence of flow in the endometrial and subendometrial zones on day of hCG indicates total failure of implantation.[15]

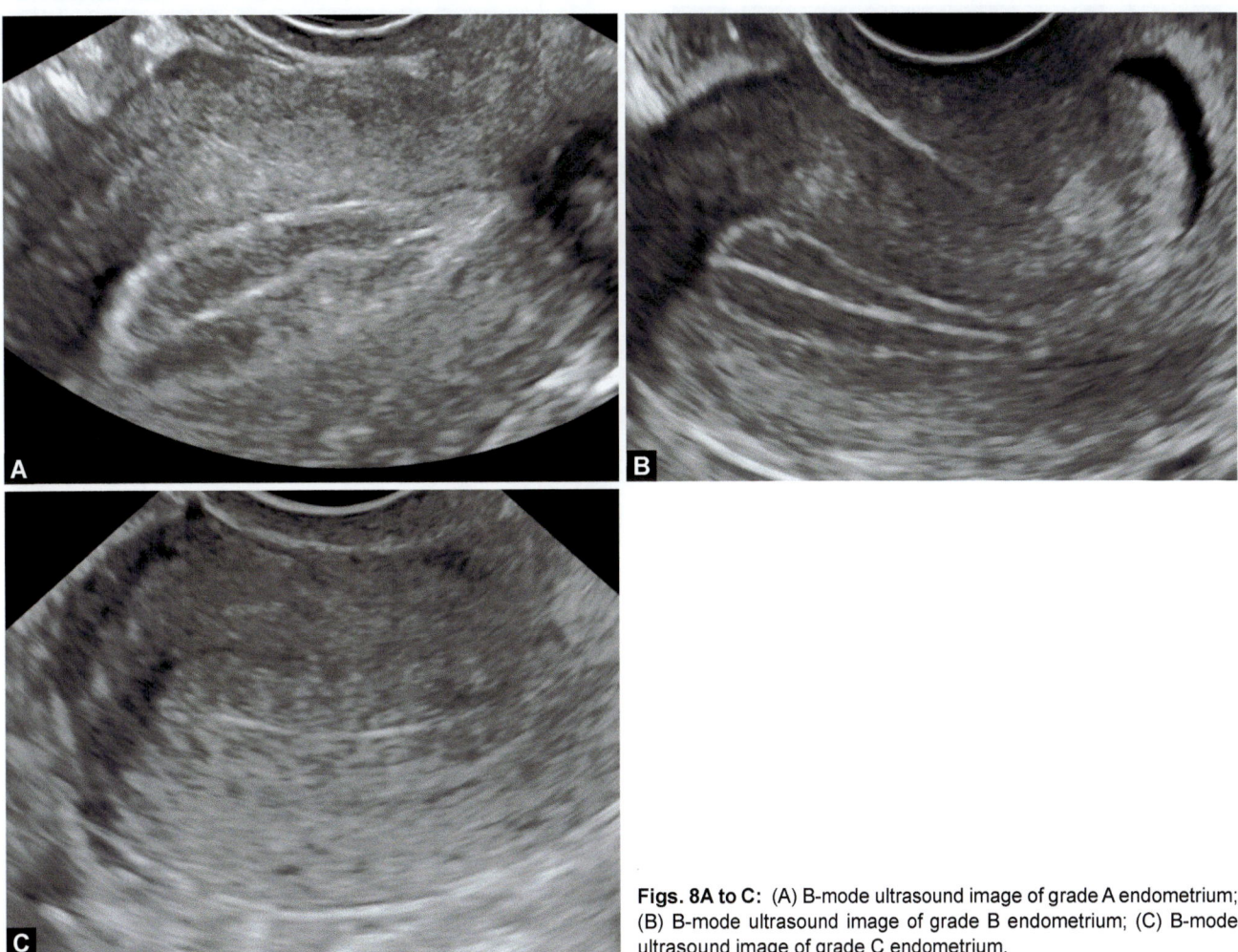

Figs. 8A to C: (A) B-mode ultrasound image of grade A endometrium; (B) B-mode ultrasound image of grade B endometrium; (C) B-mode ultrasound image of grade C endometrium.

Table 2: Endometrial vascularity and its relation to implantation rates.

Vascularity in	Zone 1	Zone 2	Zone 3	Zone 4
Percentage of patients	6.69%	20.73%	58%	14.47%
+beta human chorionic gonadotropin (βhCG)	19%	21.87%	39.77%	70.14%
Gestational sac	9.6%	14.58%	36.8%	68.65%
Abortions	50%	23.8%	5.6%	1.5%

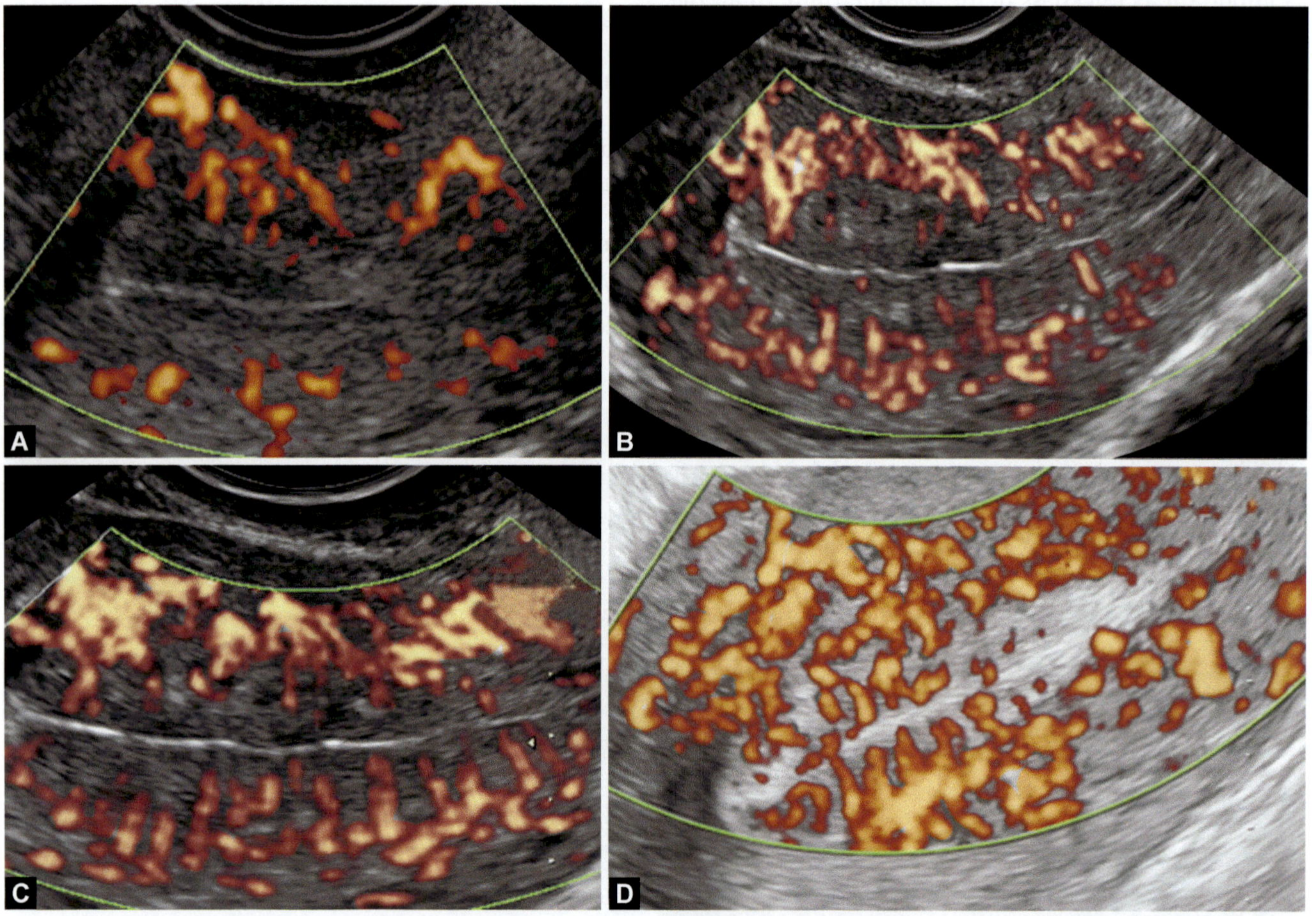

Figs. 9A to D: Power Doppler images of the zones 1–4 endometrium endometrial vascularity, respectively from Figures A to D.

The zones of vascularity are defined according to Applebaum[16] as (Figs. 9A to D): Zone 1 when the vascularity on power Doppler is seen only at endometrio-myometrial junction, zone 2 when vessels penetrate through the hyperechogenic endometrial edge, zone 3 when it reaches intervening hypoechogenic zone, and zone 4 when they reach the endometrial cavity.

On pulse Doppler, these arteries should have an RI of <0.6 and should cover 5 mm² area of the endometrium to have adequate receptivity.

Moreover, uterine artery pulsatility index (PI) should be <3.2 (Fig. 10).

Several authors have shown that the optimum uterine receptivity was obtained when average PI of the uterine artery was between 2 and 3 on the day of trigger.[17,18]

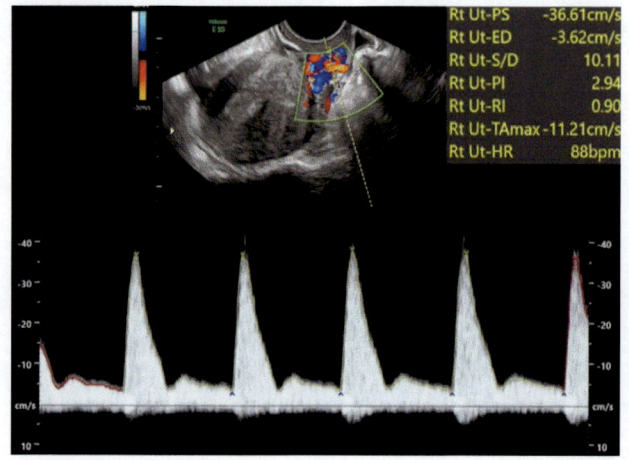

Fig. 10: Pulse Doppler image showing high-resistance uterine artery flow waveform.

Endometrial volume by 3D ultrasound volume calculation of the endometrium may help to correlate the cycle outcome with quantitative parameter rather than endometrial thickness.[19]

A study by Raga et al.[20] shows pregnancy and implantation rates were significantly lower when endometrial volume <2 mL, while no pregnancy was achieved when endometrial volume was <1 mL.

To summarize (refer Table 3).

SECRETORY PHASE ASSESSMENT

Rupture of the follicle leads to formation of corpus luteum. Corpus luteum is responsible for progesterone production. The functional efficacy of the corpus luteum can be assessed by Doppler by assessing the pericorpus luteal vascularity. Since there is a clear correlation between RI of corpus luteum and plasma progesterone levels, RI of the corpus luteum can be used as an adjunct to plasma progesterone assay as an index of luteal function.[21]

A corpus luteum that is functionally normal and produces adequate amount of progesterone shows corpus luteal flow: RI 0.35–0.50 and PSV 10–15 cm/s (Figs. 11A and B).

Endometrium starts showing fluffy margins as the progesterone exposure starts, followed by hyperechogenicity starting from the periphery in the luteal phase. Endometrium becomes completely hyperechoic in the midluteal phase. With adequate progesterone levels, that are achieved in the midluteal phase, the spiral arteries show RI of 0.48–0.52 (low-resistance flow) and uterine artery shows PI of 2.0–2.5 cm/s. Inadequate progesterone production and, therefore, corpus luteal inadequacy are suggested by high resistance flow in corpus luteal vessels.[21] High spiral artery resistance would suggest inadequate response of endometrium to progesterone. This is because of inadequate

Table 3: Optimum ultrasound parameters for pretrigger follicle and endometrium.

	Follicle	Endometrium
Size/thickness	16–18 mm	8–10 mm
Morphology	Thin wall, no internal echoes, halo	Grade A/B
Vascularity	Three-fourths of circumference	Zones 3–4
Resistance index (RI)	0.4–0.48	<0.5
PSV	>10 cm/s	–
Uterine artery PI	–	<3.2
Volume	3–7 cc	3–7 cc
3D morphology	Cumulus	Intact endometrio-myometrial junction
3D PD	More symmetrical the better	Higher the better

(PD: pulse Doppler; PI: pulsatility index; PSV: peak systolic velocity)

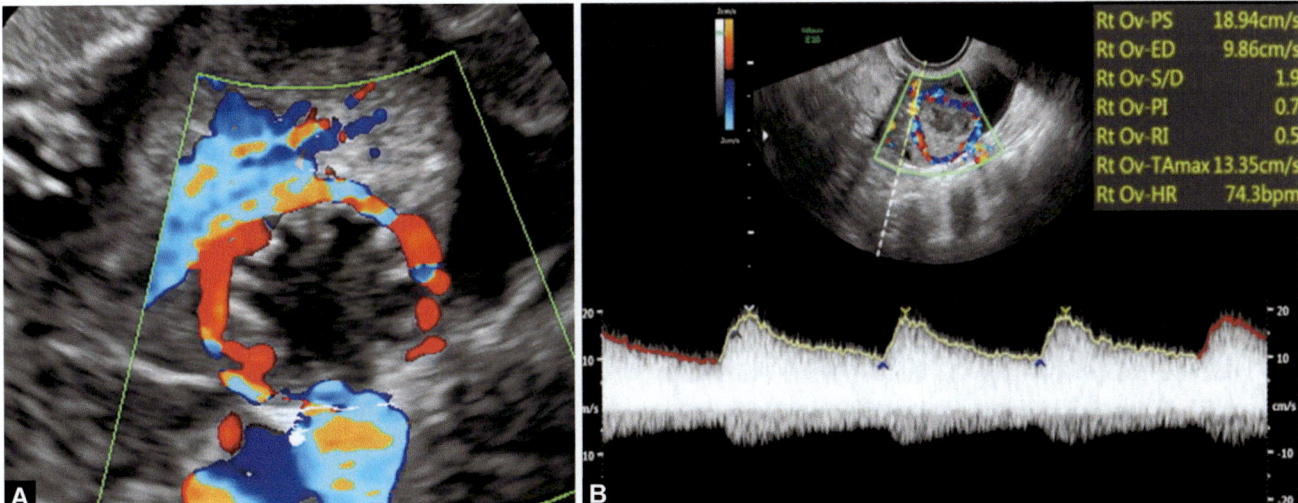

Figs. 11A and B: Normal corpus luteal flow seen on color Doppler and pulse Doppler.

progesterone receptors in the endometrium or because of local endometrial cause, like endometrial injury or chronic endometritis.

In luteal phase defect because of low progesterone levels, the resistance in the pericorpus luteal vessels is high.

CONCLUSION

Ultrasound is an excellent tool for assessment of the menstrual cycle. Hormonal changes occurring day-to-day during the menstrual cycle reflects as morphological and vascular changes in the ovary and the uterus. Assessing these changes by transvaginal ultrasound and Doppler and correctly interpreting can explain the hormonal basis of these changes. Ultrasound with Doppler can, thus, be used as the only modality for cycle assessment in patients undergoing assisted reproduction technology and may be of help to reduce the cost of the cycle by avoiding certain hormonal assessments and still maintaining close and accurate watch on the hormonal changes occurring during treatment cycle.

REFERENCES

1. Kupesic S, Kurjak A. Predictors of IVF outcome by three-dimensional ultrasound. Hum Reprod. 2002;17:950-5.
2. Popovic-Todorovic B, Loft A, Lindhard A, et al. A prospective study of predictive factors of ovarian response in 'standard' IVF/ICSI patients treated with recombinant FSH. A suggestion for recombinant FSH dosage nomogram. Hum Reprod. 2003;18:781-7.
3. Freiesleben NL, Lossl K, Bogstad J, et al. Predictors of ovarian response in intrauterine insemination patients and development of a dosage nomogram. Reprod Biomed Online. 2008;17:632-41.
4. Krishnakumar J, Agarwal A, Nambiar D, et al. Comparison of antral follicle count, antimullerian hormone and day 2 follicle stimulating hormone as predictor of ovarian response and clinical pregnancy rate in patient with an abnormal ovarian reserve test. Int J Reprod Contracept Obstet Gynecol. 2016;5:2762-7.
5. Zaidi J, Barber J, Kyei-Mensah A, et al. Relationship of ovarian stromal blood flow at baseline ultrasound to subsequent follicular response in an in vitro fertilization program. Obstet Gynecol. 1996;88:779-84.
6. Engmann L, Saldkevicius P, Agrawal R, et al. Value of ovarian stromal blood flow velocity measurement after pituitary suppression in the prediction of ovarian responsiveness and outcome of in vitro fertilization treatment. Fertil Steril. 1999;71:22-9.
7. Lam PM, Johnson IR, Rainne-Fenning NJ. Three-dimensional ultrasound features of the polycystic ovary and the effect of different phenotypic expressions on these parameters. Hum Reprod. 2007;22:3116-23.
8. Panchal S, Nagori CB. Ultrasound-based decision making on stimulation protocol for superovulated intrauterine insemination cycles. Int J Infertil Fetal Med. 2016;7:7-13.
9. Panchal S, Nagori CB. Ultrasound-based decision-making on stimulation protocol in IVF. DSJUOG. 2016;10:330-7.
10. Van Blerkom J, Antezak M, Schrader R. The developmental potential of human oocyte is related to the dissolved oxygen content of follicular fluid: association with vascular endothelial growth factor levels and perifollicular blood flow characteristics. Hum Reprod. 1997;12:1047-55.
11. Panchal SY, Nagori CB. Can 3D PD be a better tool for assessing the preHCG follicle and endometrium? A randomized study of 500 cases. J Ultrasound Obstet Gynecol. 2006;28:504.
12. Vlaisavljevic V, Reljic M, Gavric-Lovrec V, et al. Measurement of perifollicular blood flow of the dominant preovulatory follicle using three dimensional power Doppler. Ultrasound Obstet Gynecol. 2003;22:520-6.
13. Bourne TH, Jurkovic D, Waterstone J, et al. Intrafollicular blood flow during human ovulation. Ultrasound Obstet Gynecol. 1991;1:53-9.
14. Nagori C, Panchal S. Endometrial vascularity: its relation to implantation rates. Int J Infertil Fetal Med. 2012;3:48-50.
15. Zaidi J, Campbell S, Pittrof R, et al. Endometrial thickness, morphology, vascular penetration and velocimetry in predicting implantation in an in vitro fertilization program. Ultrasound Obstet Gynecol. 1995;6:191-8.
16. Applebaum M. The 'steel' or 'teflon' endometrium—ultrasound visualization of endometrial vascularity in IVF patients and outcome. Presented at the third World Congress of Ultrasound in Obstetrics and Gynecology. Ultrasound Obstet Gynecol. 1993;3:10.
17. Zaidi J, Pittrof R, Shaker A, et al. Assessment of uterine artery blood flow on the day of human chorionic gonadotrophin administration by transvaginal colour Doppler ultrasound in an in vitro fertilization program. Fertil Steril. 1996;65:377-81.
18. Steer CV, Campbell S, Tan SL, et al. The use of transvaginal colour flow imaging after in vitro fertilization to identify optimum uterine conditions before embryo transfer. Fertil Steril. 1992;57:372-6.
19. Wittmack FM, Kreger DO, Blasco L, et al. Effect of follicular size on oocyte retrieval, fertilization, cleavage and embryo quality in in vitro fertilization cycles: a 6 year data collection. Fertil Steril. 1994;62:1205-10.
20. Raga F, Bonilla-Musoles F, Casan EM, et al. Assessment of endometrial volume by three dimensional ultrasound prior to embryo transfer: clues to endometrial receptivity. Hum Reprod. 1999;14:2851-4.
21. Glock JL, Brumsted JR. Colour flow pulsed Doppler ultrasound in diagnosing luteal phase defect. Fertil Steril. 1995;64:500-4.

6

Imaging in Endometriosis

Glossy Sabharwal, Meenu Agarwal, Liselotte Mettler

INTRODUCTION

Endometriosis is defined as the presence of functional endometrial glandular tissue and stroma outside the uterus.[1] This ectopic endometrial tissue induces chronic, inflammatory reaction which may result in pelvic pain and infertility. Endometriosis primarily occurs in the pelvis manifesting as ovarian endometriomas, pelvic peritoneal implants and/or deep pelvic endometriosis. Endometriosis at extrapelvic sites may occur rarely. This enigmatic condition is most commonly seen in the reproductive age group. Although, benign in nature, endometriosis can be aggressive and invasive resulting in severe morbidity among females of reproductive age group. The etiology and pathogenesis of endometriosis are still unclear and probably are multifactorial.

While some women with endometriosis experience painful symptoms, others have no symptoms at all. Symptoms are related to the site of endometrial deposits. Common sites of endometrial deposits are within the pelvis affecting the ovaries (typically presenting as endometriomas), fallopian tubes, uterosacral ligaments, and pouch of Douglas. Endometriosis can also exist in previous cesarean-section scar. Common symptoms include cyclical pelvic pain, dysmenorrhea, periovulatory pain, chronic noncyclical pelvic pain, dyspareunia (due to involvement of the uterosacral ligaments), dyschezia (due to rectosigmoid infiltration), and dysuria with or without cyclical hematuria (secondary to the bladder and/or ureteric implants). Uncommon symptoms include cyclical nasal bleeding, cyclical umbilical bleeding, cyclical hemoptysis, cyclical constipation, and urinary urgency.

Exact prevalence of endometriosis is unknown:
- It has an estimated prevalence of 6.1% of women in reproductive age.[2]
- Prevalence of 25–50% has been reported among women presenting with infertility.[3]
- Nearly 90% of women with chronic pelvic pain would have the diagnosis of endometriosis.[4]
- Women with affected first-degree relative have 10 times higher risk of developing endometriosis.[4]

Diagnosis of endometriosis is based on combination of clinical suspicion, noninvasive, and invasive diagnostic techniques:
- *Clinical suspicion*: Medical history, the symptoms and signs, and physical examination.
- *Noninvasive diagnostic tests*: Transvaginal ultrasonography (TVS), transrectal ultrasonography (TRS), three-dimensional (3D) ultrasound, and magnetic resonance imaging (MRI).[5,6]
- *Invasive diagnostic tests*: Laparoscopy—when combined with biopsy and histological examination, laparoscopy is the "gold standard" for the diagnosis of endometriosis. It can be diagnostic as well as therapeutic in situations where surgical resection of endometriotic deposits is required.

The noninvasive diagnostic tests such as ultrasonography and MRI are ideal initial tests, and have largely replaced diagnostic laparoscopy. US is the first imaging test in suspected endometriosis. MRI is an excellent tool when US is not definitive. Due to excellent soft tissue resolution, MRI is highly sensitive and specific for the diagnosis of endometriosis and provides critical preoperative information when surgical excision or debulking is being contemplated. Computerized tomography (CT) scan is not used for the diagnosis of endometriosis. However, due to the extensive use of CT scan in clinical practice, it is important to understand the appearance of endometriosis on CT.

CLINICAL EXAMINATION

This includes the speculum and bimanual vaginal and rectal examination. Unfortunately, due to varying nature of endometriotic lesions, physical examination is mostly unrevealing. Few lesions can be palpated along the rectovaginal septum or in the cul-de sac, especially before menses. The clinician may appreciate uterine or adnexal fixation. Pelvic examination has a poor predictive value.[7]

SERUM MARKERS

Cancer antigen 125 (CA-125) is the serologic marker most often used for diagnosing endometriosis. However, its diagnostic value CA-125 is limited. Increased levels are seen in advanced stages of endometriosis,[8] as well as in epithelial ovarian cancers.[9]

DIAGNOSTIC IMAGING MODALITIES

Imaging is mandatory to ascertain the diagnosis and assess internal organs before start of the treatment. Radiological imaging aims at describing the precise location, depth, and number of endometriotic lesions, so that the condition is treated completely. Currently, TVS is the preferred test for the diagnosis and initial assessment of both endometriomas and deep pelvic endometriosis. However, TVS even with adequate bowel preparation and use of high-frequency probes has important limitations, because of the relatively small field-of-view and operator dependency.[10,11]

ULTRASOUND SCAN

Transvaginal ultrasonography is the first-line imaging study in suspected endometriosis. It is readily available, simple, has no ionizing radiation, quicker, and cost-effective. Moreover, it is a dynamic study with real-time feedback from patients for areas of concern. It is particularly recommended for ovarian cysts and bladder endometriosis.

The best time to do this scan for suspected endometriosis is during the menstrual phase of the cycle when the endometriotic implants grow and are easier to detect. Mais et al. reported that TVS has a sensitivity of 88% in differentiating endometrioma from other ovarian masses with a specificity of 90%.[12]

Endometriomas are seen on US/TVS as cysts containing homogeneous low-level echoes (Figs. 1A and B). Endometriomas may be either unilateral or bilateral and may contain internal partial septations and fluid levels. Malignant transformation is most commonly seen in postmenopausal women with larger endometriomas (>9 cm). These lesions can be differentiated from retractile clots within the endometrioma by using Doppler US.

Adhesions between the ovaries and uterus can cause the ovaries to be pulled medially into the pouch of Douglas, so that they abut one another, described as "kissing ovaries".

Ultrasonography is a dynamic test and can allow the detection of adhesions between the uterus and ovaries and between the uterus and bowel. Fibrotic retroflexion may also be seen on ultrasound and should lead to careful assessment of the retrouterine and retrocervical regions. When applying pressure to the uterine fundus, the uterus should be able to move smoothly anterior to the rectosigmoid, described

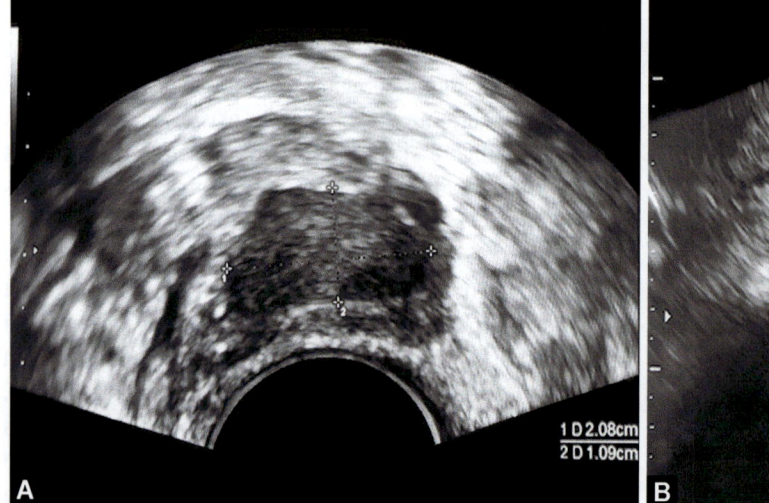
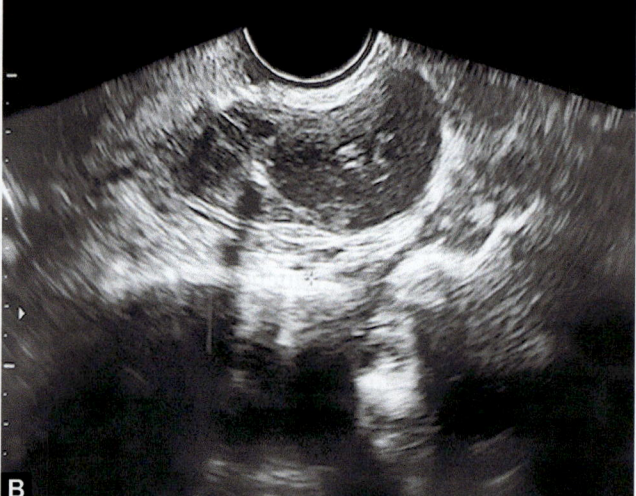

Figs. 1A and B: (A) Transvaginal ultrasonography shows a diffusely homogeneous ground-glass appearance cyst in the right ovary consistent with endometriotic cyst; and (B) Transvaginal ultrasonography shows atypical endometriotic cyst with heterogeneous internal echoes and calcification.

as the "sliding sign". This appearance disappears when there are adhesions between the uterus and bowel. The anterior surface of the rectum and distal sigmoid should be systematically reviewed to identify serosal endometriotic deposits, which are typically hypoechoic nodules and plaques.

In patients with urinary symptoms associated with suspected endometriosis, TVS combined with color Doppler can show the flow of urine through the ureters to the bladder (seen as ureteric jet) showing patency of the ureter. TVS must be combined with transabdominal ultrasonography (TAS) scan to check the kidneys for hydronephrosis secondary to ureteral obstruction caused by endometriotic involvement of lower ureters.

In young girls or women who have never been sexually active, when TVS is not possible, TAS and TRS may be used. For TAS, the urinary bladder should be fully distended. For TRS, it is preferred to have the bowel preparation a night before the scheduled scan. Alternatively, a single dose of ready-to-use enema can be given to the patient 30 minutes before the scan to cleanse the terminal bowel loops. However, a recent study has found that bowel preparation does not improve the diagnostic performance of TVS in detecting rectosigmoid endometriosis and in assessing characteristics of endometriotic nodules.[13]

Limitations of Ultrasonography/Transvaginal Ultrasonography

- Limited field of view. Lesions in proximal/midsigmoid colon, cecum, appendix, and small bowel are impossible to see with TVS.
- Operator dependent. Experience with thorough updated knowledge is needed to look for the disease.

MAGNETIC RESONANCE IMAGING

MRI is a second-line imaging technique which is used when US/TVS is not definitive. MRI is lesser operator dependent than TVS and more sensitive for detecting foci of deeply infiltrating endometriosis. MRI has ability to completely survey the anterior and posterior compartments of the pelvis. It has a large field of view, provides excellent anatomical mapping preoperatively, and template reporting improves report accuracy and reproducibility. However, its diagnostic accuracy in superficial peritoneal lesions, and ovarian foci is still controversial.[12,14-17]

A dedicated MR protocol is essential for diagnosis and presurgical planning of endometriosis. MRI at 3 Tesla is preferred due to superior resolution. The scan is done with patient lying in supine position. In claustrophobic patients, prone position may reduce the anxiety and improve scan acceptability.

Recently, the European Society of Urogenital Radiology (ESUR) published specific guidelines focusing on patient preparation:[18]

- Fasting (at least 6–8 hours before the scan)
- Administration of antiperistaltic agents for better image quality
- Urinary bladder should be moderately filled
- MR imaging at 1.5 or 3 Tesla is preferred due to superior resolution with use of pelvic phased-array coils
- *MR sequences*:
  - Sagittal T2-weighted image (T2WI)
  - Axial T2WI
  - Coronal or oblique T2WI
  - Axial T1-weighted image (T1WI)
  - Axial T1WI with fat suppression
  - *Consider (if complex endometrioma)*: Axial diffusion-weighted imaging (DWI) and axial T1WI with fat suppression postintravenous gadolinium.
- Bowel preparation can be done with an oral laxative a day before imaging. A single dose of ready-to-use enema is given 30 minutes before the examination. To avoid motion artifacts caused by bowel peristalsis, scan is done after intramuscular injections of muscle relaxant. Although bowel preparation is useful to look for deeply infiltrating implants, it is not routinely done in all centers.[15]

MRI features of endometriotic foci with histology correlation:

- *Endometriomas in ovaries*: These appear as bright signal on T1WI and low signal on T2WI.
- *Ectopic endometrial glands*: These have variable signal (depending on the age of hemorrhage) on T1W and T2W images.
- *Subacute bleeding*: Usually has high signal on T1WI and relatively low signal on T2WI.
- *Fibrotic (chronic) endometriotic deposits*: Appear as low signal on both T1W and T2W images.
- *Adhesions*: Pose a low signal bands between pelvic organs.

Disadvantages of MRI

- Expensive and time-consuming
- Not suitable for patients with claustrophobia

COMPUTED TOMOGRAPHY SCAN

Multislice CT scan offers the opportunity to evaluate the depth of the lesions with excellent precision. However, there are two major drawbacks of CT scan, first; exposure to high ionizing radiation and second; use of IV contrast agent for better characterization of the lesions.

LAPAROSCOPY AND BIOPSY WITH HISTOLOGICAL EXAMINATION

Laparoscopy is the gold standard for the diagnosis of endometriosis. One-step surgery is essential for successful treatment of endometriosis. There should be systematic checking of: (1) the uterus and adnexa, (2) the peritoneum of ovarian fossae, vesicouterine fold, pouch of Douglas, and pararectal spaces, (3) the rectum and sigmoid (isolated sigmoid nodules), (4) the appendix and cecum, and (5) the diaphragm on laparoscopic evaluation in cases of endometriosis.

Direct visualization during laparoscopy shows the peritoneal spread of endometriosis in different stages. Therefore, allowing for disease staging especially in cases of deep infiltrating endometriosis (DIE). However, it is very important for the operating surgeon to know about the various appearances of DIE deposits, so that no lesion is left untreated. Removal of all disease present must be done in the same procedure. The disadvantages of laparoscopy are that it is an invasive procedure and may not delineate the full extent of the disease. Adhesions within the pouch of Douglas, a common result of endometriosis, will often make laparoscopic assessment challenging and underestimate the extent of disease particularly within the rectovaginal septum.

DIAGNOSTIC ALGORITHM

Sites of endometriosis and their imaging characteristics on different imaging modalities are described in Table 1.

RECENT ADVANCED IN THE IMAGING TECHNIQUES FOR ENDOMETRIOSIS

Positron Emission Tomography Scan

Positron emission tomography (PET)-CT with 16α-[18F]-fluoro-17β-estradiol ([18F]FES)—a recent study showed that PET-CT with [18F]FES was feasible and had greater accuracy than MRI, particularly in patients with previous surgery. Further studies are needed, however, to investigate its role in bowel endometriosis in sites other than recto-sigmoid junction, nerve localization, and subcentimetric disease.[19]

Table 1: Sites of endometriosis and their imaging characteristics on different imaging modalities.

Sites of endometriosis	TVS	MRI	CT scan	Other imaging modalities
Typical ovarian endometriomas	Hypoechoic cysts with low-level internal echoes giving ground-glass appearance (Figs. 1A and B)	Homogeneous high signal on T1-weighted (T1W) and T1 fat-saturated images and relatively low signal on T2-weighted (T2W) images or variable signal	Fluid density cysts in ovaries with surrounding fat stranding and sometimes with hyperdense hemorrhagic foci within	–
Deep peritoneal implants	Hypoechoic irregular-shaped foci seen in retrouterine and retrocervical regions and at other sites (Figs. 2A to C)	Most are fibrous tissue with low signal intensity lesions on T1W and T2W images. When these sites have bleeding foci, the MRI shows high-intensity signal on T1W and T2W images or even greater with fat-suppressed T1W image	Hypodense or hyperdense solid nodular lesions (more frequent), thickening of soft tissues—parametrial infiltration and adjacent fat stranding	Positron emission tomography–computed tomography with 16α-[18F]-fluoro-17β-estradiol[21]
Abdominal/pelvic wall scars	Solid heterogeneous hypoechoic mass with echogenic spots or thick fibrotic strands and showing internal vascularity on power Doppler examination (Fig. 3)	Hyperintense heterogeneous nodule on both T1W and T2W images due to subacute hemorrhage. Postgadolinium contrast there is usually significant enhancement seen in at least some part of the nodule	Soft tissue isodense or hyperdense mass in deep subcutaneous tissue with mild-to-moderate enhancement on postintravenous contrast scans	US-guided fine-needle aspiration cytology (FNAC) may help to establish the diagnosis. Because needle tract endometriosis has been reported, it is advised to site of FNAC in the surgical resection field
Primary/secondary umbilical endometriosis	Solid or cystic mass in the umbilicus (Figs. 4A to D)	Hyperintense heterogeneous nodule on both T1W and T2W images due to subacute hemorrhage	Solid well-circumscribed umbilical mass	–
Urinary bladder endometriosis	Localized bladder wall thickening or focal echogenic nodular lesions in bladder	Low intensity thickened bladder walls on T2W images with muscle detrusor lesions showing more enhancement than the normal muscle on contrast series	Thickened nodular isodense bladder walls showing enhancement on intravenous contrast CT images	Cystoscopic evaluation

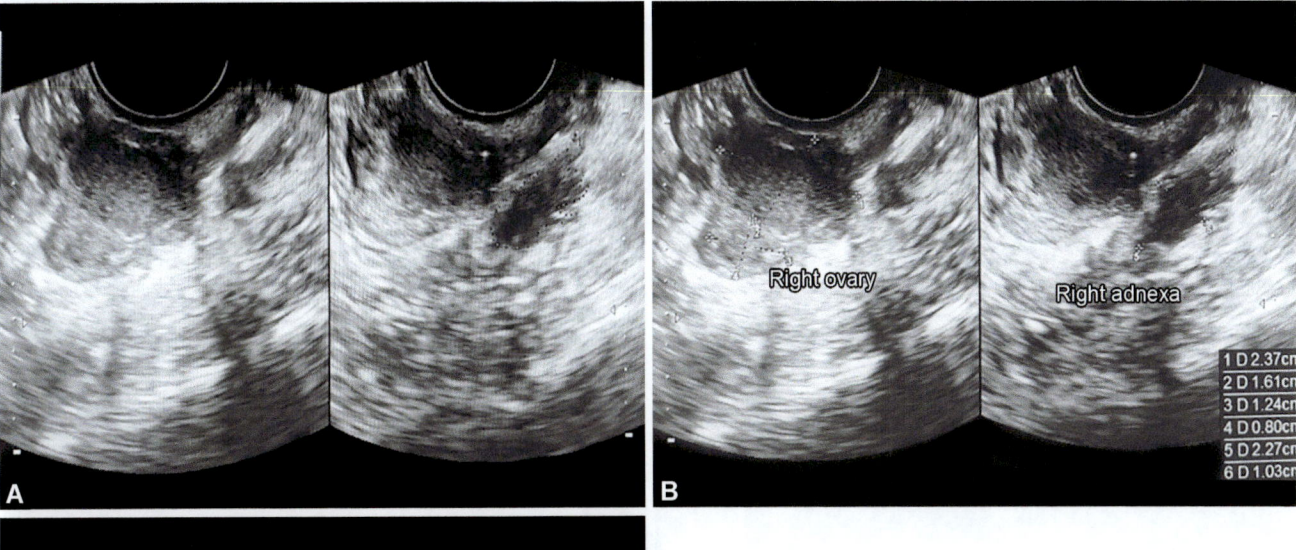

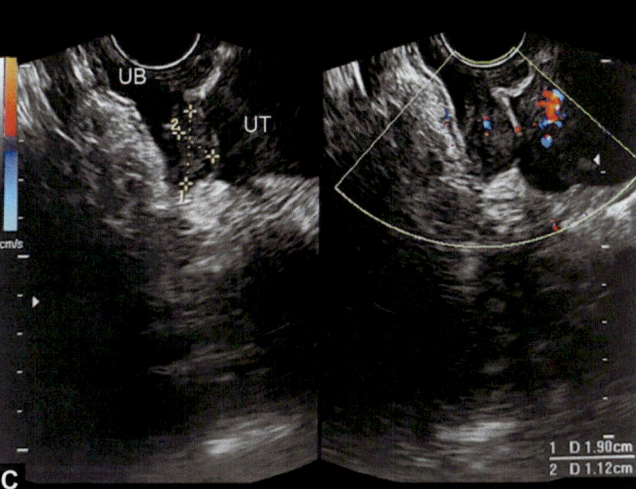

Figs. 2A to C: (A) Transvaginal ultrasonography shows a nodular irregular-shaped hypoechoic solid lesion in the uterosacral ligament in favor of deep infiltrating endometriosis (DIE); (B) Same patient shows two endometriotic cysts in the right ovary; and (C) Another patient, known case of DIE, showing a hypoechoic nodule abutting the urinary bladder and uterine walls.

diagnosis of endometriosis due to the wide spectrum of presentations. The appearance of endometriotic implants at US and MRI depends on the phase of the patient's menstrual cycle and the amount of acute bleeding. TVS is the first imaging in the diagnosis and evaluation, however MRI is the modality of choice for presurgical evaluation and surgical planning in patient with DIE.

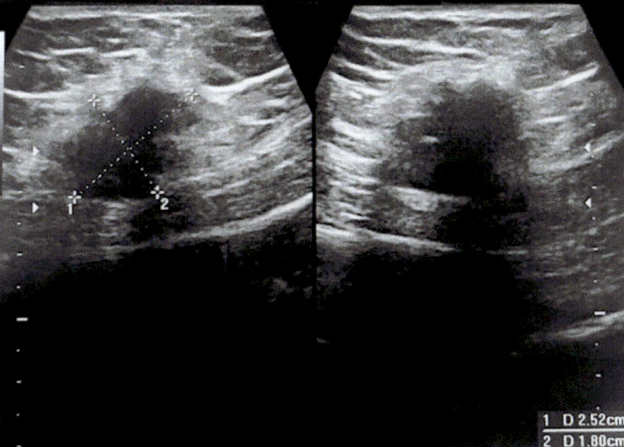

Fig. 3: A subcutaneous nodule is seen with irregular margins, heterogeneous echotexture, proven on fine-needle aspiration as previous cesarean scar endometriosis.

CONCLUSION

Endometriosis is a common disease with high recurrence and significant associated morbidity. Ultrasound (TVS and TRS), CT scan, and MRI have important roles in the

REFERENCES

1. Junior AC, Bittencourt LK, Pires CE, et al. MR imaging in deep pelvic endometriosis. Radiographics. 2011;31:549-67.
2. Fuldeore MJ, Soliman AM. Prevalence and symptomatic burden of diagnosed endometriosis in the United States: national estimates from a cross-sectional survey of 59,411 women. Gynecol Obstet Invest. 2017;82:453-61.
3. Imaoka I, Wada A, Matsuo M, et al. MR imaging of disorders associated with female infertility: use in diagnosis, treatment, and management. Radiographics. 2003;23:1401-21.
4. Chamie LP, Blasbalq R, Pereira RM, et al. Findings in pelvic endometriosis at transvaginal US, MR imaging and laparoscopy. Radiographics. 2011;31:E77-100.
5. Chapron C, Fauconnier A, Vieira M, et al. Anatomical distribution of deeply infiltrating endometriosis: surgical

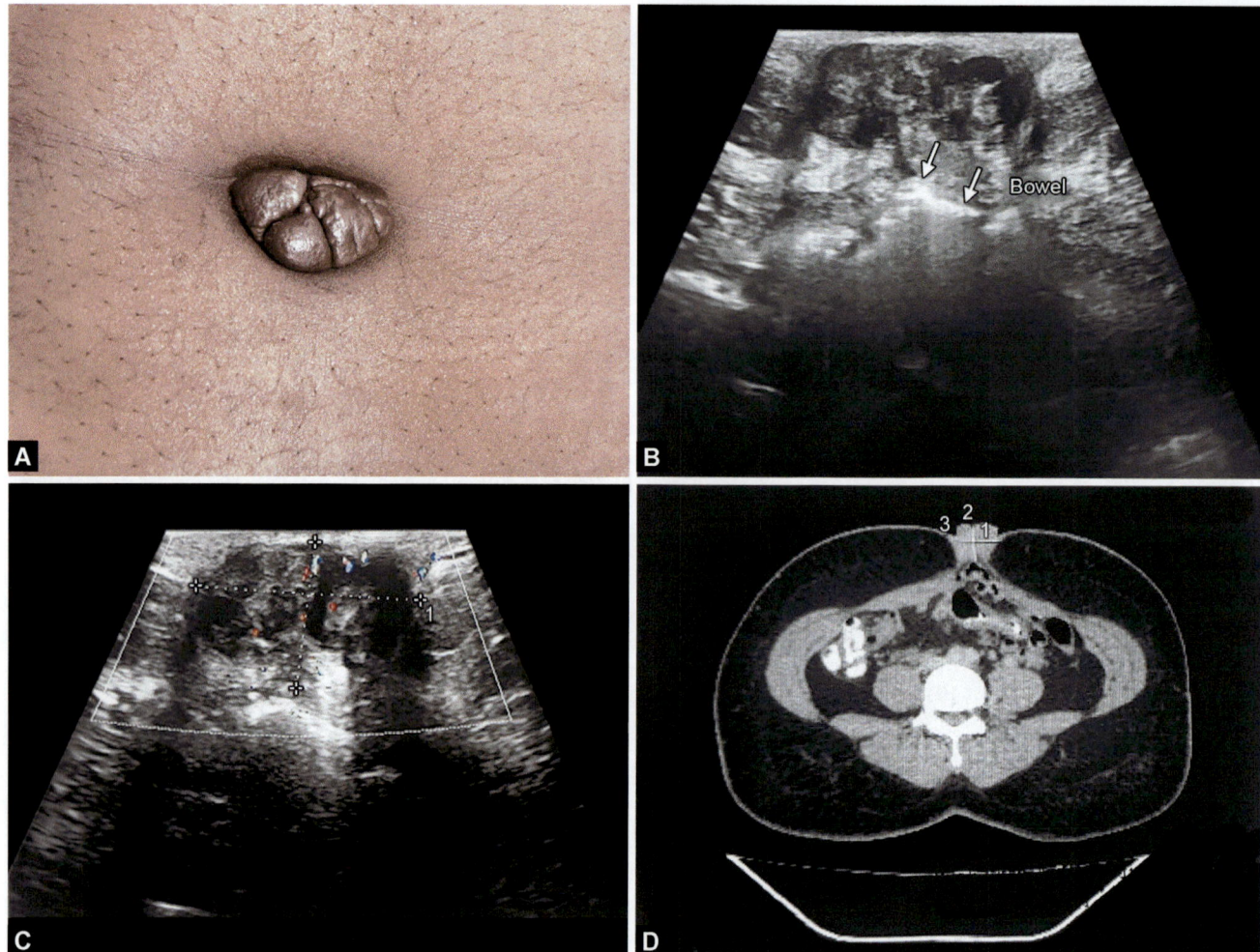

Figs. 4A to D: (A) Clinical picture of a 40-year-old woman who presented with painful umbilical swelling that used to bleed during menstruation. On clinical examination, a 4 × 3 cm dark-colored firm nonreducible nodular lesion involving whole of the umbilicus; (B) Transabdominal ultrasonography showed a 32 mm predominantly hypoechoic complex soft-tissue lesion at the umbilicus, approximately 5 mm below the skin surface (arrows); (C) On color Doppler study, significant intralesional vascularity is seen; and (D) Contrast-enhanced CT scan of the abdomen confirmed the finding of ultrasound, showing an enhancing hyperdense umbilical nodule with rest of the abdominal viscera being normal.

implications and proposition for a classification. Hum Reprod. 2003;18:157-61.
6. Woodward PJ, Sohaey R, Mezzetti TP. Endometriosis: radiologic-pathologic correlation. Radiographics. 2001;21:193-216.
7. Nezhat C, Santolaya J, Nezhat FR. Comparison of transvaginal sonography and bimanual pelvic examination in patients with laparoscopically confirmed endometriosis. J Am Assoc Gynecol Laparosc. 1994;1:127-30.
8. Barbieri RL, Niloff JM, Bast RC, et al. Elevated serum concentrations of CA-125 in patients with advanced endometriosis. Fertil Steril. 1986;45:630-4.
9. Bon GG, Kenemans P, Dekker JJ, et al. Fluctuations in CA 125 and CA 15-3 serum concentrations during spontaneous ovulatory cycles. Hum Reprod. 1999;14:566-70.
10. Dunselman GA, Vermeulen N, Becker C, et al. ESHRE guideline: management of women with endometriosis. Hum Reprod. 2014;29:400-12.
11. Bazot M, Bharwani N, Huchon C, et al. European society of urogenital radiology (ESUR) guidelines: MR imaging of pelvic endometriosis. Eur Radiol. 2017;27:2765-75.
12. Mais V, Guerriero S, Ajossa S, et al. The efficiency of transvaginal ultrasonography in the diagnosis of endometrioma. Fertil Steril. 1993;60:776-80.
13. Ferreo S, Scala C, Stabilini C, et al. Transvaginal sonography with vs without bowel preparation in diagnosis of rectosigmoid endometriosis: prospective study. Ultrasound Obstet Gynecol. 2019;53:402-9.
14. Zawin M, McCarthy S, Scoutt L, et al. Endometriosis: appearance and detection at MR imaging. Radiology. 1989;171:693-6.
15. Togashi K, Nishimura K, Kimura I, et al. Endometrial cysts: diagnosis with MR imaging. Radiology. 1991;180:73-8.
16. Balleyguier C, Chapron C, Dubuisson JB, et al. Comparison of magnetic resonance imaging and transvaginal ultrasonography in diagnosing bladder endometriosis. J Am Assoc Gynecol Laparosc. 2002;9:15-23.
17. Siegelman ES, Oliver ER. MR imaging of endometriosis: ten imaging pearls. Radiographics. 2012;32:1675-91.
18. Biscaldi E, Ferrero S, Remorgida V, et al. Bowel endometriosis: CT-enteroclysis. Abdom Imaging. 2007;32:441-50.
19. Cosma S, Salgarello M, Ceccaroni M, et al. Accuracy of a new diagnostic tool in deep infiltrating endometriosis: positron emission tomography-computed tomography with 16α-[18F]fluoro-17β-estradiol. J Obstet Gynaecol Res. 2016;42:1724-33.

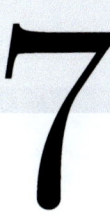

Ultrasound in Gynecology

Aarti Deenadayal Tolani, Hema Desai, Mamata Deenadayal

INTRODUCTION

Ultrasound in gynecology is not any more a luxury. It has become a very reliable diagnostic modality in day-to-day practice, enabling a quick and accurate management, and reducing the necessity of invasive procedures. Because of its safety, high patient acceptance, and relatively low cost, ultrasonography (USG) has become a common diagnostic modality in gynecology today. A proper history and clinical examination of the woman is a prerequisite before any ultrasound evaluation. Noting the menstrual and obstetrics history adequately enables to establish an accurate ultrasound diagnosis. Ultrasound in gynecology has become a necessity flowing history and examination. This chapter summarizes the basic standards necessary in performing ultrasound in gynecology in today's practice. These parameters will enable the gynecologists to perform USG of the female pelvis.

REQUIREMENTS

For a good quality ultrasound, a good ultrasound machine with appropriate probes is a must. Transabdominal scan (TAS) requires a convex curvilinear probe of frequency range 3.5–5 MHz. For transvaginal scan (TVS), an endocavitary probe with frequency range of 5–7.5 MHz is essential. Three-dimensional (3D) scan requires a volume probe of frequency 5–9 MHz. This probe can serve the purpose for both 2D and 3D scans.

TECHNIQUES

Ultrasound in gynecology is a specialization by itself. Being limited to the female pelvis, it gives the clear picture of the deep-seated internal organs, adding to a vaginal examination.

In the unmarried, TAS is the only modality possible.

In the married women, consenting for TVS, TAS followed by TVS is the best way to perform the scan as they together complement each other.

Systematic approach to scan the pelvis is to be applied. Starting with scanning the uterus (endometrium, myometrium, serosa, and cervix), the ovaries, cul-de-sac, and last but not the least, the kidneys.

Transabdominal scan: TAS is done with a full bladder, adequate enough to just reach over the uterus. The bladder must be just adequate, not more (causes discomfort to the patient) or less (impair proper vision of the pelvic organs). Sagittal and transverse views of uterus and ovaries are noted. TAS gives a panoramic view of the entire pelvis and enables to improve on the TVS. It is very useful in midposition uterus, postmenopausal and unmarried women, bulky uterus, etc.

Transvaginal scan: Having completed screening the pelvis on TAS with a full bladder, the bladder is emptied and TVS done for the married women consenting for it. Proximity of the structures to the probe in TVS enables clearer view, improved texture of structures, and a visual palpation of the pelvic organs (Table 1).

Special Maneuvers

Sliding sign: On TVS, gentle probe movements cause the adjacent structures to slide along the walls of the uterus, cervix, vagina, and bladder. This sliding sign is absent in cases of adhesions of organs to each other, like in endometriosis.

Crescent sign (Fig. 1): An ovarian cyst usually shows some ovarian tissue stretched over the cyst wall, giving it a crescent shape.

Table 1: Comparison between TAS and TVS modalities.	
Transabdominal scan (TAS)	Transvaginal scan (TVS)
Low frequency (3.5–5 MHz)	High frequency (5–9 MHz)
Panoramic view of the abdomen	Targeted view of pelvic organs
Requires full bladder	Requires empty bladder
Poor resolution of image	Good resolution of image
Useful in the unmarried	With consent in the married

Splitting sign: Cysts adjacent to the ovary are differentiated from ovarian cysts, by eliciting this sign. Gentle probe pressure splits the paraovarian cyst away from the ovary and splits the two structures, called splitting sign.

Timing of Scan

- Polyps are best picked up in the proliferative phase (days 10–12).
- Uterine anomalies and submucous fibroid (SMF) on 3D are clearly seen in the secretory phase.
- Ovarian cysts are best ruled out in the immediate postmenstrual period.

SETTINGS

The B-mode settings.

Gain

General/Targeted Gain Control

General gains increase the gain of the whole screen. When we require adjustment of the gain in a specific region only, then targeted gain control (TGC) is used.

Angle of Insonation

A full angle gives a complete picture of the region; however, reducing the angle improves the image quality.

Depth

More the depth of the image, less is the frame rate and less is the clarity. Also, the image size reduces and giving limited information of the region of interest (ROI).

Focus

Focus is to be used to enhance the image clarity of a particular region.

Zoom (Pan Zoom and High-definition Zoom)

Pan zoom enlarges the entire image, while a high-definition (HD) zoom enlarges only a selected part of the image.

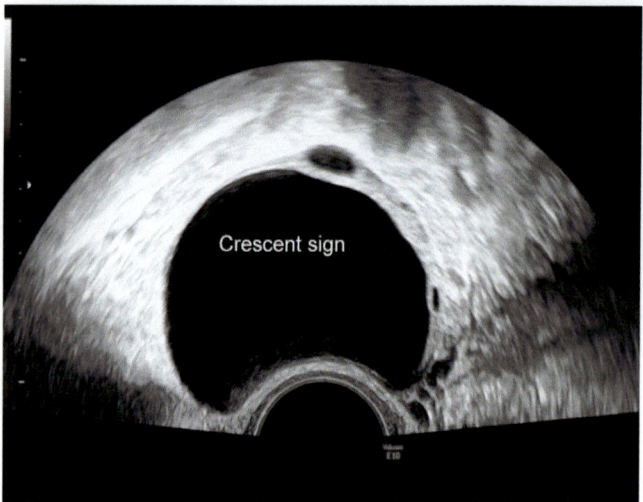

Fig. 1: Ultrasound image clearly depicts the cyst in the ovary, pushing the normal ovarian tissue to the periphery, appearing as a crescent sign.

MODALITIES OF ULTRASOUND

Two-dimensional/Grayscale/B-mode

Grayscale imaging is the base for a proper gynecological scan. It gives the complete picture of the pelvic organs and the inner realities. The other modalities can only fine tune the 2D image. Without a clear 2D ultrasound, neither 3D nor Doppler is possible. On grayscale/2D, structures perpendicular to the transmitting ultrasound beam are well-visualized. Structure parallel to the beam is not seen clearly (Figs. 2A and B).

Three-dimensional

Three-dimensional USG is the study of all the three dimensions of a volume of the tissue, giving a depth perception as well. It involves the coronal plane of the uterus and deciphers the shape of the uterine cavity, the regularity of endomyometrial junction (EMJ) in adenomyosis (Figs. 3A and B), in fibroid mapping, to exactly locate lesions, displaced intrauterine contraceptive devices (IUCDs), etc. It gives the external fundal contour as well as the shape of the endometrial cavity on a single image, just like an MRI or a laparohysteroscopy, yet, being a noninvasive, highly cost-effective modality of diagnosis.[1]

Doppler

It enables to know blood flows in the tissues on grayscale imaging. Doppler flows establish the abundance and resistance in the blood vessels of tissues and lesions. It also gives the site of origin of a lesion. Low-resistance flows

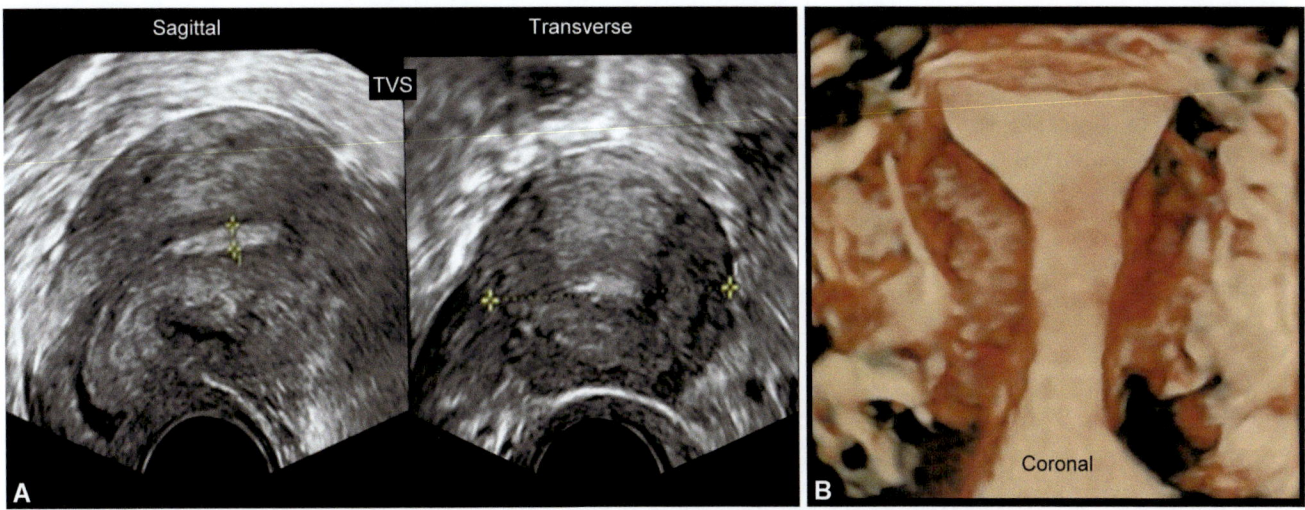

Figs. 2A and B: Ultrasound of the uterus in its three planes—sagittal, transverse, and coronal.

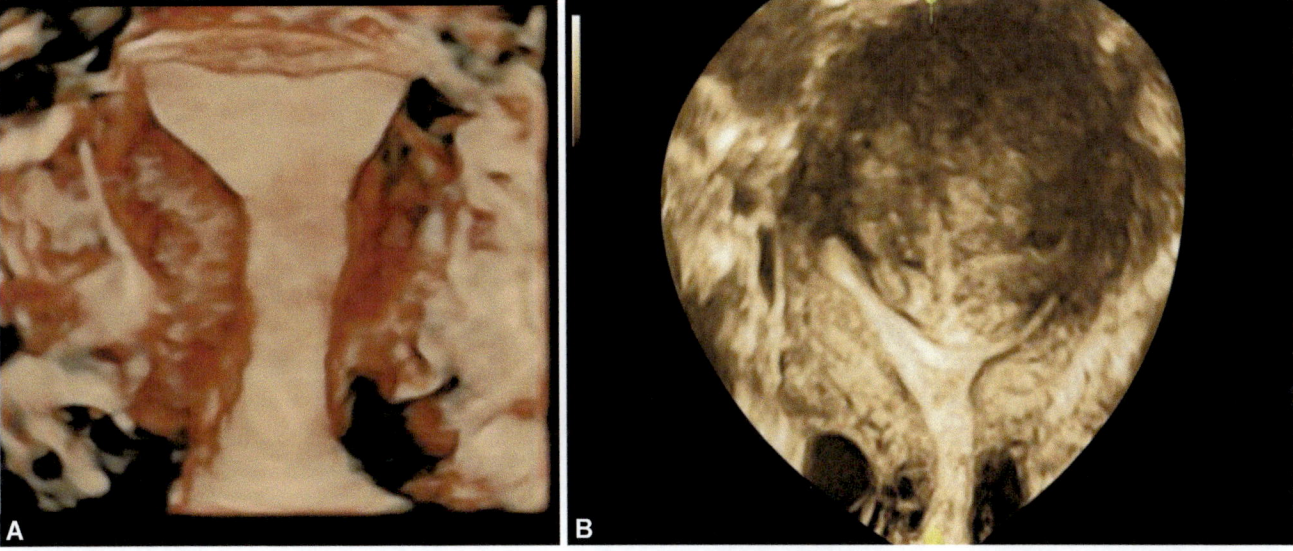

Figs. 3A and B: 3D coronal plane enables to know the details of endomyometrial junction (EMJ) and exact impact of fibroid on the endometrial echo.

indicate benign lesions while high resistance may suggest infections or malignancies. On Doppler, flows parallel to the beam are well seen and vessels perpendicular to the beam are not seen clearly.[2]

Scoring

Color score (CS) is based on subjective, semiquantitative assessment of flows in the tissues of interest. The pulse repetition frequency (PRF) in gynecological scans is always adjusted to 0.6 or 0.3 on power or color Doppler:
- No flow—CS 1
- Minimal flow—CS 2
- Moderate flow—CS 3
- Abundant flow—CS 4 (Fig. 4)

Color Doppler is useful in high velocity vessels to know the direction of blood flow (Fig. 5).

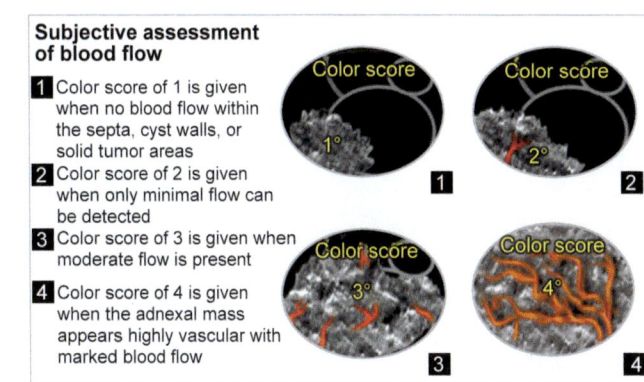

Fig. 4: Pictorial depiction of color score of various blood flows.

Power Doppler is used in low velocity tissues and depicts the amount of blood flow. This is best suitable in gynecological scans (Figs. 6A to C).

High-definition Doppler is useful in low-velocity flows and also to study their direction (Fig. 7).

Pulse wave/spectral Doppler is for quantitative assessment of the flow (Fig. 8).

Three-dimensional color Doppler is used to quantify the velocity of flow in vessels—vascularization index (VI), flow index (FI), and vascularization-flow index (VFI) (Fig. 9).

Below are the descriptions of the use of ultrasound in the common gynecological entities.

CONGENITAL UTERINE ANOMALIES

Congenital uterine anomalies are seen when there is a developmental defect in the Müllerian ducts during embryogenesis. They are usually associated with renal anomalies as well. These women present with the complaints of recurrent pregnancy losses. With the increased use of 3D in daily practice, these patients are diagnosed accurately on scan. However, preceding 2D scan must be suspicious of an anomaly.[3]

Ultrasound details necessary to classify uterine anomalies are:
- External fundal contour—normal (convex) or concave with indentation
- Shape of the endometrial cavity

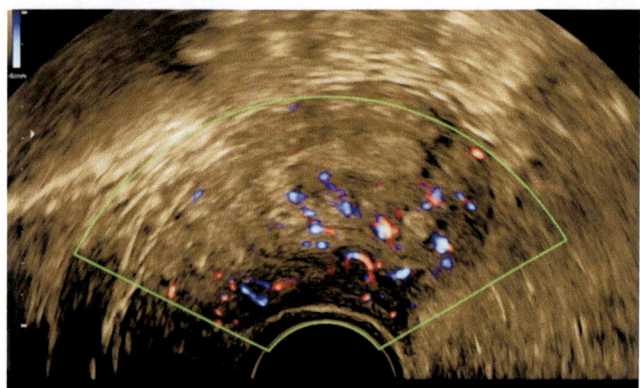

Fig. 5: Ultrasound color Doppler flow in the uterus.

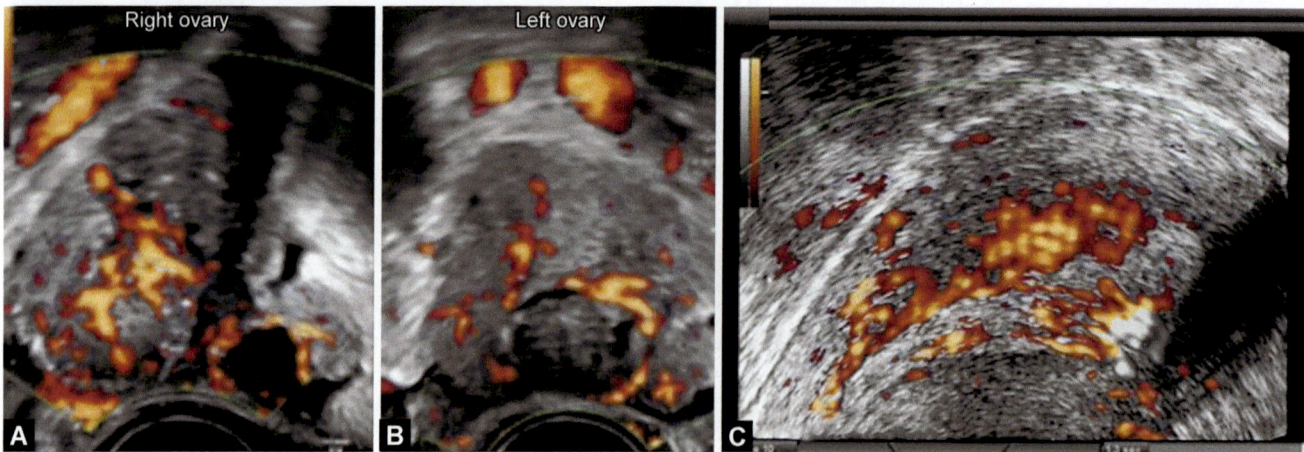

Figs. 6A to C: Power Doppler in uterus and ovaries.

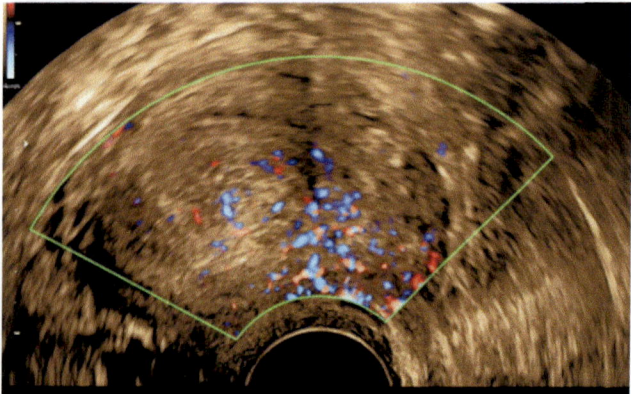

Fig. 7: High-definition flow of the uterus.

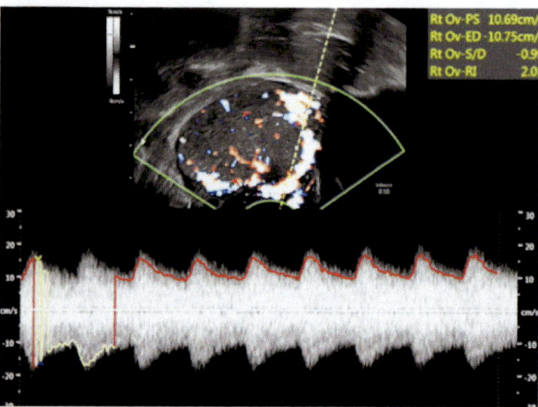

Fig. 8: Spectral Doppler flow is very well-depicted in a highly vascular lesion.

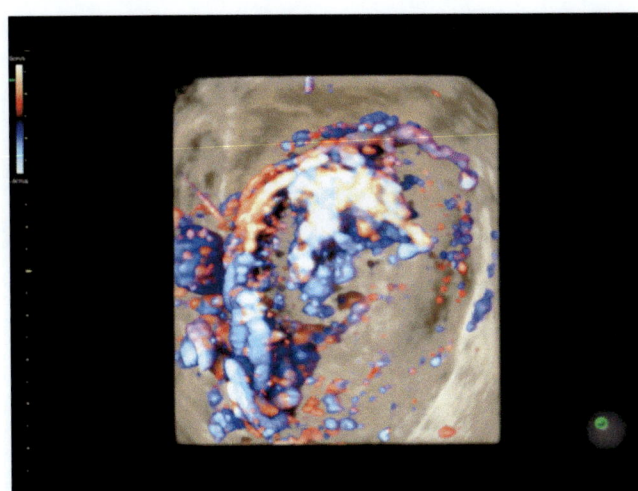

Fig. 9: 3D color Doppler flow is seen in this image, clearly showing the vascular structure.

- Depth and angle of the indentation
- Intercornual distance
- Associated anomalies of cervix, vagina, or kidneys

Under development is seen as either agenesis or hypoplastic uterus. This is usually seen in the genetic disorders such as Turner syndrome, Kallmann syndrome, Mayer-Rokitansky-Küster-Hauser (MRKH) syndrome, etc.

Agenesis of the uterus—on TAS, uterus is not seen or may be seen as a tiny uterine bud. TVS may not be possible if vagina is absent. Blind vaginal pouch allows a TVS.

Hypoplastic uterus on scan is seen as very small uterus, with infantile uterine dimensions. The uterine body and cervix are seen equal in size (1:1 ratio) as compared to the adult ratio of 2:1.

Fusion defects: On scan, these defects are seen as either didelphys uterus, complete or partial bicornuate, and unicornuate with or without a rudimentary horn.

Didelphys uterus is seen as two separate uterine bodies, with or without two cervices and vaginas. This is better picked up on TAS due to its broad dimensions and splaying of the bodies, which may be possible on TVS. The external fundal contour is indented inward. Same is seen in bicornuate uterus. A noncommunicating rudimentary horn may be misdiagnosed for a subserous pedunculated fibroid, unless its origin and vascularity are scanned.

Unicornuate uterus appears as a banana-shaped endometrial cavity deviated toward one side with single cornua (Figs. 10A to D).

Resorption defects: They are seen on scan as complete or partial septum, arcuate uterus. On 2D, these defects are seen as a split in the endometrial echo on the transverse view, giving it an owl's eye appearance. The external fundal contour on 3D is normal, while the endometrial cavity is indented inward with an acute angle in *septate uterus* and obtuse angle in an *arcuate uterus*.

MORPHOLOGICAL UTERUS SONOGRAPHIC ASSESSMENT

Myometrium is looked for the echogenicity, contour, wall thickness, cysts, masses, etc. The two most common pathologies seen in the myometrium are the fibroids and adenomyosis:

1. *Fibroids*: Well-demarcated solid hypoechoic mass with linear internal fan-shaped echoes and edge shadows. There is loss of uterine contour and disturbed endometrial echo. The vascularity is mostly circumferential and may be calcified or degenerated and cystic in appearance.

   Mapping of the fibroids is done both on 2D and 3D USG along with Doppler flows to establish accurately the location and origin of the fibroids. Depending on the proximity of the fibroid to the endometrium, they are graded from 0 to 7 as submucosal to subserous with a uterine location and grade 8 being nonuterine locations.

2. *Adenomyosis*: Globular enlargement of the uterus, symmetrical or asymmetrical myometrial hypertrophy and fan-shaped internal echoes, thickened EMJ, myometrial cysts, buds, and spots. It shows intralesional vascularity. Adenomyosis is best seen on 3D ultrasound on volume contrast imaging (VCI) mode. In adenomyosis, the uterine contour and endometrial echo are always maintained (Figs. 11A to D and Table 2).[4]

INTERNATIONAL ENDOMETRIAL TUMOR ANALYSIS GROUP

Standardized systematic evaluation and reporting of endometrium.

Measurement of the Endometrium

Endometrium is measured in sagittal plane at its thickest, perpendicular to the endometrial echo. In endometrial lesions, except in submucous myoma and fluid in the cavity, the thickness of endometrium must include the lesion.

Endometrial pathologies are best seen in preovulatory phase (days 10–12).

Normal thickness of the endometrium in the reproductive women ranges from 5 mm to 15 mm. The thickness should not exceed 5 mm in the menstrual phase or in the postmenopausal years (Fig. 12).

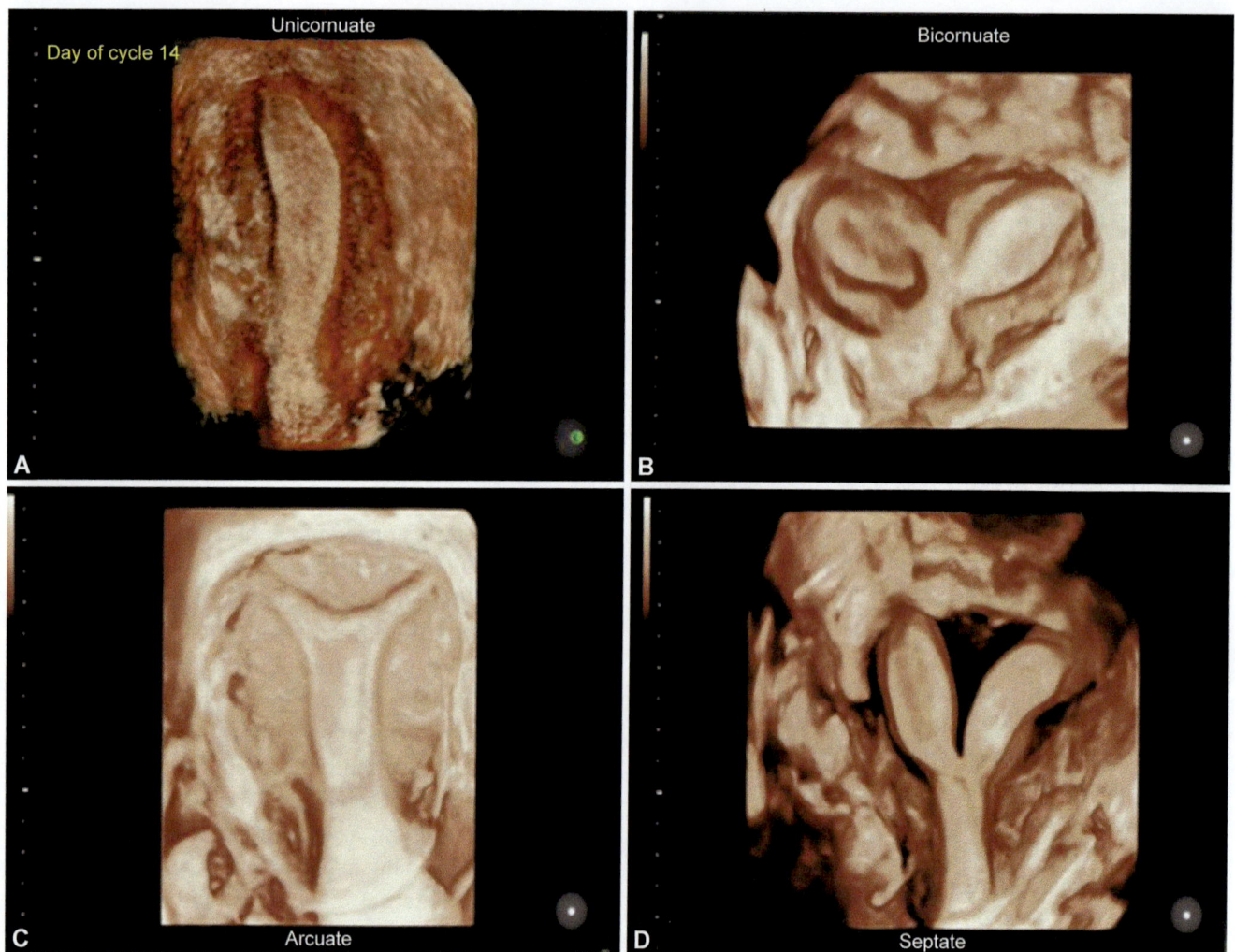

Figs. 10A to D: Various congenital uterine anomalies on ultrasound.

Endometrial Polyps

These are seen as hyperechoic, well-circumscribed, and endometrial lesions with a hyperechoic line all around on 2D and a regular EMJ. A vascular feeder vessel crossing the EMJ (*pedicle sign*) on color Doppler is usually seen. Polyps are better visualized when there is fluid around it. On 3D sweep, the polyps are very well-picked up with their exact size, number, and location (Figs. 13A to D).

Endometrial Hyperplasia

Thickened endometrium is usually seen in the high estrogenic endometrium of women with polycystic ovary syndrome (PCOS) and those exposed to unopposed estrogens. A heterogeneous echotexture is seen with cystic spaces and a regular EMJ. There is excessive vascular flow at the EMJ; however, the vessels appear linear and parallel to each other and of same capacity.

Asherman's Syndrome/Intrauterine Adhesions

Intrauterine adhesions (IUAs) are seen as postinfections (such as tuberculosis), postsurgical, or traumatic events. IUA is a common cause for infertility and recurrent pregnancy loss (RPL) in women.

Ultrasonography Features of Intrauterine Adhesion

On 2D—irregular endometrial outline with break in the continuity, interrupted by hypoechoic areas of fibrotic scars.

On 3D—irregular endometrial margins with synechiae seen running across the endometrial echo. Saline infusion enables delineation of the bands accurately.

Fluid in the Endometrial Cavity (Fig. 14)

Fluid in the cavity is commonly during the menstrual phase and in the atrophic uterus of the postmenopausal women.

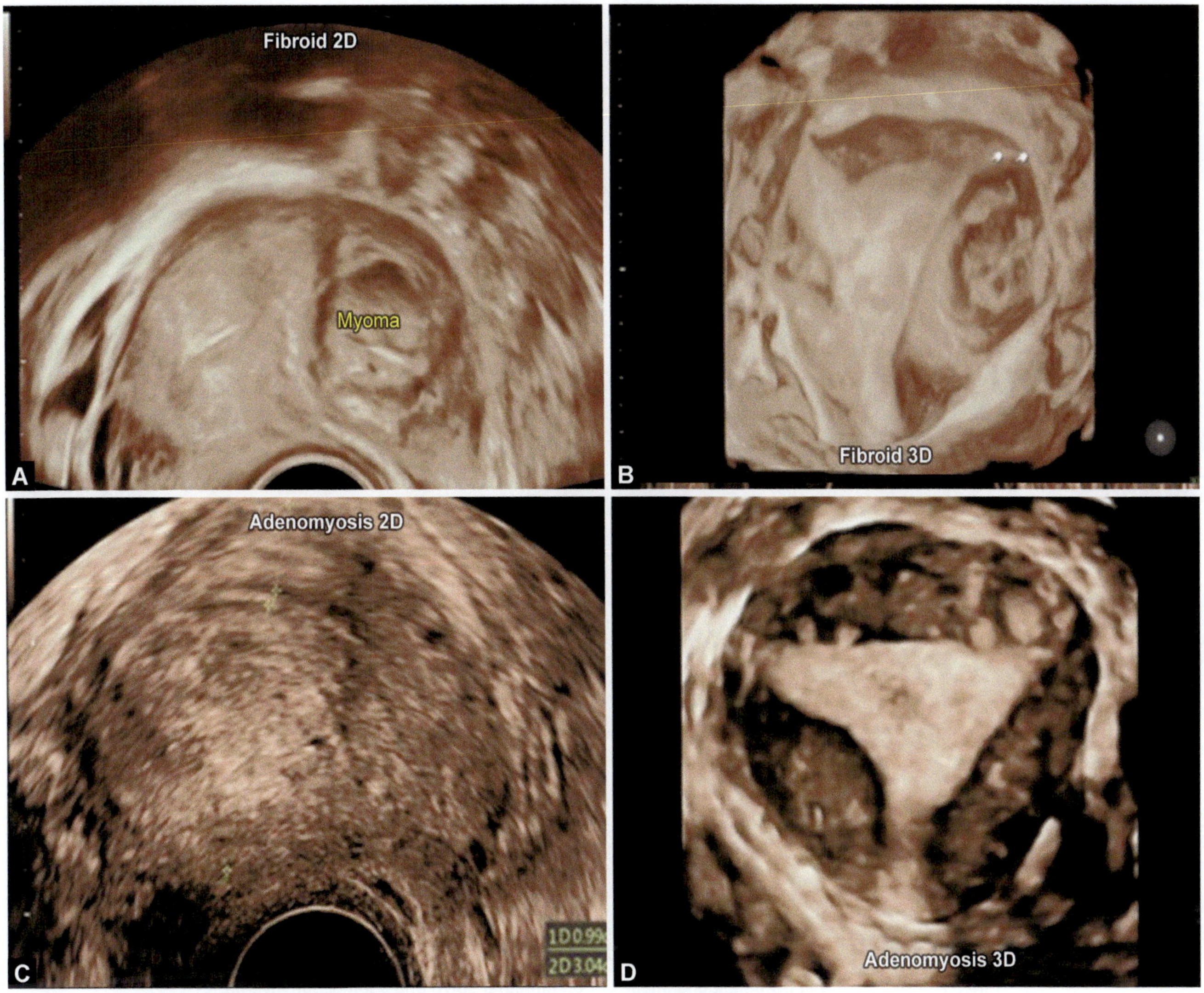

Figs. 11A to D: 2D and 3D modalities in myometrial lesions—fibroids and adenomyosis.

Table 2: Ultrasound features of fibroid and adenomyosis.	
Fibroid	Adenomyosis
Uterus lobulated	Uterus regular, globular
Internal linear shadows with edge shadows	Only internal linear shadows
Distorted endometrium	Central endometrium, well-visualized
Junctional zone (JZ) well-defined and regular	JZ ill-defined, irregular, and thickened
Vascularity mainly circumferential	Vascularity is mainly intralesional
Fibroids are well-circumscribed lesions	Ill-defined, generalized lesion

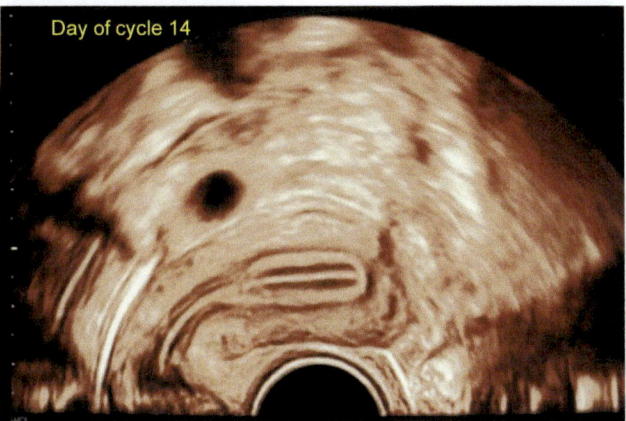

Fig. 12: Endometrium of the uterus on longitudinal view at its thickest.

The endometrial thickness measurement must exclude any fluid and hence measured in two layers. In cases of excessive fluid, volume may be calculated by measuring the three dimensions of the fluid in two perpendicular planes.

The presence of fluid in the endometrial cavity is alarming when it is hemorrhagic (*hematometra*) suggestive of any bleed or obstruction to outflow or infections (*pyometra*) in the postmenopausal or any

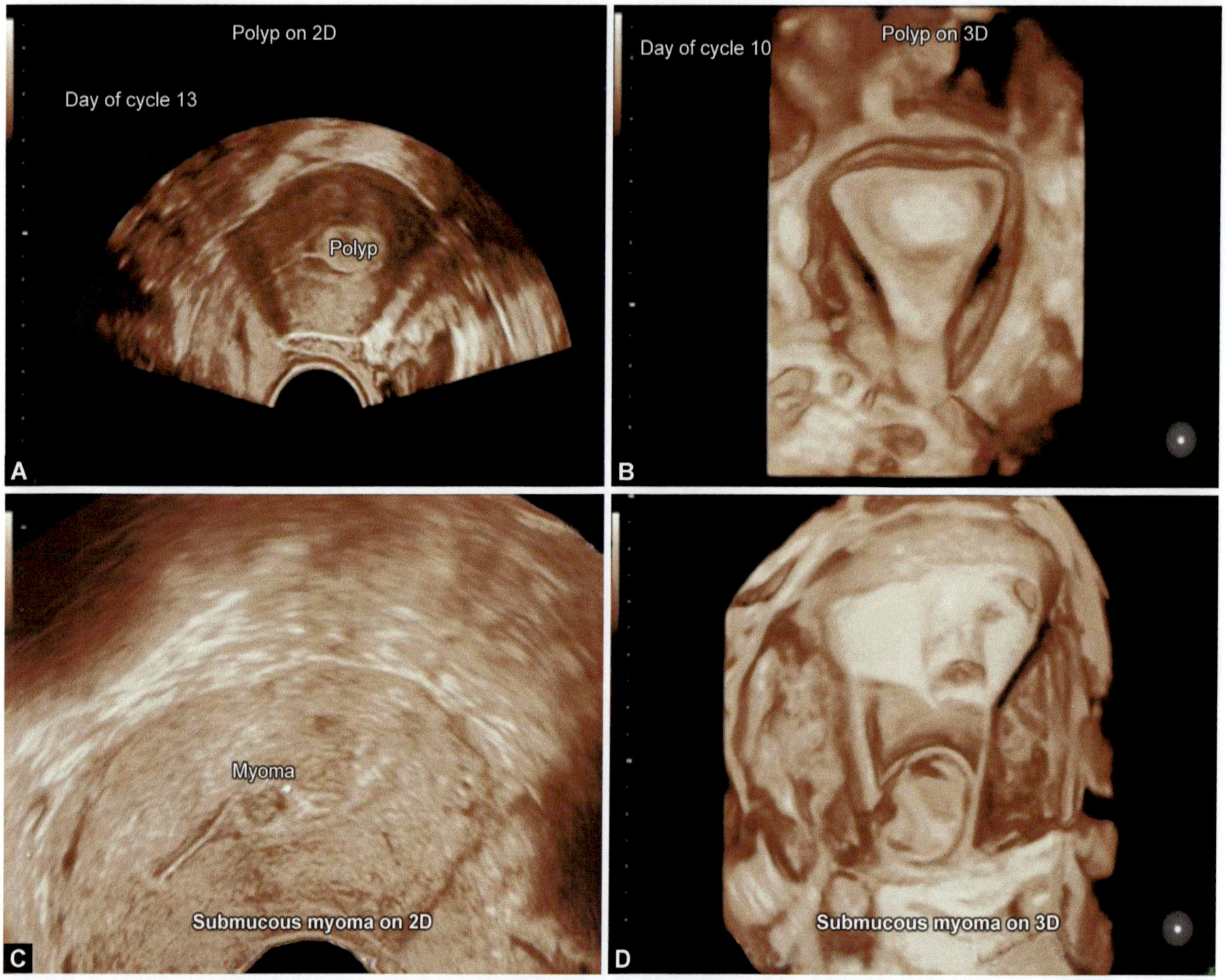

Figs. 13A to D: 2D and 3D ultrasound images of endometrial polyp and submucous myoma.

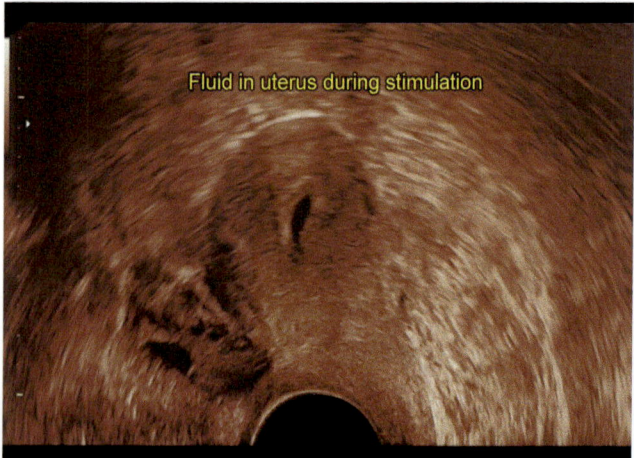

Fig. 14: Fluid in the endometrial cavity appears as anechoic echo in the cavity.

foreign bodies. Fluid in the cavity may be an indicator of fallopian tube carcinomas as well.

Ultrasound in Endometrial Carcinoma (Fig. 15)

The endometrium is very thick (>20 mm), appears heterogeneous in echotexture with or without fluid. The EMJ is irregular with loss of the endometrial borders, suggestive of myometrial invasion of the endometrial carcinoma. It exhibits high vascularity with randomly dispersed vessels running across the EMJ. These vessels have low-resistance flows and of varied sizes and shapes.[5]

OVARIES

Ovaries are deep seated and best visualized on TVS with an empty bladder. The ovarian volume is measured in two perpendicular dimensions and in three orthogonal planes in their largest dimensions. They are best assessed in the menstrual phase for antral follicle count (AFC), and for any persisting cysts. The stimulated ovaries are then monitored

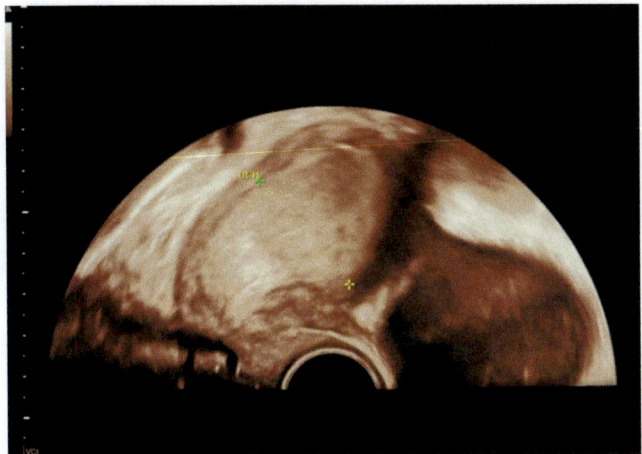

Fig. 15: An endometrial thickness of 33.8 mm in a case of endometrial carcinoma.

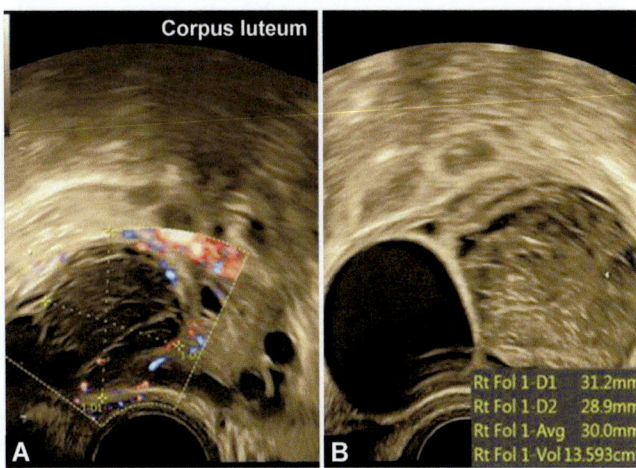

Figs. 16A and B: Corpus luteum postovulatory with vascular circumferential flow and internal echoes (cobweb pattern).

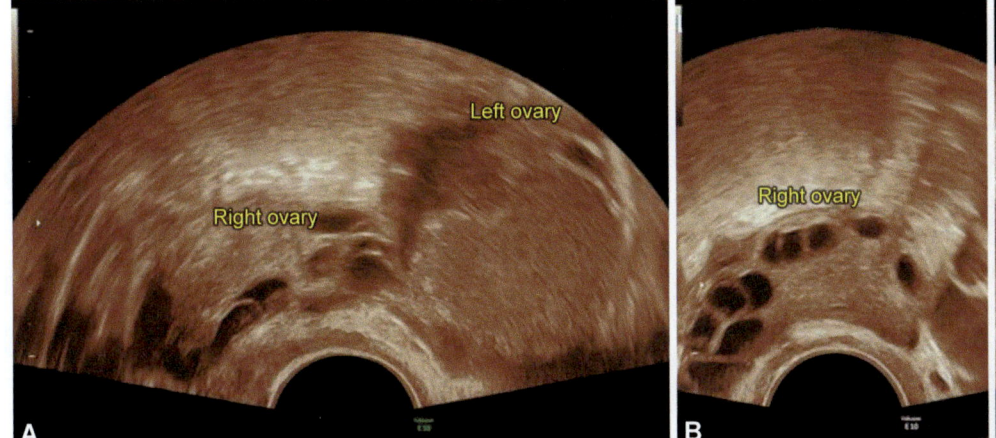

Figs. 17A to C: Endometriomas on ultrasound with a ground-glass appearance.

on TVS for the follicular development and to plan the treatment cycle.

Follicle: A follicle is thin walled, regular, and anechoic.

Corpus Luteum

Postovulation corpus luteum (CL) has varied appearance on ultrasound. It may be completely collapsed, thick walled, or present a "cobweb pattern" within (Figs. 16A and B). In hemorrhagic cysts, the hemorrhagic contents may be seen as heterogeneous echoes with clots and fibrin within.

Endometrioma

Endometriosis in the ovaries is called endometriomas or endometriotic cysts. They are well-defined, hypoechoic cysts with low-level internal echoes and a typical low-level internal echoes (*ground-glass appearance*) (Figs. 17A to C).[6]

Ovarian adnexal pathologies usually seen are dermoid cysts. Nonovarian adnexal lesions are paraovarian cysts.

Ovarian Masses

The various less common ovarian masses include inflammatory (abscess), neoplastic, torsed ovary, or ovarian ectopic. These can be assessed by ultrasound and are beyond the scope of this chapter.

Infertility

Detailing of the use of ultrasound in infertility is beyond the scope of this chapter. However, awareness of its use as a minimally invasive diagnostic tool in this field, starting with pretreatment assessment of the pelvic organs, follicular monitoring, oocyte retrieval, and embryo transfer to the diagnosis of complication and their outcome monitoring.

Polycystic ovary syndrome is a syndrome with hormonal and metabolic derangements. It consists of polycystic ovarian sonomorphology along with anovulation and/or hyperandrogenism. It has four phenotypes with various

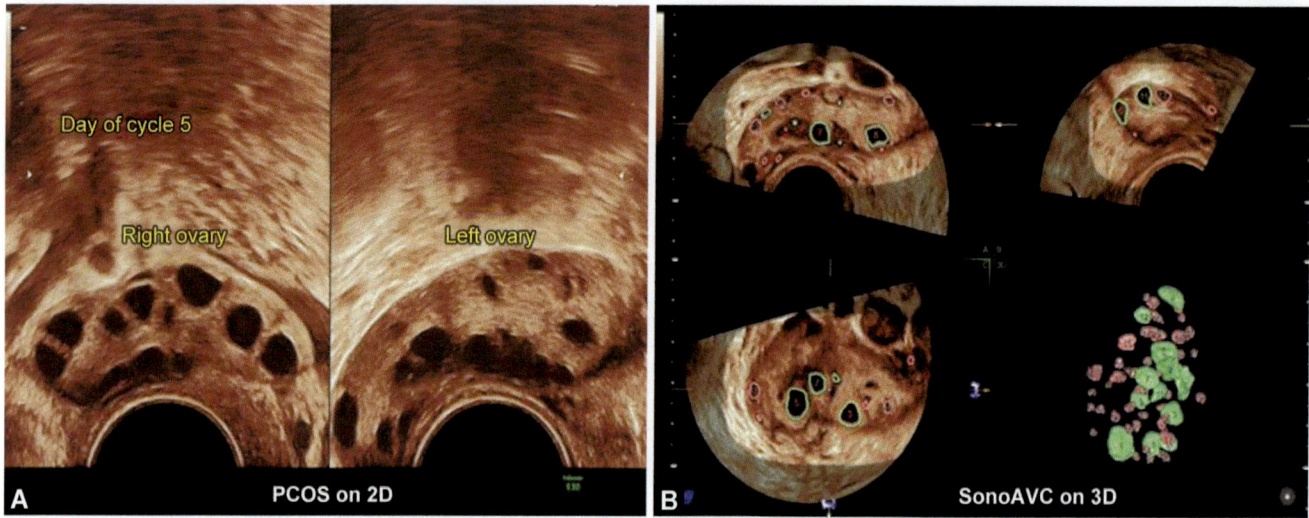

Figs. 18A and B: Ovarian polycystic sonomorphology both on 2D and 3D ultrasound.
(PCOS: polycystic ovary syndrome; SonoAVC: sonography-based automated volume count)

combinations. Rotterdam's criteria: Ovarian volume of >10 cc, follicle number per ovary (FNPO) of 26, increased stroma, hyperechoic, and vascular stroma are typical ovarian features of PCOS on ultrasound. AFC on D2 of cycle is diagnostic. Sonography-based automated volume count (SonoAVC) on 3D is advantageous to count the excessive follicles and know their sizes (Figs. 18A and B).

INTERNATIONAL OVARIAN TUMOR ANALYSIS COLLABORATION

The International Ovarian Tumor Analysis (IOTA) guidelines are based on objective evaluation of the adnexal masses worldwide for the benefit of all womankind. It standardizes the ultrasound features and terms used to describe the morphology, origin, consistency, and vascularity of various ovarian masses.[7]

The ovaries or the cysts are measured for their volume in three orthogonal planes. This enables to know the regression in follow-up visits.

Morphological Classification

Based on this classification, the likelihood ratio for malignancy is as follows:
- Unilocular cyst—1.3%
- Multilocular cyst with no solid area—10%
- Unilocular solid (includes papillae)—37%
- Multilocular solid—43%
- Solid (≥80%)—65%

Significance: Solid area in a cyst itself increases the chances of malignancy.

Table 3: Benign and malignant features of simple rules.

Malignant (M-rules)	Benign (B-rules)
Irregular solid tumor (≥80% solid)	Unilocular
Ascites	Solid components (<7 mm)
At least four papillary structures	Acoustic shadowing
Irregular multilocular solid tumor (≥10 cm)	Smooth multilocular tumor (<10 cm)
Color score 4	Color score 1

Simple Rules

Ten simple rules for malignant and benign ovarian masses are given in Table 3:
- One or more of "M" feature signifies mass as malignant.
- One or more of "B" feature implies it to be a benign mass.
- Mass with both the features of M and B is inconclusive and requires further evaluation by other modalities.
- By this method, 77% of masses can be classified into either benign or malignant types.

Simple Descriptors

The simple descriptors are used for masses which have certain specific features that are easy to recognize. They do not need any further evaluation for their diagnosis. They include:
- *Benign descriptors*:
  - *Endometriotic cyst*: Typical ground-glass appearance
  - *Dermoid cyst*: Unilocular, mixed echogenic cyst with posterior acoustic shadow
  - *Hemorrhagic cyst*: Regular cyst with internal clots and fibrin strands
  - *Cyst adenoma*: Unilocular anechoic cyst with regular wall and <10 cm in largest diameter.

- *Malignant descriptors*:
  - Age > 50 years and CA 125 > 100 mIU/mL
  - Postmenopausal with ascites and CS of 3 or 4.

ENDOMETRIOSIS

It is the presence of ectopic endometrial glands in the ovaries, pelvic peritoneum, uterosacrals, rectosigmoid, bladder, and extrapelvic organs.

Endometriosis in the ovaries are seen as endometriomas (single or multiple), unilateral, or bilateral. The cysts are well-defined hypoechoic with ground-glass appearance. The cyst wall is usually avascular unlike a CL. Endometriomas are usually benign in the premenopausal. Periovarian adhesions and loculated fluid are a common feature with hyperechogenic bright spots in the cyst walls, suggestive of cholesterol deposits.

Deep Infiltrative Endometriosis

The endometriotic deposits on the rectosigmoid and the uterosacrals are seen as hypoechoic, ill-defined, fusiform, firm, and tender areas with poor vascularity. The uterus in deep infiltrative endometriosis (DIE) is retroflexed at midcorpus and is seen as a comma or S-shaped fixed structure often accompanied with posterior wall adenomyosis.

PREGNANCY

Early pregnancy scan in the low-risk women is best done at 7 weeks. This reduces the false diagnosis of pregnancy of unknown location (PUL) at 5 weeks and pregnancy of unknown viability at 6 weeks. Intrauterine pregnancy can be picked up on TVS with a beta-human chorionic gonadotropin (βhCG) values of about 1,200 and on TAS at βhCG of about 6,500.

Ultrasonography findings: A round, regular, and hypoechoic area in either endometrial layer is seen with an echogenic ring of chorionic reaction all around. The sac wall shows color on Doppler.

Retained Products of Conception

The retained products are most often seen as hyperechoic or mixed echogenic, heterogeneous mass in the endometrial cavity, with or without vascularity (Fig. 19).

Gestational Trophoblastic Disease

Gestational trophoblastic disease (GTD) seen in its common benign form as a molar pregnancy. On USG, it is seen as a hyperechoic mass in the endometrial cavity with cystic areas and very high serum βhCG values. Color Doppler shows multidirectional low-velocity flows.

Ectopic

Any pregnancy located outside the endometrial cavity is considered ectopic. Tube is the most common site for an ectopic (Fig. 20).

Features of Ectopic

- Absent intrauterine gestation sac at a βhCG of >1,000
- Pseudogestational sac in the endometrial cavity
- Adnexal hyperechoic well-circumscribed mass with a peripheral ring of vascularity, usually on the same side as the CL
- Probe tenderness with hemorrhage in the pouch of Douglas and Morison's pouch.

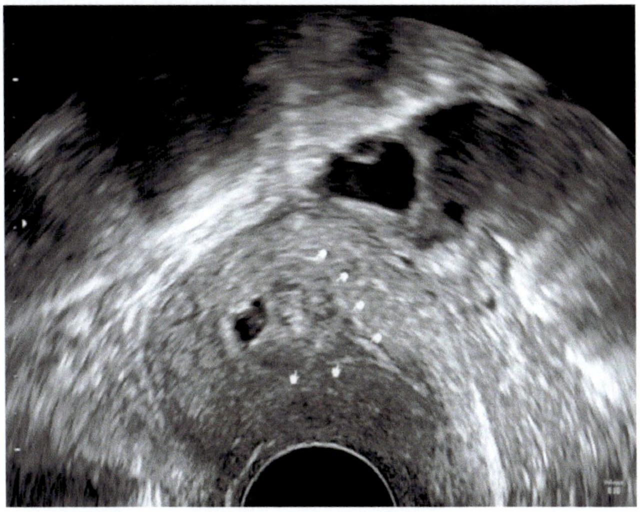

Fig. 19: The retained products of conception are seen as hyperechogenic area in the endometrial cavity, outlined by the arrows.

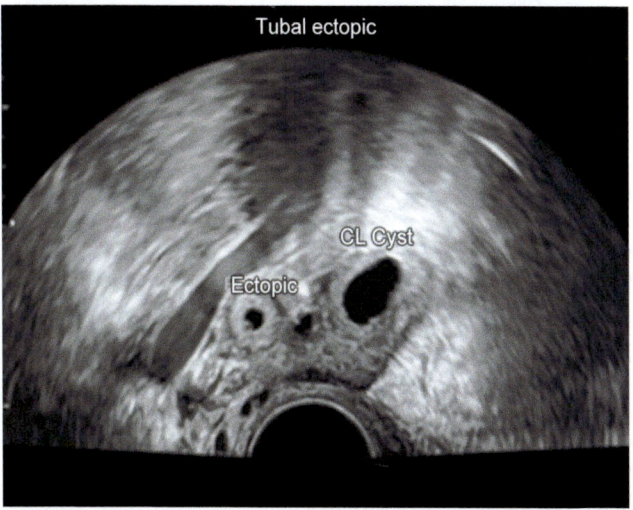

Fig. 20: The scan image shows the tubal ectopic on the same side as the corpus luteum in the ovary.

TORSION

Torsion of the ovary or adnexa is a diagnostic dilemma with an emergency. It is a diagnosis of clinical suspicion and ultrasound features.[8]
- Common and less specific features—enlarged, edematous ovary.
- More specific features—Whirlpool sign in the pedicle, follicular ring sign, and abnormal blood flows.
- Whirlpool sign—on 2D, it is seen as a round adnexal mass, separate from the ovary, either heterogeneous with cystic area or hyperechoic (*target sign*).
- On Doppler, it exhibits a crisscross of blood flows in the twisted pedicle of the ovary.
- Follicular ring sign (FRS)—the follicles are peripherally arranged around the edematous stroma. These follicles exhibit thick hyperechoic margins. FRS is an early, simple, easy, specific, and frequently seen feature of ovarian torsion.

REPORTING PELVIC ULTRASOUND

The reporting pelvic ultrasound is described in Box 1.

CONCLUSION

Real-time USG, more specifically, transvaginal USG, interfaces well with the pelvic examination and offers the potential for enhanced diagnostic accuracy of gynecologic conditions. The knowledge of anatomy, maximizing image details, and correlation with the patient's history and physical examination offer a comprehensive evaluation of the patient. The role of gynecologic scanning will continue to expand. The correlation of palpable pelvic findings with visual images of tissue texture should enhance the diagnostic acumen of the clinical gynecologist. Prerequisites to the use of this technique are a thorough knowledge of gynecologic, physiologic, and pathologic features; the ability to access or obtain a thorough gynecologic history and physical examination; and experience in acquisition, display, and documentation of USG images. The basis for ultrasound in gynecology is to orient oneself to the image, develop the skill to optimize the image quality by adjusting the available ultrasound settings, and improve on performing and deciphering the ultrasound data. Always use a systematic approach to scan the pelvis and simultaneously report every detail visualized on ultrasound. Attention to continuing education through reading periodicals and taking postgraduate courses is necessary for the gynecologist to stay abreast of this rapidly expanding field.

REFERENCES

1. Coyne L, Jayaprakasan K, Raine-Fenning N. 3D ultrasound in gynecology and reproductive medicine. Women's Health (Lond). 2008;4(5):501-16.
2. Kurjak A, Kupesic S, Anic T, et al. Three-dimensional ultrasound and power Doppler improve the diagnosis of ovarian lesions. Gynecol Oncol. 2000;76(1):28-32.
3. Ghi T, Casadio P, Kuleva M, et al. Accuracy of three-dimensional ultrasound in diagnosis and classification of congenital uterine anomalies. Fertil Steril. 2009;92(2):808-13.
4. Exacoustos C, Brienza L, Di Giovanni A, et al. Adenomyosis: three-dimensional sonographic findings of the junctional zone and correlation with histology. Ultrasound Obstet Gynecol. 2011;37(4):471-9.
5. Smith-Bindman R, Kerlikowske K, Feldstein VA, et al. Endovaginal ultrasound to exclude endometrial cancer and other endometrial abnormalities. JAMA. 1998;280(17):1510-7.
6. Mais V, Guerriero S, Ajossa S, et al. The efficiency of transvaginal ultrasonography in the diagnosis of endometrioma. Fertil Steril. 1993;60:776-80.
7. Alcàzar JL, Mercé L, Laparte C, et al. A new scoring system to differentiate benign from malignant adnexal masses. Am J Obstet Gynecol. 2003;188(3):685-92.
8. Lee EJ, Kwon HC, Joo HJ, et al. Diagnosis of ovarian torsion with color Doppler sonography: depiction of a twisted vascular pedicle. J Ultrasound Med. 1998;17(2):83-9.

Box 1: Reporting pelvic ultrasound.

- *Uterus*:
    - *Shape*:
        - Normal, regular, and pear shaped
        - Distorted, lobular with fibroids
        - Globular, as in adenomyosis
    - *Size*:
        - Enlarged (symmetrically or asymmetrically)
        - Hypoplastic
        - Atrophic
    - *Position*:
        - Anteversion/Retroversion
        - Anteflexed/Retroflexed
        - Midposition
- *Endometrium*—appearance, thickness, and lesions
- *Myometrium*—thickness of the walls, echotexture, lesions, and vascularity
- *Cervix*—normal, nabothian cysts, lesions (any pathology)
- *Ovaries*—ovarian volume, size, AFC, cysts, vascularity, and any other pathology
- *Adnexa*—any pathology
- *POD*—free fluid, adherence
- The mobility and adherence of various structures
- Probable ultrasound diagnosis and the main features leading to it
- Next follow-up scan if required
- Differential diagnosis if any
- Required additional tests to enable establish accurate diagnosis

Ultrasound of Ectopic Pregnancy

Punam Dixit, Aashita Shrivastava

INTRODUCTION

Ectopic pregnancy is a common condition with significant maternal mortality and morbidity. The first successful noninvasive diagnosis of tubal ectopic pregnancy was described by Kobayashi in 1969. This was a very important milestone; however, the reported sensitivity and specificity of transabdominal ultrasound is around 50%. Transvaginal ultrasound helps in early diagnosis of ectopic pregnancy. Transabdominal views are important to screen for hemoperitoneum and to visualize ectopic pregnancies beyond the range of vaginal probe, i.e., presence of fibroids or adhesions.

DIAGNOSIS

Clinical suspicion of ectopic pregnancy is based on history and symptoms. History of infertility, intrauterine contraceptive device (IUCD), previous ectopic, tubal surgery, or sterilization is important risk factors. Ectopic pregnancy is suspected when a woman presents with pain, bleeding per vaginum, and positive pregnancy test. Next step is evaluation by transvaginal ultrasound in stepwise approach. Pregnancy test is positive in majority of ectopic pregnancies, except in chronic ectopic. Serum human chorionic gonadotropin (hCG) estimation helps in confirming diagnosis of ectopic pregnancy in indeterminate cases. Serum hCG rise is less than 60% in ectopic pregnancy in 48 hours whereas in normal intrauterine pregnancy, hCG level doubles in 48 hours.[1]

First step is evaluation of endometrial cavity, and presence of gestational sac practically rules out ectopic pregnancy. Heterotopic pregnancy occurs in 1:7000 pregnancies and incidence is much higher in assisted reproductive technology (ART) pregnancies so in such pregnancies, adnexa should be carefully evaluated.

Gestational sac, which is the first sign of early pregnancy on ultrasound, is seen between 4th and 5th week and corresponds to chorionic cavity of the embryo, yolk sac appears at 5th week followed by amnion between 5th and 6th week, and the embryo by 6th week. Gestational sac has a thick rim of echogenic tissue, eccentrically located within the endometrium which differentiates it from pseudosac. Pseudosac is collection of blood or fluid in endometrial cavity.[2]

Next step is evaluation of cul-de-sac for presence of free fluid (Fig. 1). Presence of small amount of fluid is a normal finding and part of normal menstrual cycle.

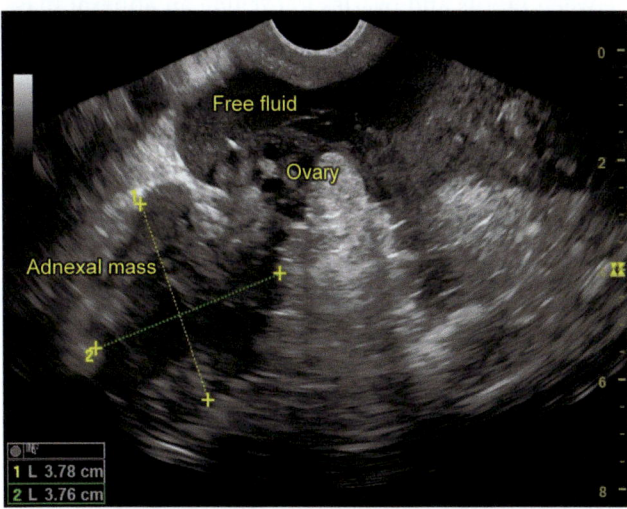

Fig. 1: *Ectopic pregnancy:* Adnexal mass near ovary and free fluid in cul-de-sac.

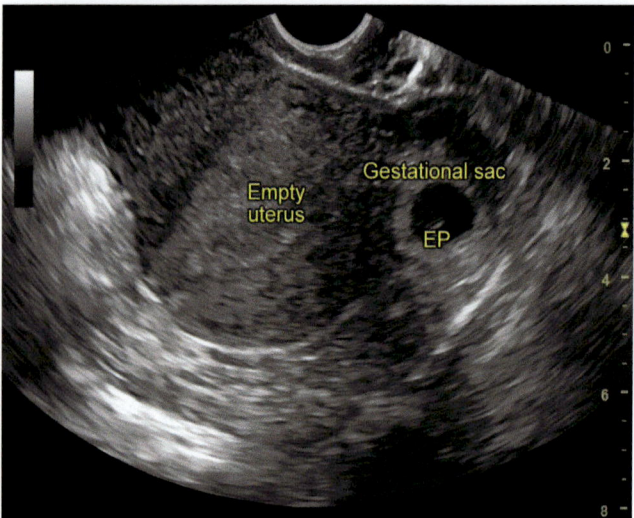

Fig. 2: Ectopic pregnancy (EP).

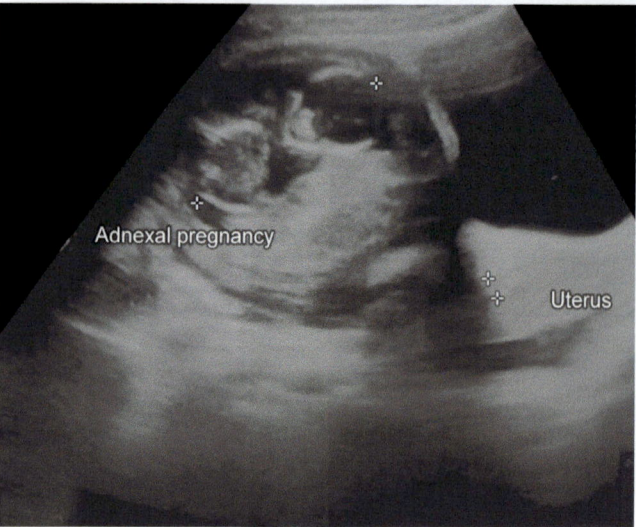

Fig. 3: Adnexal pregnancy of 12 weeks.

Hemoperitoneum appears as echogenic. Amount of fluid should be assessed by transvaginal sonography (TVS) and classified as mild, moderate, or severe which helps in planning management of ectopic pregnancy. Mild hemoperitoneum is defined as presence of echogenic fluid in pouch of Douglas, moderate hemoperitoneum is defined as presence of blood clots within pouch of Douglas and uterovesical fold, and severe hemoperitoneum is defined as presence of blood clots within pouch of Douglas and uterovesical fold/or in Morison's pouch *(Video clip)*.

ASSESSMENT OF ADNEXA

Tube is the most common location for ectopic pregnancy, so it is important to scan above and below the ovaries and between uterus and ovaries to exclude an adnexal mass. Presence of extrauterine gestational sac with or without fetal pole confirms the diagnosis (Fig. 2). Ultrasonography picture can vary and five morphological types can be found. Positive predictive value of TVS for diagnosis of ectopic pregnancy is 99.4% with sensitivity of 98.5% in expert hands.

DIFFERENT MORPHOLOGICAL TYPES OF ECTOPIC PREGNANCY

- *Type 1*: Gestational sac containing embryo and yolk sac with visible cardiac activity
- *Type 2*: Gestational sac containing embryo and yolk sac without cardiac activity
- *Type 3*: Gestational sac containing only yolk sac
- *Type 4*: Empty gestational sac with no structures
- *Type 5*: Solid inhomogeneous mass (blob or bagel sign).

Majority of ectopics are ampullary or isthmic. Rare forms are cornual, cervical, and abdominal scar ectopics.

Cornual or interstitial ectopics have higher rate of mortality and morbidity as it presents late. Diagnosis is suggested when intrauterine pregnancy is not surrounded in all planes by 5 mm of myometrium (Fig. 3).

Cervical ectopic pregnancies occur in less than 1% of all ectopic pregnancies and are diagnosed by presence of gestational sac with peritrophoblastic flow or live embryo within the cervix.

Scar ectopic, implantation occurs within the prior cesarean scar. Once a rare entity is becoming increasingly more common. Rising cesarean section rate and better modality of diagnosis may be the reason for increased incidence in last decade.[3]

CRITERIA FOR DIAGNOSIS OF SCAR ECTOPIC

- Gestational sac located anteriorly at the level of internal os within a visible myometrial defect (thin or absent myometrium at the site of previous lower segment cesarean scar).
- Evidence of functional trophoblastic/placental circulation on color Doppler examination characterized by high velocity (peak velocity > 20 cm) and low impedance (pulsatility index < 1) blood flow.
- Negative sliding sign defined as inability to displace the gestational sac on gentle pressure applied by transvaginal probe.

- Vascularity of ectopic is assessed and score is given from 1 to 4. Score of 1 is given when no blood flow is found surrounding the pregnancy, score 2 when minimal flow is detected, score 3 when moderate flow is present, and score 4 when the pregnancy appears highly vascular with marked blood flow.

Scar ectopic can be managed by ultrasound-guided evacuation, Foley's tamponade, or Shirodkar suture can be used to control postprocedure hemorrhage.[4] Laparoscopic excision and suturing of defect can be done to treat scar ectopic.

CONCLUSION

Ectopic pregnancy can have variable presentations and features on ultrasound. Proactive and systematic approach helps in early detection of unruptured ectopics. Ultrasound helps not only in diagnosis but planning the treatment. For example, cornual and cervical ectopics can be treated by direct instillation of methotrexate into the gestational sac. Estimation of serum hCG helps in diagnosis and follow-up after conservative or expectant management.

Video title: Right sided ectopic pregnancy

Description: Uterus is empty and on right side gestational sac is seen with yolk sac within it. Considerable amount of blood present in pouch of Douglas (POD) and anterior to uterus. Although patient was hemodynamically stable, presence of significant amount of blood requires urgent intervention. We did laparoscopic salpingectomy for this patient and it was incomplete tubal abortion.

REFERENCES

1. Callen PW. Ultrasonography in Obstetrics and Gynecology, 5th edition. Philadelphia: Saunders Elsevier; 2007. pp. 1020-47.
2. Abuhamad A. Ultrasound in Obstetrics and Gynecology: A Practical Approach, 1st edition. New York: GLOWM Publishers; 2014. pp. 286-306.
3. Dooley WM, Chaggar P, De Braud LV, et al. Effect of morphological type of extrauterine ectopic pregnancy on accuracy of preoperative ultrasound diagnosis. Ultrasound Obstet Gynecol. 2019;54(4):538-44.
4. Jurkovic D, Knez J, Appiah A, et al. Surgical treatment of cesarean scar ectopic pregnancy: efficacy and safety of ultrasound-guided suction curettage. Ultrasound Obstet Gynecol. 2016;47(4):511-7.

9
Ultrasound of Adnexa

Punam Dixit, Jhillmill Kumari

INTRODUCTION

The term adnexa conventionally describes accessory or adjoining anatomical parts as ovaries, fallopian tubes, and uterine ligaments such as broad and round in relation to the uterus.

Any adnexal pathology which may be benign or malignant must be evaluated properly. Proper transvaginal sonography (TVS) in gynecological outpatients can help us diagnose most of adnexal pathologies. As gynecologist, we can easily correlate with symptoms and clinical signs.

Pelvic ultrasound is the preferred imaging modalities for adnexal masses in symptomatic and asymptomatic women of reproductive and menopausal age.[1] The benefits of ultrasonography (USG) is the assessment of morphological features of an adnexal mass as solid, cystic, or complex, its location, and vascularity. USG is less expensive than computed tomography and magnetic resonance imaging.

COMMON INDICATIONS OF ULTRASOUND OF ADNEXA

Asymptomatic cases of adnexal masses are discovered during routine pelvic examination. Symptomatic adnexal masses are evaluated by age of presentation and typical ultrasound appearance.[2] Proper evaluation helps the clinician to reach the correct diagnosis and guiding management: conservative follow-up with interval scans versus surgical intervention:

- *Age*: Adnexal masses can occur at any age. In reproductive age group, benign adnexal cysts are most common whereas in postmenopausal age, there is higher risk for malignancy.
- *Symptoms*:
    - Pelvic pain
    - Pelvic mass
    - Bleeding at the site of the cyst or mass
    - Backache
    - Irregular periods
    - Difficulty with urination
    - Frequent urination
    - Abdominal distension with gastrointestinal complaints and weight loss
- *Others*: Personal or family history of breast and ovarian cancer.

COMMON CAUSES OF BENIGN ADNEXAL MASSES

In reproductive age group:
- Simple cyst
- Polycystic ovarian disease
- Hemorrhagic cyst
- Endometrioma
- Dermoid cyst
- Hydrosalpinx
- Paratubal cyst
- Tubo-ovarian abscess (TOA)
- Peritoneal inclusion cysts
- Adnexal torsion

Simple cyst: A simple cyst is unilocular, smooth walls, with anechoic content, no internal echoes, good distal enhancement, and is almost always benign (Fig. 1). On gray-scale ultrasound, a normal ovarian follicle is a physiological cyst which normally disappears in secretory phase of normal menstrual cycle. If the follicle fails to rupture in midcycle, it becomes a follicular cyst of size >3 cm in diameter, self-limited which resolves spontaneously in several months.

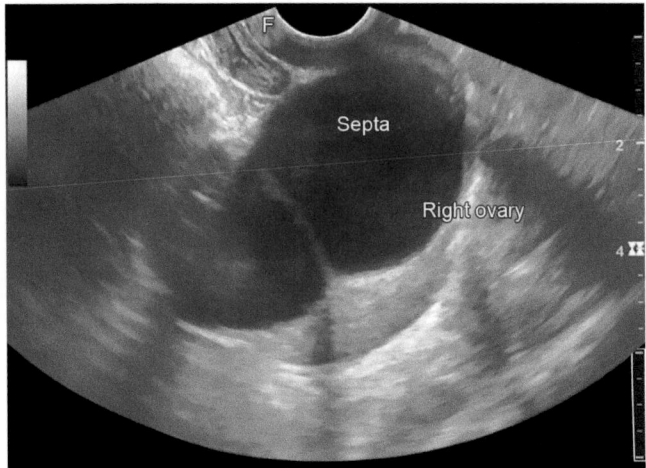

Fig. 1: Simple cyst.

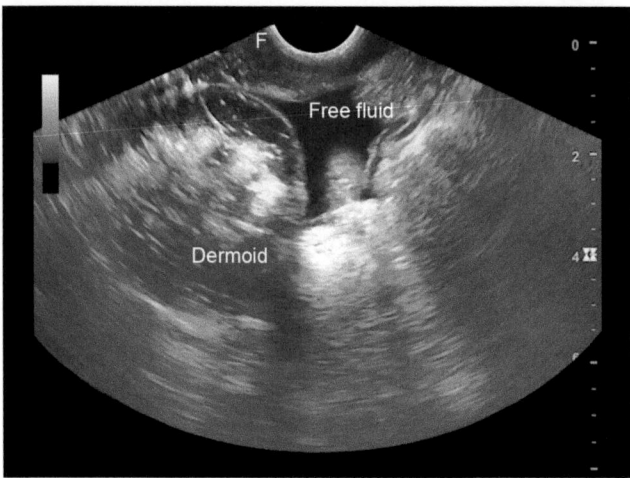

Fig. 2 Dermoid cyst.

Benign persistent cysts of epithelial origin (serous cystadenoma) may be unilocular or multilocular with thick septas and large anechoic areas greater than 5 cm. Malignant ovarian cysts are >7.5 cm in diameter, with nodules in cyst wall, and contains mixed cystic and solid tissues.[3]

Polycystic ovary: Polycystic ovary is the most common cause of infertility due to failure of ovulation and irregular menstrual cycle. In unilateral or bilateral presence of polycystic ovary, there are multiple small follicles (25 or more per ovary) arranged peripherally with stromal hyperplasia resulting in increased size of the ovary. The morphological criteria for diagnosis of polycystic ovaries have changed over the years. The current consensus is follicular number of 25 or more by TVS and when transabdominal sonography (TAS) is used, ovarian volume of greater than 10 mL has been suggested for diagnosis of polycystic ovaries.

Hemorrhagic cyst: Hemorrhagic cyst occurs from bleeding within a corpus luteum cyst. In reproductive age, women present with acute pain in the right or left lower quadrant of the abdomen. The hemorrhagic cyst resolves in 6–8 weeks of duration. It passes from bleeding to clot formation, clot lysis, clot retraction, and clot resolution phases. On ultrasound, appearance of the hemorrhagic cyst depends on the stage of resolution of the cyst's content. In early stage, cyst appears as solid masses with smooth thin walls and variable echogenic content with characteristic thin linear reticular strands. Later on when the clot retracts, a fluid layer develops within the cyst with an echogenic structure inside it, which moves with transducer ballottement. Finally, during clot lysis with fibrin thread, formation appears as an avascular cyst containing irregular fine lines resembling a "cobweb pattern", "reticular pattern", or "lace-like pattern".

Resolving stage of hemorrhagic cyst can be differentiated from malignant pathology by Doppler sonography. There is absence of capillary flow within the cyst and contains thin lines which do not extend across the entire cyst diameter.

Endometrioma: An endometrioma is a thin-walled chocolate fluid-filled cyst resulting from ectopic location of endometrial tissue within the peritoneal cavity and on the surface of abdominal and pelvic organs and pelvic ligaments. The ectopic endometrial tissue undergoes cyclical changes and bleeds during the menstrual cycle. On USG, in most of the cases, endometriotic collections present as unilocular with multiple internal echoes giving it ground-glass appearance.

Dermoid cyst (mature cystic teratoma): Dermoid cysts are the most common benign type of germ cell tumors in young adolescents and reproductive age group. These are slow growing tumors and bilateral in 10% cases. Dermoid cyst is a complex cyst with solid and cystic components. These cysts contain sebaceous material (hypoechogenic) and solid components may comprise of hair, fat, bones, and calcification (hyperechogenic). On ultrasound, this mixed component gives a "tip of the iceberg" effect, i.e., a white echogenic "ball" (Rokitansky nodule) which typically corresponds to the sebum and hair content, long and short echogenic linear strands which correspond to the hair in the fluid content of the cystic components and significant acoustic shadow (Fig. 2). When the hair component of the cyst disperses in the fluid, it gives a mesh-like appearance. When dermoid contains bone or teeth, it appears as a solid hyperechoic area. Bright components due to fat are less echogenic than calcification. When there is fat, it gives a fat-fluid level, i.e., upper bright (fat) and lower dark (fluid) components.

Sometimes, it may give a pseudokidney appearance with central bright area (such as renal sinus) due to fat.

When benign cystic teratoma is seen in peri- or postmenopausal women with cyst size large >10 cm, malignancy of dermoid cysts may be suspected.

Hydrosalpinx: On TVS, normal fallopian tube is rarely seen. Hydrosalpinx is a condition when fluid is trapped in fallopian tubes with distal obliteration. Mostly seen in cases of postmenopausal women with past history of pelvic inflammatory disease (PID). On USG, it gives a fluid-filled sausage shaped or tubular structure with incomplete septations and a "cogwheel appearance" on cross-section. Hydrosalpinx is seen adjacent to ovary tapering near the uterine origin (*waist sign*) and there is absence of peristalsis, which differentiate it from bowel loops. To differentiate it from a simple cyst, the ultrasound probe must be rotate at 90° angle. In chronic cases, small mural nodules seen resembling "beads of string" appearance. On follow-up scan, there is no change in appearance.

Paratubal cyst: Also known as paraovarian cysts. On grayscale USG, it appears as small unilocular, thin-walled anechoic cysts with smooth margins, separate from the ovary. In adolescent, it is one of the most common pathology for acute pelvic pain due to torsion.

Tubo-ovarian abscess: PID spreads to ovary and fallopian tubes by ascending route from lower genital tracts or hematogenous spread. In acute condition, patient presents with fever, pelvic pain, and tenderness in adnexal area. On USG, TOA presents as multilocular mass with thick walls, thick incomplete septae, echogenic fluid content giving ground-glass appearance, and involvement of the ovary. Chronic cases are asymptomatic or mild pain presents.

Peritoneal inclusion cysts (pseudocysts): This is localized fluid collection in peritoneal cavity due to entrapment of fluid secreted from ovary. Mostly seen following pelvic surgeries, trauma, PID, and endometriosis cases. On USG, it gives picture of entrapped ovary by loculated cystic masses giving a *spider web appearance*. There is multiple thin septations which are attached to the pelvic organs.

Adnexal torsion: Adnexal torsion presents with acute pelvic pain, tenderness on abdominal, and bimanual palpation along with nausea and vomiting. Mostly it occurs when ovary is enlarged, rarely torsion may be seen in normal ovaries. Ultrasound findings of torsion are enlarged edematous ovary with peripherally arranged follicles. There is probe tenderness. Right side is affected more than the left side.

SOLID MASSES OF ADNEXA

Complete solid adnexal mass is less common than cystic masses. In younger patients, the presence of such a lesion often indicates dysgerminoma, which is malignant:

- *Ovarian fibroma*: Most common benign solid neoplasm. It presents as solid adnexal mass with a vascular pedicle. Sonographic features of fibromas are solid tumor with regular striped echogenicity, venetian blind shadowing, and not freely move in adnexa.
- *Thecoma*: Benign theca cell tumor like ovarian fibroma on USG, it gives appearance of an echogenic mass with distal acoustic attenuation.

MALIGNANT ADNEXAL MASSES

Clinical features suggestive of malignancy include large painless or painful solid irregular mass, presenting before menarche or after menopause. On USG, features suggestive of malignancy include thick septa (>2–3 mm in width), solid components, and cyst wall thickening with papillary projections. Doppler shows neovascularization.

The International Ovarian Tumor Analysis (IOTA) simple rule model (Table 1) includes five ultrasound features suggestive of benignity (B features) or malignancy (M features).[4] If one or more B features are present in the absence of M features, the mass is classified as benign and vice versa. If both B and M features exist and if none of the 10 features are present, simple rules yield inconclusive result. Next recommended step is subjective assessment by expert.

The IOTA simple rule model has been validated in many centers and helps in differentiating benign masses from malignant.[5]

The ADNEX model is next step and was developed by the IOTA group based on clinical and ultrasound data from almost 6,000 women in 24 centers in 10 countries.[6] The ADNEX model uses nine predictors. There are three clinical variables such as age, serum CA 125 level, and type of center (oncology referral vs. others) and six ultrasound variables.

Table 1: International Ovarian Tumor Analysis (IOTA) guidelines.

Benign	Malignant
B1—Unilocular cyst	M1—Irregular solid
B2—Presence of solid components (<7 mm)	M2—Ascites
B3—Shadowing	M3—Papillary projections
B4—Smooth multilocular with diameter < 10 cm	M4—Irregular multilocular with diameter ≥ 10 cm
B5—No flow	M5—High color content

Maximal diameter of lesion, proportion of solid tissue more than 10 cyst lobules, and number of papillary projections.

Metastatic disease of ovary occurs from stomach and colon cancers. Such lesions are referred to as Krukenberg tumors associated with ascites. On Doppler, there is marked vascularity.

CONCLUSION

Wide spectrum of pathologies is found in adnexal region. Ultrasound is invaluable in diagnosis of lesions and differentiation of benign from malignant. In younger woman, conservative management can be done and when surgery is needed, laparoscopic surgery and fertility-sparing surgery can be done. Malignant ovarian masses require extensive surgery in specialized centers. So careful evaluation by clinician guides in proper management and counseling of patient. Essential basic knowledge helps in interpretation of ultrasound and better management of gynecological problems.

One stop solution is current trend in woman healthcare and having an ultrasound machine in outpatients helps us achieve it.

REFERENCES

1. Smorgick N, Maymon R. Assessment of adnexal masses using ultrasound: a practical review. Int J Womens Health. 2014;6:857-63.
2. Palmer PES, Breyer B, Bruguera CA, et al. Manual of Diagnostic Ultrasound, 7th edition. Geneva: World Health Organization; 1995. pp. 196-222.
3. Abuhamad A. Ultrasound in Obstetrics and Gynecology: A Practical Approach, 1st edition. New York: GLOWM Publishers; 2014. pp. 253-85.
4. Alcazar JL, Pascual MA, Graupera B, et al. External validation of IOTA simple descriptors and simple rules for classifying adnexal masses. Ultrasound Obstet Gynecol. 2016;48: 397-402.
5. Hartge DR, Bembenek N, Gembicki MA, et al. Applying IOTA simple rules and ADNEX model in daily routine. Ultrasound Obstet Gynecol. 2017;509:154-256.
6. Van Calster B, Van Hoorde K, Valentin L, et al. Evaluating the risk of ovarian cancer before surgery using the ADNEX model to differentiate between benign, borderline, early and advanced stage invasive, and secondary metastatic tumours: prospective multicentre diagnostic study. BMJ. 2014;349:g5920.

10
Ultrasonography for Bleeding in Obstetrics

PK Shah, Keshav Pai

INTRODUCTION

Vaginal bleeding during pregnancy is a scary prospect for any pregnant woman irrespective of the trimester. It could be a harbinger of untoward obstetric outcome. It is noteworthy that at early stages of pregnancy, physical evaluations have major pitfalls and beta-human chorionic gonadotropin (βhCG) assay is not comprehensive in the elucidation of the etiology of vaginal bleeding.[1] Also, a seemingly innocuous pervaginum examination in conditions like placenta previa and vasa previa for bleeding during late trimesters of pregnancy could have catastrophic outcome both for the mother and the baby. The ultrasound technology is not only the best noninvasive method for detecting the cause of bleeding, thereby helping the treating physician, but also allays the fear and anxiety of the couple. A simple ultrasound examination of pregnant woman who is bleeding can go a long way in preventing maternal morbidity and mortality.

CAUSES OF BLEEDING IN OBSTETRICS

First Trimester

Vaginal bleeding during first trimester is estimated to occur in 16–20% of all pregnant women. Bleeding during first trimester increases the chances of miscarriage. Rarely, it can be extrauterine pregnancy, which can have life-threatening consequences if undiagnosed.

Implantation Bleeding

It is the small amount of spotting associated with implantation of embryo into the uterine wall. It is frequently confused with routine periods. It is usually not associated with any adverse outcome.

Threatened Abortion

Threatened miscarriage (or threatened abortion) is mainly a clinical term, used when a pregnant woman in first 20 weeks of gestation presents with spotting, mild abdominal pain, and contractions, with a closed cervical os.

It occurs in 20–25% of pregnancies and is associated with an increased rate of fetal loss (15–50%, compared to 2–7%).

Ultrasound features: Cervix is closed, and there is a live intrauterine gestation.

In many cases, the ultrasound will be either completely normal, or with a subchorionic hemorrhage (SCH).

Some features suggestive of a poor outcome are:
- *Fetal bradycardia*: <80–90 bpm
- Small mean gestational sac diameter
- Large and calcified yolk sac of >7 mm
- *Small or irregular gestational sac*: Mean sac diameter (MSD)/crown-rump length (CRL) <5 mm
- Large SCH more than two-thirds of gestational sac
- Expanded amnion sign (an abnormally large amniotic cavity)
- Absent or poor decidual reaction

Subchorionic Hemorrhage

Choriodecidual hemorrhage leading to hematoma is seen as an echo-free area indistinguishable from a second sac of twin pregnancy (Figs. 1A and B). Subjective hematoma size based on the fraction of gestational sac size correlates

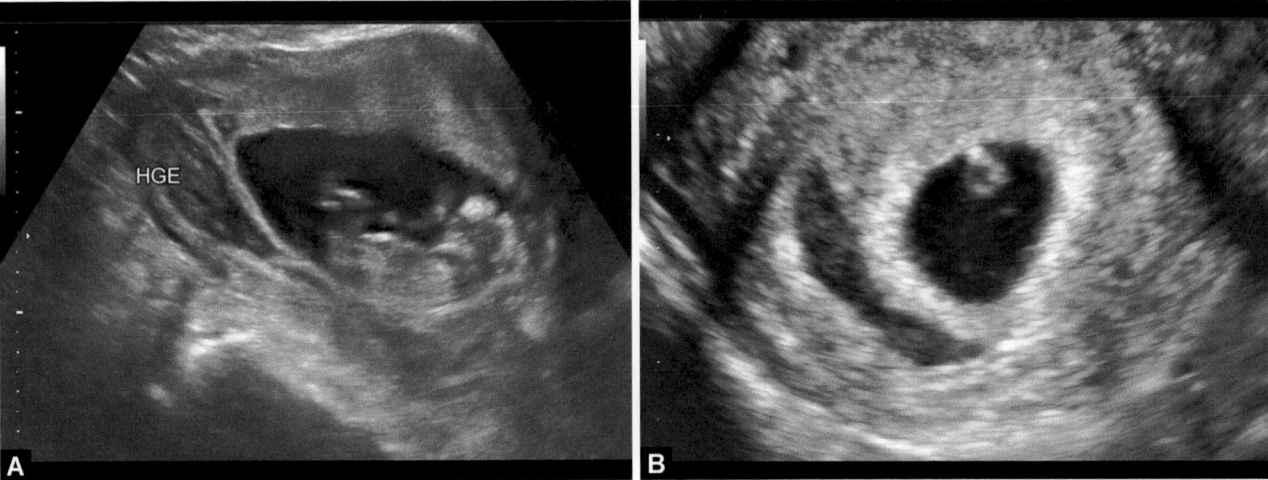

Figs. 1A and B: Subchorionic hematoma seperating gestation sac from uterine wall.

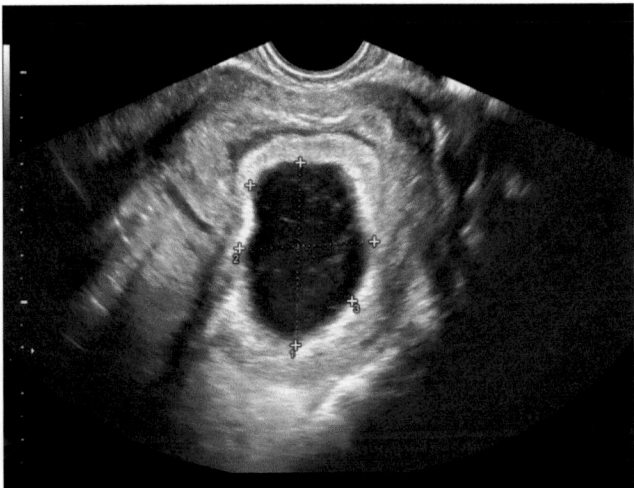

Fig. 2: Blighted ovum showing mean sac diameter (MSD 27 mm) with no embryo or yolk sac and has irregular walls.

best with first-trimester pregnancy outcome. The earlier in pregnancy an SCH is detected, the higher the rate of subsequent pregnancy failure.[2] The pregnancy outcome is generally poor when the hematoma volume exceeds more than 60 mL.

Anembryonic Pregnancy

Anembryonic pregnancy is a form of a failed early pregnancy, where a gestational sac develops, but the embryo does not form. The term blighted ovum is synonymous with this, but is falling out of favor and is best avoided (Fig. 2).

Ultrasound features: An anembryonic pregnancy may be diagnosed:
- When there is no embryo seen on endovaginal scanning in a gestational sac with MSD ≥ 25 mm.
  Or
- There is no embryo on follow-up endovaginal scan:
  - ≥11 days after scan showing gestational sac with yolk sac, but no embryo, or
  - ≥2 weeks after scan showing gestational sac without yolk sac or embryo.

Assessment of interval MSD growth has been shown to be insufficiently accurate in the diagnosis of anembryonic pregnancy, due to an overlap of gestational sac growth rates of viable and nonviable pregnancies.

Other ancillary features have been described, and may be considered poor prognostic factors, but do not contribute to the formal diagnosis of a failed pregnancy. These include:
- Absent yolk sac when MSD > 8 mm on transvaginal ultrasound (TVUS)
- *Poor decidual reaction*: Often <2 mm
- Irregular gestational sac shape
- Abnormally low sac position.

Incomplete and Complete Abortion

Diagnosis mainly rests on history and clinical findings. Nevertheless, transvaginal sonography (TVS) is useful for diagnosing when clinical findings are inconclusive. The placental remnants left in the uterine cavity and cervical canal usually produce dense irregular echoes. An empty uterine with cavity seen as an echogenic line less than 4 mm thickness obviates the need of curettage. Thus, an ultrasound can help avoid unnecessary hospitalization and surgery.

Missed Abortion (Fig. 3)

A *missed abortion* is a situation when there is a nonviable fetus within the uterus, without symptoms of a miscarriage.

Ultrasound features: Ultrasound diagnosis of miscarriage should only be considered when either a mean gestational

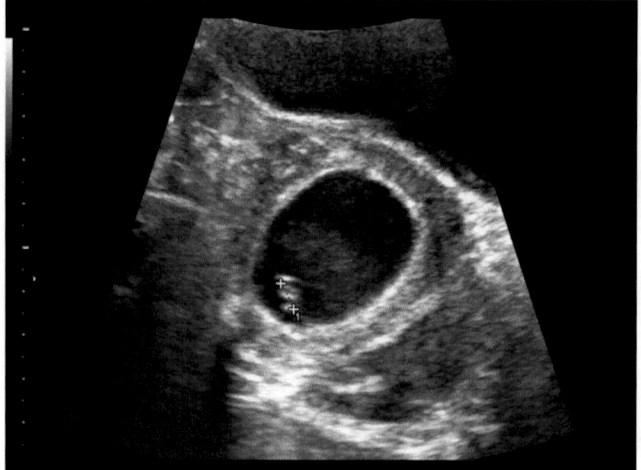

Fig. 3: Missed abortion showing small fetal pole (>7 mm) with no cardiac activity and shows disparity between the size of fetal pole and gestation sac.

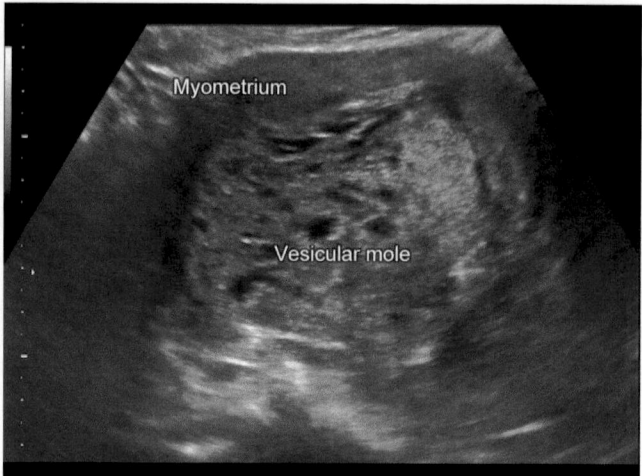

Fig. 4: Complete vesicular mole.

sac diameter is ≥25 mm with no obvious yolk sac or a fetal pole with a CRL of ≥7 mm without evidence of fetal cardiac activity. TVUS is the mainstay in the diagnosis of miscarriage. Once the diagnosis of miscarriage is made based on the above ultrasound criteria, the patient can then be offered different types of management depending on their clinical status and patient's choice.

Trophoblastic Diseases

Trophoblastic diseases can be classified as hydatidiform mole—complete, partial, or invasive mole, choriocarcinoma, placental site trophoblastic tumor (PSTT), and epithelioid trophoblastic tumor:

- Complete hydatidiform mole comprises 80% of gestational trophoblastic diseases (GTDs) (Fig. 4). Patients present with vaginal bleeding, pelvic discomfort, and hyperemesis gravidarum:
  - *Ultrasound features*: They appear as hyperechoic lesion filling up the entire uterus, when the cysts are very small and then when the cysts enlarge, it shows multiple small anechoic areas giving a snowstorm appearance or a honeycomb appearance on B-mode ultrasound. At this stage, the gestational sac is not seen if it is a complete vesicular mole. This may also be known as molar pregnancy. Typically, active corpus luteum or theca lutein cysts are seen.
- *Partial hydatidiform mole (Fig. 5)*: It is the partial conversion of chorionic villi into molar vesicles:
  - *Ultrasound features*: The gestational sac is seen, embryo/fetus is also seen, but the trophoblastic layer appears very thick and edematous in some parts of the trophoblast. The molar part of the placenta shows the same B-mode and Doppler features like a complete mole. This can be better appreciated by three-dimensional (3D) ultrasound than by B-mode. Detailed scans are required to exclude fetal anomalies as these are fairly common in pregnancies with partial mole.

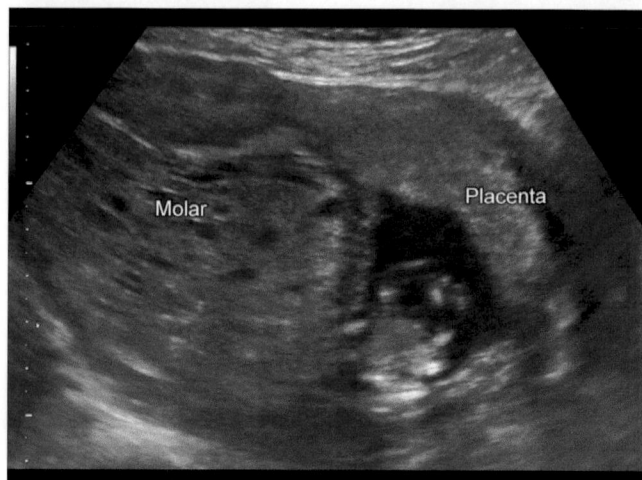

Fig. 5: Partial vesicular mole showing molar changes of placenta along with fetal pole.

- *Invasive hydatidiform mole (Fig. 6)*: It refers to invasion of molar vesicles into the myometrium after the evacuation of complete or partial mole or during pregnancy.
  - *Ultrasound features*: Enlarged mass is filled with solid looking hyperechoic mass with anechoic areas. The endomyometrial junction is not identifiable. It is a highly vascular tumor with low-resistance flow in vessels.

Extrauterine Pregnancies

The overall incidence has increased over the last few decades and is currently thought to affect 1–2% of pregnancies.

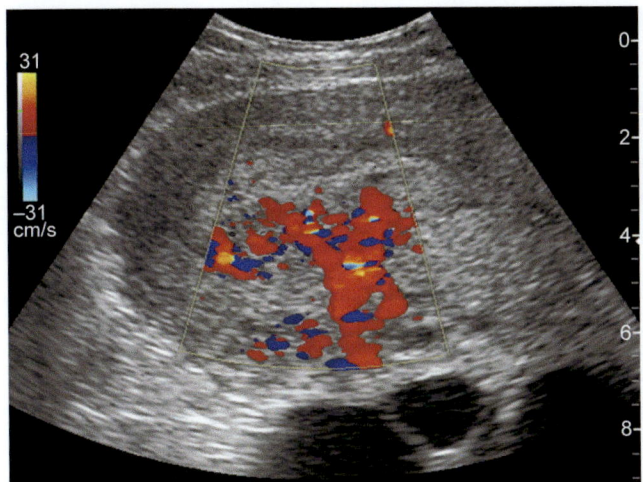

Fig. 6: Doppler findings in invasive mole showing penetration of molar tissue into myometrium with low resistance in vessels.

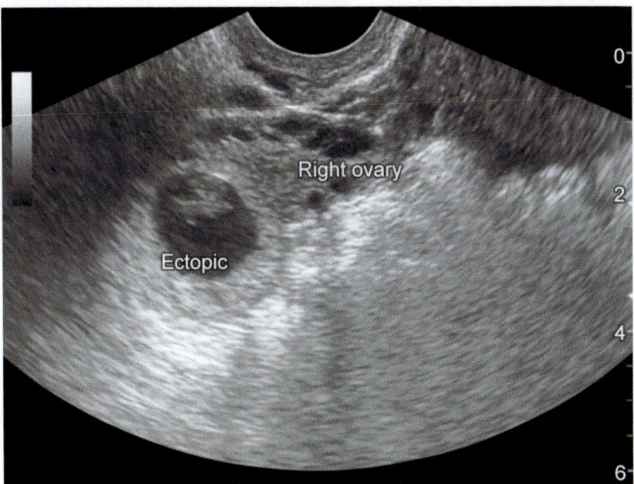

Fig. 7: Tubal ectopic showing unruptured live tubal ectopic close to right ovary.

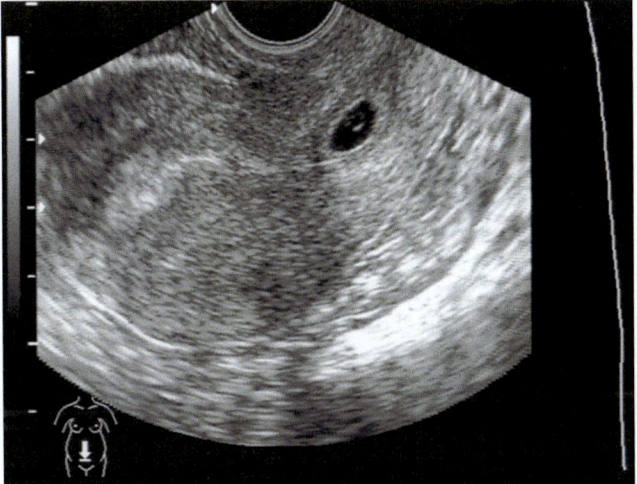

Fig. 8: Cervical pregnancy showing gestation sac with yolk sac in cervical canal.

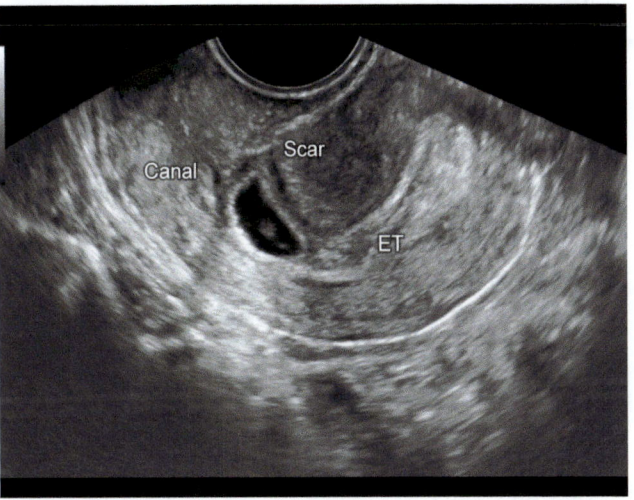

Fig. 9: Scar ectopic showing ectopic tissue penetrating isthmic portion of uterus anteriorly.

The risk is as high as 18% for first trimester pregnancies with bleeding.[3] There is an increased incidence associated with in vitro fertilization (IVF) pregnancies.

In the vast majority of cases, the ectopic implantation site is within a fallopian tube.

- *Tubal ectopic (Fig. 7)*: 93–97%
  - *Ampullary ectopic*: Most common ~70% of tubal ectopics and ~65% of all ectopics
  - *Isthmal ectopic*: ~12% of tubal ectopics and ~11% of all ectopics
  - *Fimbrial ectopic*: ~11% of tubal ectopics and ~10% of all ectopics.
- *Interstitial ectopic/cornual ectopic*: 3–4%; also essentially a type of tubal ectopic
- *Ovarian ectopic*: Ovarian pregnancy; 0.5–1%
- *Cervical ectopic*: Cervical pregnancy; rare <1% (Fig. 8)
- *Scar ectopic (Fig. 9)*: Site of previous cesarean section scar; rare
- *Abdominal ectopic*: Rare ~1.4%

It is useful to know a quantitative βhCG prior to scanning as this will guide what you expect to see. At levels <2,000 IU, a normal early pregnancy may not be visible.

The most reliable sign of ectopic pregnancy is the visualization of an extrauterine gestation, but this is not seen in 15–35% of ectopic pregnancies.

Ultrasound features: The ultrasound examination should be performed both transabdominally and transvaginally. The transabdominal component provides a wider overview of the abdomen, whereas a transvaginal scan is important for diagnostic sensitivity.

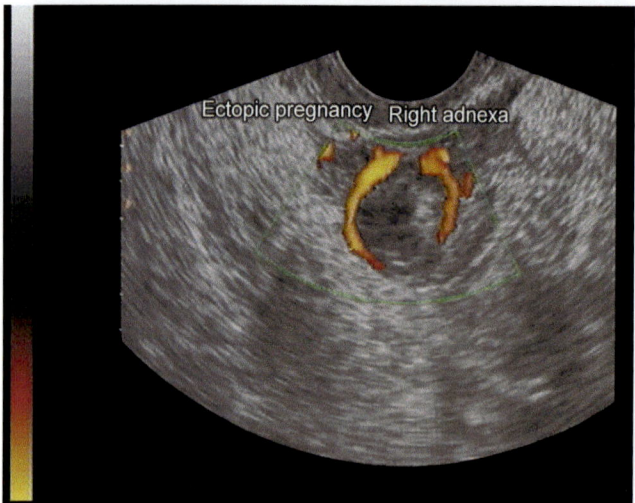

Fig. 10: Doppler findings in tubal ectopic gestation showing ring of fire.

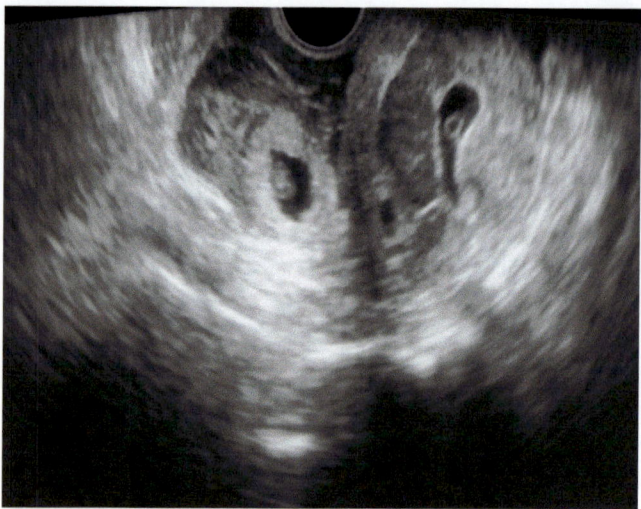

Fig. 11: Heterotopic pregnancy showing intrauterine pregnancy as well as extrauterine pregnancy.

Positive sonographic findings include:
- *Uterus*:
  - An empty uterine cavity or no evidence of an intra-uterine pregnancy (IUP):
    - An exception to this is a rare heterotopic pregnancy
  - *Pseudogestational sac or decidual cyst*: It may be seen in 10–20% of ectopic pregnancies:
    - Current evidence suggests that one should not initiate treatment for an ectopic pregnancy in an hemodynamically stable woman on the basis of a single hCG value
  - Decidual cast
  - Thick echogenic endometrium.
- *Tube and ovary*:
  - *Simple adnexal cyst*: 10% chance of an ectopic
  - *Complex extra-adnexal cyst/mass*: 95% chance of a tubal ectopic (if no IUP):
    - An intra-adnexal cyst/mass is more likely to be a corpus luteum
  - Solid hyperechoic mass is possible but non-specific
  - *Tubal ring sign*:
    - 95% chance of a tubal ectopic if seen
    - Described in 49% of ectopics and in 68% of unruptured ectopics
  - *Ring of fire sign*: It can be seen on color Doppler in a tubal ectopic, but can also be seen in a corpus luteum (Fig. 10)
  - An absence of color Doppler flow does not exclude an ectopic
  - *Live extrauterine pregnancy (i.e., extrauterine fetal cardiac activity)*: 100% specific, but only seen in a minority of cases.
- *Peritoneal cavity*:
  - Free pelvic fluid or hemoperitoneum in the pouch of Douglas:
    - The presence of free intraperitoneal fluid in the context of a positive βhCG and the empty uterus is:
      - ~70% specific for an ectopic pregnancy
      - ~63% sensitive for an ectopic pregnancy
      - Not specific for ruptured ectopic (seen in 37% of intact tubal ectopics)
  - *Free fluid in the hepatorenal recess*:
    - Interrogation of the right upper quadrant for free fluid reduces time to diagnosis
    - Free fluid in Morison's pouch in the context of an ectopic pregnancy is highly suggestive that operative management will be necessary
  - *Live pregnancy*: 100% specific, but only seen in a minority of cases
- In patients receiving IVF, it is important not to be completely reassured by the presence of a live IUP,[4] as there is a possibility of a coexisting ectopic pregnancy in ~1–3:100 (i.e., heterotopic pregnancy). In patients not receiving IVF, the risk of heterotopic pregnancy is minuscule (1:30,000) (Fig. 11).

BLEEDING IN LATE PREGNANCY

Placenta Previa (Fig. 12)

Routine ultrasound scanning at 20 weeks of gestation should include placental localization. Transvaginal scans improve the accuracy of placental localization that is safe, so the suspected diagnosis of placenta previa at 20 weeks of gestation by abdominal scan must be confirmed by

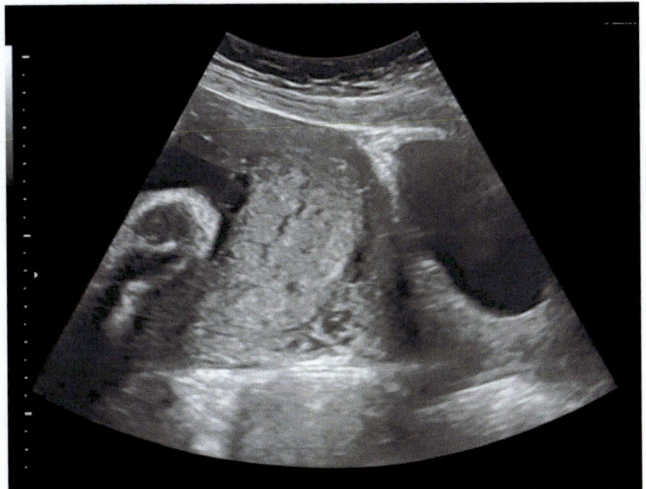

Fig. 12: Complete placenta previa showing placental tissue covering internal os and lower segments of uterus anteriorly and posteriorly.

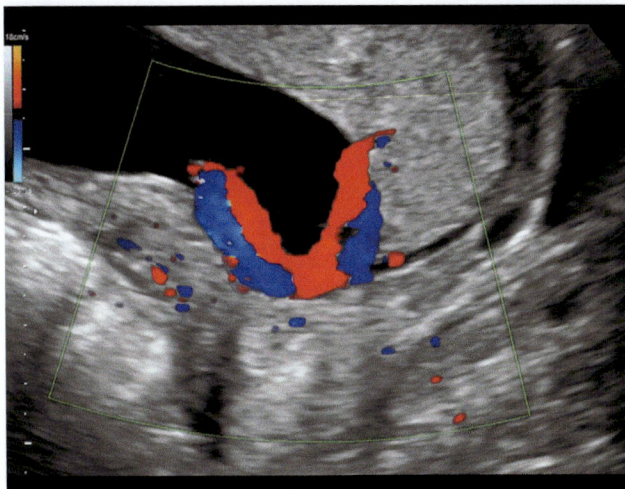

Fig. 13: *Vasa previa*: Color Doppler showing placental vessels crossing internal os in a case of succenturiate lobe of placenta.

TVS. In the second trimester, TVS will reclassify 25–60% of cases where the abdominal scan diagnosed a low-lying placenta, meaning fewer women will need follow-up. In the third trimester, TVS changed the transabdominal scan diagnosis of placenta previa in 12.5% of 32 women. Leerentveld demonstrated high levels of accuracy of TVS in predicting placenta previa in 100 women suspected of having a low-lying placenta in the second and third trimesters.

Vasa Previa (Fig. 13)

Vasa previa refers to a situation where there are aberrant fetal vessels crossing over or in close proximity to the internal cervical os, ahead of the fetal presenting part. These vessels are within the amniotic membranes, without the support of the placenta. Vasa previa is a rare, but potentially catastrophic cause of antepartum hemorrhage.

Ultrasound Features

Sonographic features are considered generally specific (~90%).

The diagnosis is often made with transabdominal color Doppler sonography demonstrating flow within vessels, which are seen overlying the internal cervical os. Non Doppler (grayscale) images may suggest the diagnosis, if there are echogenic parallel or circular lines within the placenta near the cervix.

Occasionally, a transvaginal scan is required to better visualize aberrant vessels. TVUS has a reported sensitivity of 100% and specificity of 99–99.8% when performed with color Doppler.[5]

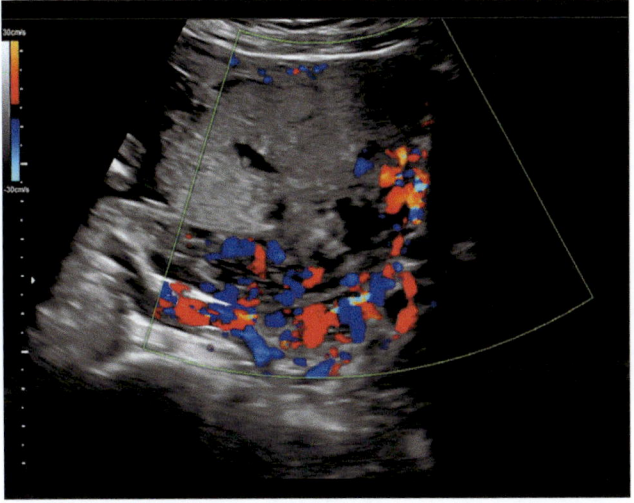

Fig. 14: Doppler findings in placenta percreta showing penetration of vascular tissue through myometrium and going beyond serosal surface.

Morbidly Adherent Placenta

Placenta accreta is both the general term applied to abnormal placental adherence and also the condition seen at the milder end of the spectrum of abnormal placental adherence. Placenta increta and placenta percreta complete the spectrum.

Ultrasound Features

According to one study,[6] ultrasound has a sensitivity of 89.5%, the positive predictive value of 68%, and a negative predictive value of 98% for the diagnosis of placenta accreta.

Several sonographic criteria for the diagnosis of placenta accreta have been reported (Fig. 14):
- Marked thinning or loss of the retroplacental hypoechoic zone

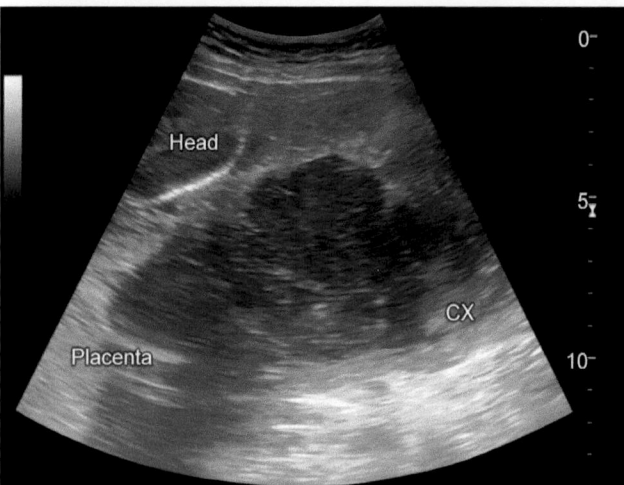

Fig. 15: Abrupture placenta showing separation of placenta from uterine wall with collection of hematoma.

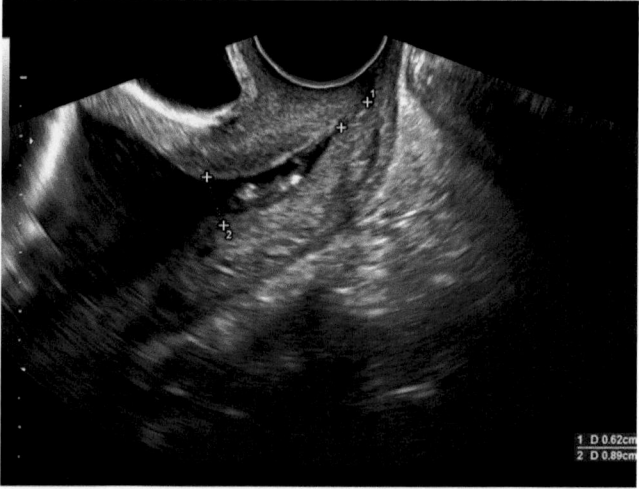

Fig. 16: Cervical insufficiency showing dilated internal os and upper cervical canal with very short cervix.

- Interruption of the hyperechoic border between the uterine serosa and bladder
- Presence of mass-like tissue with echogenicity similar to that of the placenta
- Visualization of prominent vessels or lakes within the placenta or myometrium:
  - Visualization of lacunae has the highest sensitivity in the diagnosis of placenta accreta, allowing the identification in 78–93% of cases after 15 weeks of gestation, with a specificity of 78.6%.

When a placenta accreta occurs on the posterior or lateral walls of the uterus, it may be difficult to detect by ultrasound.

Abruptio Placentae (Fig. 15)

Placental abruption (or abruptio placentae) refers to a premature separation of the normally implanted placenta after the 20th week of gestation and before the third stage of labor. It is a potentially fatal complication of pregnancy and is a significant cause of third trimester bleeding.

Ultrasound is almost always the first (and usually the only) imaging modality used to evaluate placental abruption, but an index of suspicion should be maintained for the diagnosis, since ultrasound is relatively insensitive for the diagnosis. This is partly because a retroplacental hematoma may be identified only in 2–25% of all abruptions.

The sonographic signs of placental abruption include:
- Retroplacental hematoma (often poorly echogenic)
- Intraplacental anechoic areas
- Separation and rounding of the placental edge
- *Thickening of the placenta*: Often to over 5.5 cm
- *Thickening of the retroplacental myometrium*: Usually, it should be 1–2 cm unless there is a focal myometrial contraction
- Disruption in retroplacental circulation
- Intra-amniotic echoes due to intra-amniotic hemorrhage
- Blood in the fetal stomach
- Intermembranous clot in twins.

The echogenicity of hematomas depends upon their age. Acute hematomas imaged at the time of symptoms tend to be hyperechoic or isoechoic compared to the adjacent placenta. As the hematoma is commonly isoechoic to the placenta, it may be mistaken for focal thickening of the placenta. A "normal" ultrasound does not exclude a placental abruption—particularly as the blood may have escaped through the vagina in the case of external hemorrhage.

In other cases, the retroplacental hematoma may be hypoechoic or of heterogeneous echogenicity.

Cervical Insufficiency (Fig. 16)

The cervical length (CL) is obtained by measuring the endocervical canal from the internal cervical os to the external cervical os.

The normal cervix should be at least 30 mm in length. Cervical incompetence is variably defined, however, a CL of <25 mm at or before 24 weeks is often used.

In borderline cases, transfundal pressure may be used to confirm the diagnosis.

The presence of cervical funneling is also an important finding. Greater than 50% funneling before 25 weeks is associated with 80% risk of preterm delivery.

Sonographic determination of the residual closed length of the cervix may be measured if there is:
- Known complicating preterm premature rupture of membranes

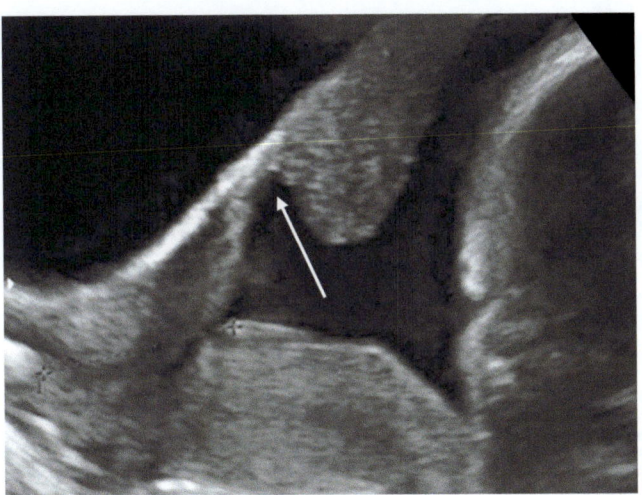

Fig. 17: Scar dehiscence showing thinned out lower segment at the level of scar (arrow).

- Known hourglass type membranes
- Active vaginal bleeding.

Scar Dehiscence and Uterine Rupture (Fig. 17)

Uterine rupture is a rare, but nevertheless potentially catastrophic complication that can occur in pregnancy.

Ultrasound Features

Reported sonographic signs of uterine rupture include:
- Identification of the protruding portion of the amniotic sac
- Endometrial or myometrial defect
- Extrauterine hematoma
- Hemoperitoneum or free fluid.

CONCLUSION

Improved ultrasound technology and high-frequency endovaginal transducers have enabled the early diagnosis of abnormal and ectopic pregnancies as well as antepartum hemorrhage, reducing maternal morbidity and mortality. Ultrasound is a valuable tool in the diagnosis of causes of bleeding in pregnancy. Ultrasound is a vital factor in the decision-making algorithm with regards to the safe continuation of the pregnancy, timely intervention for abnormal pregnancy. Judicious utilization of ultrasonography is extremely necessary. However, it should be remembered that ultrasound is merely supplementary to the pelvic examination and cannot replace obstetric history and clinical examination.

It is noteworthy that at this early stage of pregnancy, physical evaluations have major pitfalls and serum βhCG assay is not comprehensive in the elucidation of the etiology of vaginal bleeding.

REFERENCES

1. Dighe M, Cuevas C, Moshiri M, et al. Sonography in first trimester bleeding. J Clin Ultrasound. 2008;36(6):352-66.
2. Heller HT, Asch EA, Durfee SM, et al. Subchorionic hematoma: correlation of grading techniques with first-trimester pregnancy outcome. J Ultrasound Med. 2018;37(7):1725-32.
3. Histed SN, Deshmukh M, Masamed R, et al. Ectopic pregnancy: a trainee's guide to making the right call: women's imaging. Radiographics. 2016;36(7):2236-7.
4. Doubilet PM, Benson CB. Further evidence against the reliability of the human chorionic gonadotropin discriminatory level. J Ultrasound Med. 2012;30(12):1637-42.
5. Ruiter L, Kok N, Limpens J, et al. Systematic review of accuracy of ultrasound in the diagnosis of vasa previa. Ultrasound Obstet Gynecol. 2015;45(5):516-22.
6. Esakoff TF, Sparks TN, Kaimal AJ, et al. Diagnosis and morbidity of placenta accreta. Ultrasound Obstet Gynecol. 2011;37(3):324-7.

Ultrasound in First Trimester

Archana Baser, Anshu Baser, Varsha Mahajan, Mumtaz P

INTRODUCTION

The first trimester is characterized by many important landmarks with regard to the ultimate outcome of pregnancy and is mostly defined by the first 100 days of pregnancy.

First-trimester ultrasound was introduced in order to more accurately estimate gestational age,[1,2] identify multiple pregnancies and diagnose nonviable pregnancies,[3] and, more recently, to measure nuchal translucency (NT) as part of aneuploidy screening schemes.[4] With the amazing improvement of technical equipment and deepened knowledge of embryonic and early fetal development, the first trimester scan has no longer the limited purpose of confirmation of viability and gestational age but now targets ovulation status contributing to embryo, conceptus, early fetus, and the most important, early anomaly scan. This knowledge helps in diagnosis of abnormal early pregnancy, pregnancy failure, and fetal abnormalities as early as possible to enable timely decisions about management.

Routinely, the aims of the first trimester examination are:
- Determination of the location of the pregnancy inside the uterus or outside of the uterus (ectopic pregnancy)
- Presence or absence of cardiac activity
- Determination of the fetal number
- Calculation of fetal age
- Now with the advancement of technology, newer machines, and better sono-embryo-hormonal correlation, prognostication of pregnancy can also be done as discussed later in chapter.

Both transvaginal sonography (TVS) and transabdominal sonography (TAS) route may be used for first trimester scanning, but TVS is the method of choice for pregnancy assessment in early weeks.

At a serum beta-human chorionic gonadotropin (βhCG) level of 1,500 mIU/mL, which is reached at day 10–14 pc in a normal gravidity, an intrauterine chorionic sac can be detected by TVS probe with minimum 5 MHz frequency. Whereas in transabdominal ultrasound, serum βhCG values may have to be as high as 6,500 mIU/mL before an intrauterine gestational sac is detected.

The practical points to be remembered while performing first trimester scan are:

A systematic approach should be followed to ensure all structures are seen and to avoid misdiagnosis. The uterus and pelvis should be imaged in both longitudinal and transverse planes, whether a transabdominal or transvaginal probe is being used. There are several images that should be recorded which are as follows:
- *The uterus* should be imaged in the longitudinal section and shows the intrauterine gestational sac, cervix, and vaginal folds (in transabdominal views). This provides evidence that the pregnancy is intrauterine and will also show free fluid in the pouch of Douglas.
- *The gestational sac* should be imaged and measured in two planes (particularly in a pregnancy of less than 7 weeks of gestation or if fetal pole is not visible). This provides a reference for anyone scanning the same pregnancy in the future.
- *The crown-rump length (CRL)* measurements should be imaged. This provides a reference for future scans.
- *The adnexae* should be visualized in both planes and imaged, including the ovaries if they are visible to avoid missing any suspicious masses.

The key structures that are to be seen in first sonography before 8 weeks are gestational sac, yolk sac, and embryo.

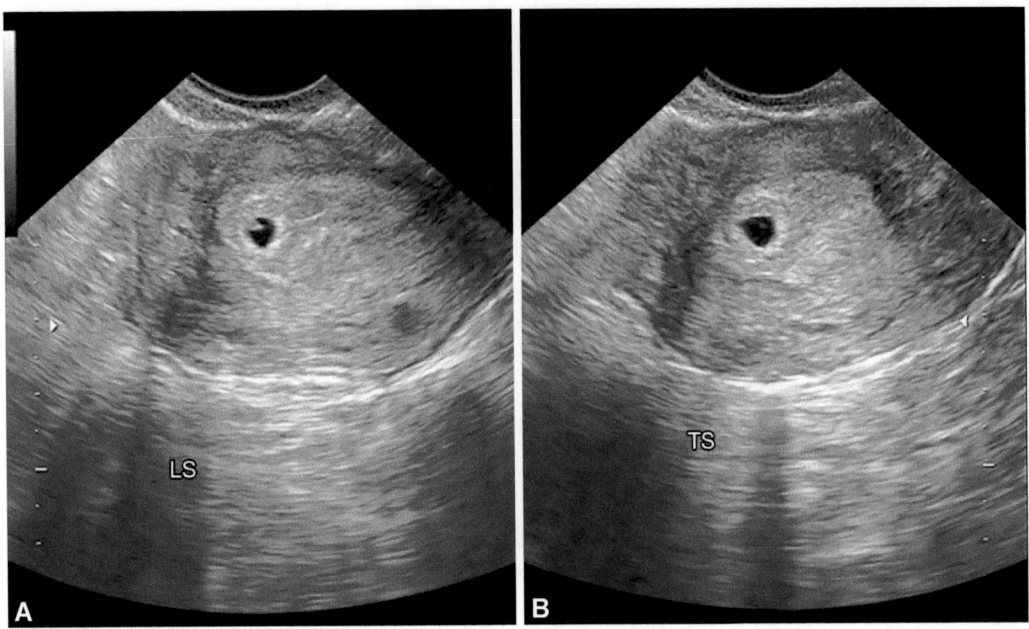

Figs. 1A and B: Gestational sac can be visible as early as 4.5–5 weeks (LS: longitudinal section; TS: transverse section).

- *The gestational sac*:
  - It is the first structure to be seen between 4.5 weeks and 5 weeks of gestation (Figs. 1A and B).
  - Appears as a circular structure, 2–3 mm diameter surrounded by thick echogenic ring.
  - Usually lies in uterine fundus and is eccentrically placed.
  - As the sac enlarges, it is surrounded by two concentric echogenic lines, giving the characteristic "double decidual sign".
  - Intervillous flow in Power Doppler assessment of the decidua around the double echogenic ring can also be seen as characteristic "comet sign" which along with visualization of a yolk sac at 5w+ confirm the impression of an intrauterine implantation.
  - Number of gestational sac should be noted.
  - The gestational sac should be measured in all three planes. The mean sac diameter (MSD) is the average of these three measurements. Anteroposterior (AP) is only measured in longitudinal section. A transverse measurement is taken in the longitudinal section and transverse section.
- *The yolk sac*:
  - It is the first element which appears inside the gestational sac at the beginning of 5 weeks. Because it is reliably seen early, it is a critical landmark identifying a true gestational sac (Figs. 2A and B).
  - It is circular in shape with well-defined echogenic periphery and sonolucent center.
  - It is usually less than 5 mm.
  - Yolk sac should be visible at MSD of 12 mm or more.
- *The embryo*:
  - The fetal pole becomes visible at later half of week 5 and measures 2–3 mm in size.
  - It is initially seen as a straight line adjacent to the yolk sac (Figs. 2A and B). As the embryo grows, it assumes a C-shape and CRL can now be measured.
  - Initial growth is at rate of 1 mm/day.
  - Crown-rump length is measured using the longest axis of fetus that can be obtained by rotating the probe and is taken from top of head (crown) to end of trunk (rump) using onscreen calipers.
  - Embryo must be visible at MSD of 25 mm or more.
  - Number of embryos to be noted in the sac.
  - Crown-rump length measures 10–17 mm and the rhombencephalon is visible, enabling distinction between the cephalad (head) and caudal (bottom) poles at 7–8 weeks.
  - Spine may be seen as double echogenic parallel lines at 8 weeks.
  - Amniotic membrane becomes visible and an umbilical cord may be seen before 9 weeks (Fig. 3).
- *Cardiac activity*:
  - Cardiac activity can be seen at 6–6.5 weeks and its frequency is also significant.
  - At 6–6.2 weeks, CRL 1–4 mm, embryo heart rate < 90 bpm is slow whereas 90–99 bpm is considered borderline.
  - At 6.3–7 weeks, CRL 5–9 mm, embryo heart rate < 110 bpm is slow and 110–119 bpm is considered borderline.

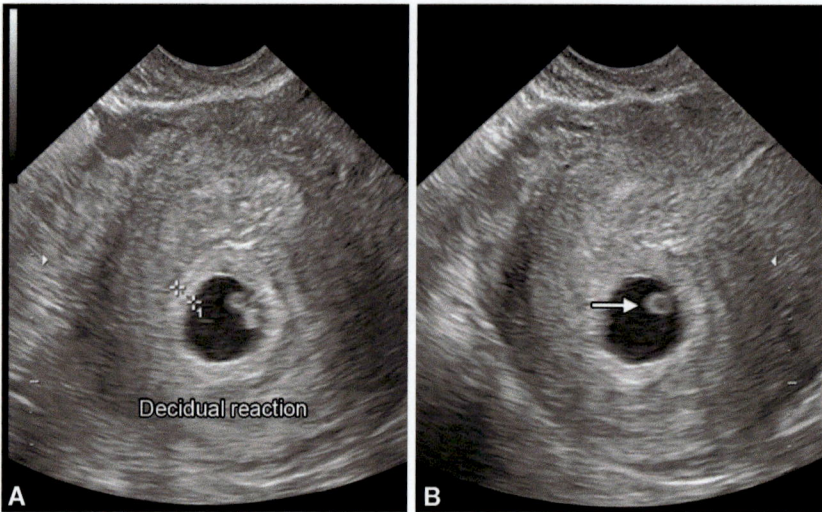

Figs. 2A and B: First structure visible inside gestational sac is yolk sac (arrow). Decidual reaction can also be observed at this stage. Figure shows good decidual reaction. Echogenic structure adjacent to yolk sac is embryo.

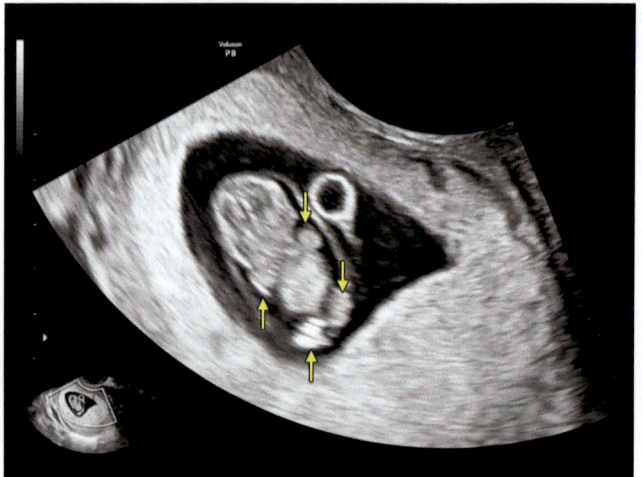

Fig. 3: Amniotic membrane visible clearly at 8 weeks with yolk sac and limb buds (arrows).

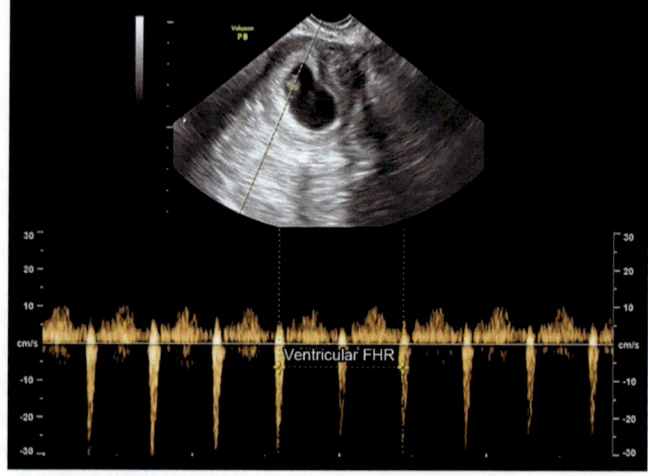

Fig. 4: Cardiac activity at 7 weeks (FHR: fetal heart rate).

- Any deviation in frequency should be considered significant and reviewed after 1 week.
- All embryos with CRL equal or above 7 mm must demonstrate cardiac activity (Fig. 4).

After 8 weeks, the following structures are noted depending on period of gestation:
- *At 8–9 weeks*:
  - Crown-rump length measures 17–23 mm and forebrain, hindbrain, and skull are visible (Fig. 5)
  - Midgut herniation occurs
  - Limb buds are visible.
- *At 9–10 weeks*:
  - Crown-rump length is 23–31 mm and limbs grow further
  - Heart rate increases to 150 bpm.

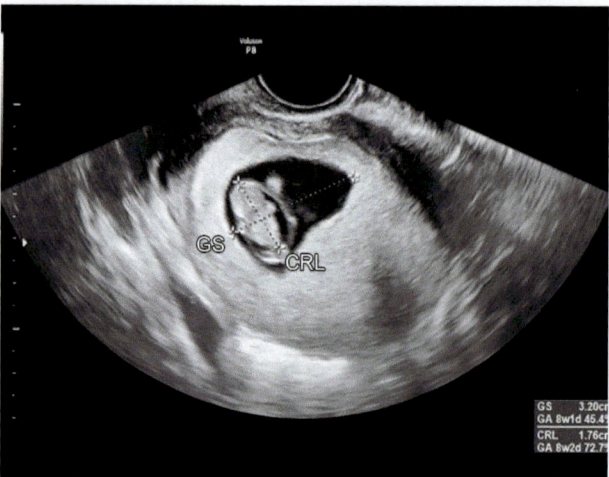

Fig. 5: CRL measurement at 8 weeks (CRL: crown-rump length; GS: gestational sac).

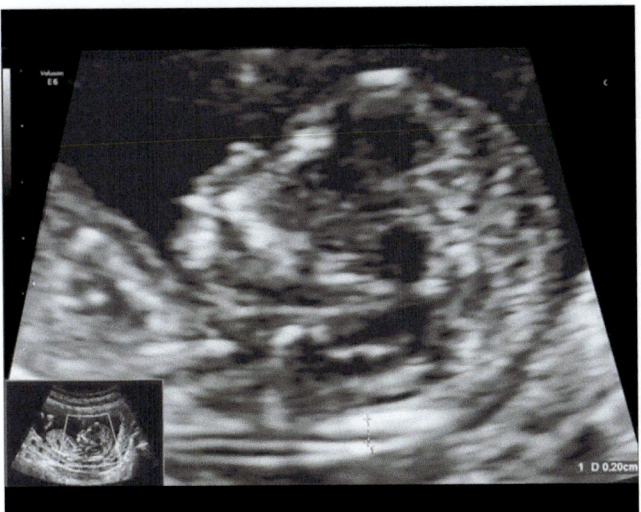

Fig. 6: NB-NT scan showing nasal bone and nuchal translucency.

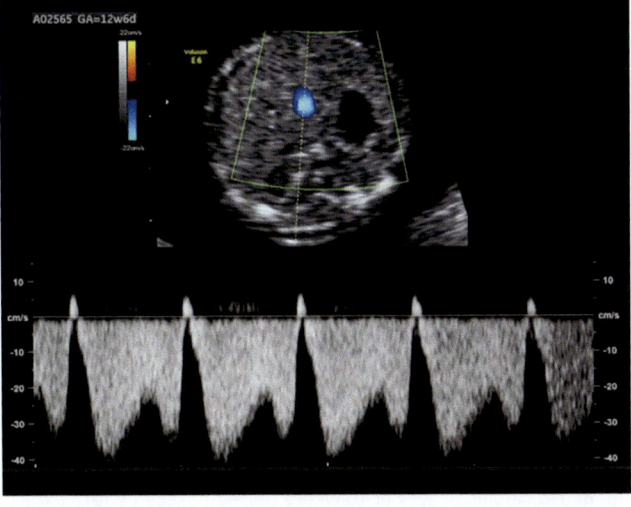

Fig. 7: Abnormal ductus venosus waveforms at the time of nuchal scan.

- *At 10–11 weeks*:
  - Crown-rump length is 32–41 mm and human features of the fetus become clearer
  - Head is still relatively large, typical fetal posture appears
  - Physiological midgut herniation disappears
  - Onset of marrow formation in the humerus marks the end of embryonic life and start of fetal life.
- *At 11–13 weeks*: This is also called early anomaly scan. Majority of the fetal defects can be picked up in this scan if done carefully. Specific features to be noted here are:
  - Presence of nasal bone (NB) and calculation of NT (Fig. 6). Calculation of NT along with fetal parameters and biochemical markers is a sensitive measure of screening of aneuploidy, which is nowadays a routine screening offered in all pregnancies.
  - Tricuspid valves are noted along with four-chamber view of heart and outflow tracts, which enable to rule the major cardiac defects, and
  - Ductus venosus (DV) blood flow used in aneuploidy screening has also been suggested to have a role as a marker for cardiac defects, similarly to NT (Fig. 7).[5-7]

There are certain specific protocols for the accurate measurement of NT which must be strictly followed:
- The gestational period must be 11–13 weeks and 6 days.
- The fetal CRL should be between 45 mm and 84 mm.
- The magnification of the image should be such that the fetal head and thorax occupy the whole screen.
- A midsagittal view of the face should be obtained. This is defined by the presence of the echogenic tip of the nose and rectangular shape of the palate anteriorly, the translucent diencephalon in the center, and the nuchal membrane posteriorly. Minor deviations from the exact midline plane would cause nonvisualization of the tip of the nose and visibility of the maxilla.
- The fetus should be in a neutral position, with the head in line with the spine. When the fetal neck is hyperextended, the measurement can be falsely increased and when the neck is flexed, the measurement can be falsely decreased.
- Care must be taken to distinguish between fetal skin and amnion.
- The widest part of translucency must always be measured.
- Measurements should be taken with the inner border of the horizontal line of the calipers placed on the line that defines the NT thickness—the crossbar of the caliper should be such that it is hardly visible as it merges with the white line of the border, not in the nuchal fluid.

CRITICAL CONDITIONS IN EARLY PREGNANCY SCAN

With the extensive use of transvaginal ultrasound, many of the abnormalities of early pregnancies can be noted and treated timely. Most common of them are:
- *Early pregnancy failure*: It is defined as a pregnancy that ends spontaneously before the embryo is detected by ultrasound at the gestational age, in which visualization of viable embryo should be possible. This is manifested commonly by vaginal bleeding.
- *Incomplete miscarriage*: Early pregnancy presented by excessive vaginal bleeding with sonographic findings suggestive of an echogenic and vascularized mass

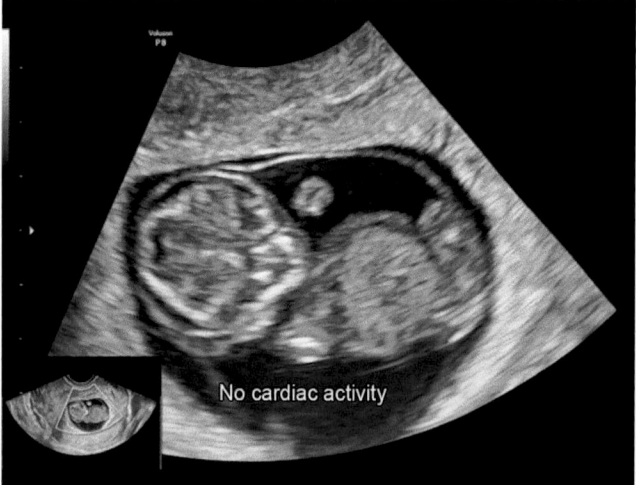

Fig. 8: No cardiac activity at 10 weeks (missed miscarriage).

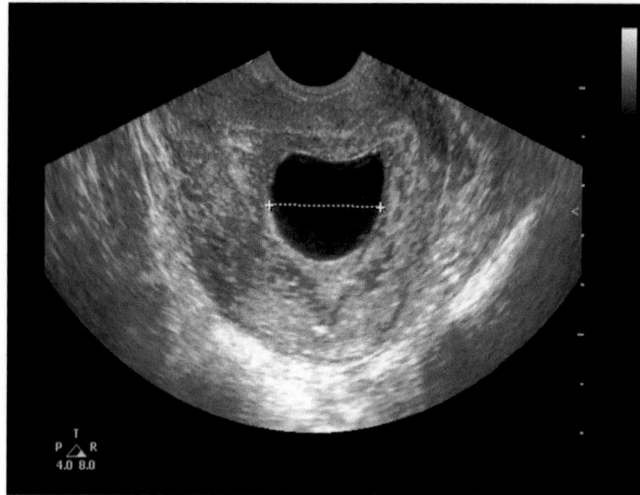

Fig. 9: Empty gestational sac, blighted ovum.

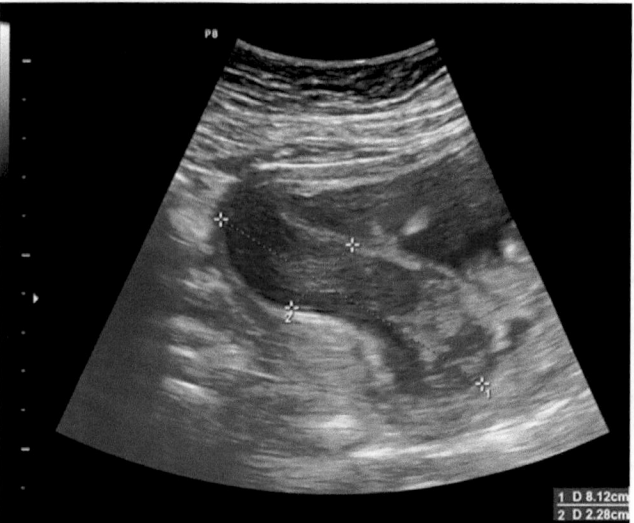

Fig. 10: Large subchorionic hematoma of 8 cm × 2 cm.

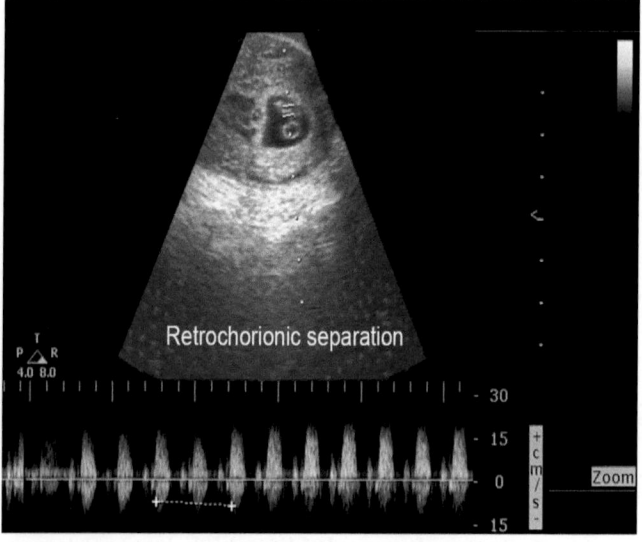

Fig. 11: Retrochorionic hematoma.

within the uterine cavity with no gestational sac and no yolk sac confirms the diagnosis of retained products of conception, i.e., incomplete miscarriage.
- *Missed miscarriage (Fig. 8)*: The diagnosis of missed miscarriage is determined by the ultrasound identification of an embryo/fetus without any heart activity when CRL is greater than 7 mm.
- *Blighted ovum (Fig. 9)*:
  – Blighted ovum (anembryonic pregnancy) refers to a gestational sac in which the embryo either failed to develop or died at a stage too early to be visualized.
  – The diagnosis of anembryonic pregnancy is based on the absence of embryonic echoes within a gestational sac, whose size is large enough to suggest a pregnancy age at which such structures should be visible, independent of the clinical data or menstrual cycle.
- *Intrauterine hematomas (Figs. 10 and 11)*:
  – Intrauterine hematomas are defined as sonolucent crescent or wedge-shaped structures between chorionic tissue and uterine wall, or fetal membranes.
  – By localization, we can divide them into retroplacental, subchorionic, marginal, and supracervical.
  – Prognostically, there are two main elements, which determine the pregnancy outcome: size and location of the hematoma.
- *Molar pregnancy (Fig. 12)*: Snowstorm appearance in uterine cavity with abnormally elevated serum βhCG levels is suggestive of molar pregnancy.

Ultrasound in First Trimester

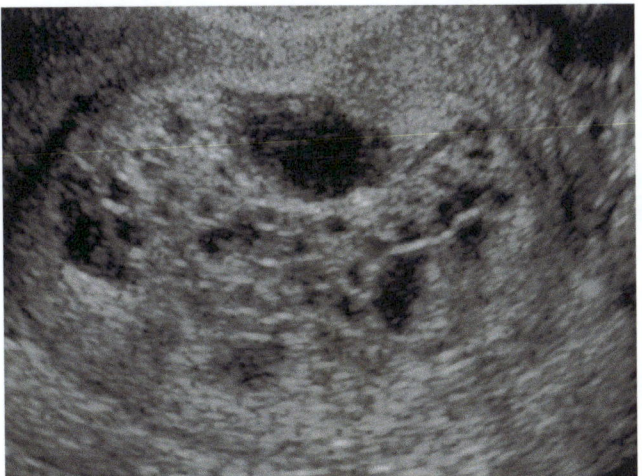

Fig. 12: Snowstorm appearance of vesicular mole.

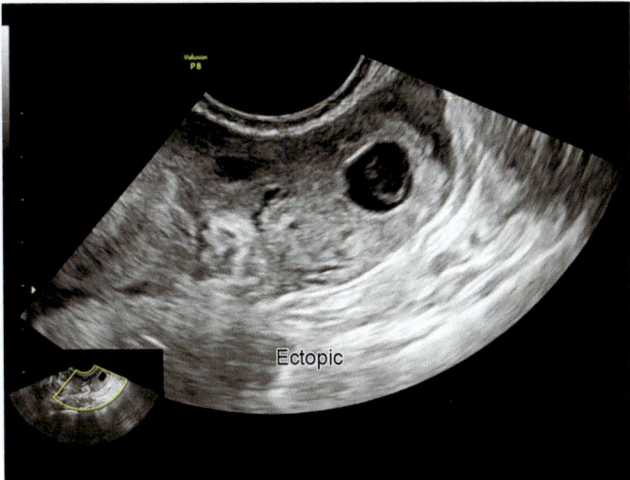

Fig. 13: Adnexal mass with empty uterine cavity and positive urine pregnancy test.

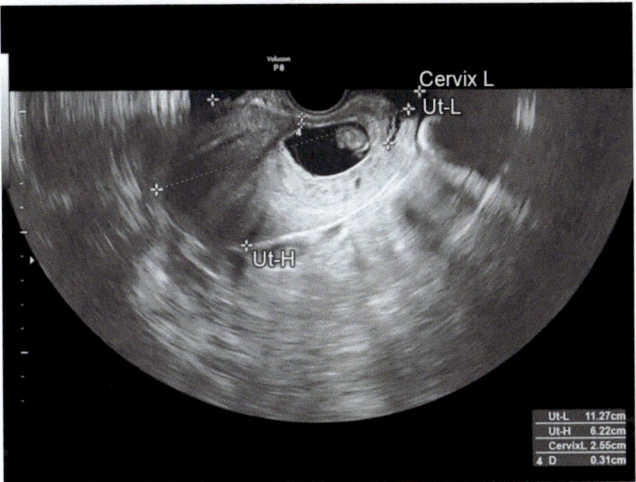

Fig. 14: Empty uterine fundus with a pregnancy at previous cesarean scar (scar pregnancy).

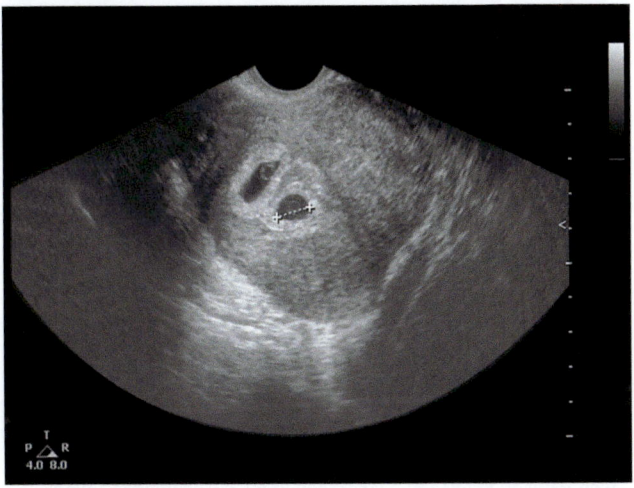

Fig. 15: Diamniotic dichorionic twin pregnancy.

- *Ectopic pregnancy (Figs. 13 and 14)*: Empty uterine cavity with adnexal mass and positive urine pregnancy test or positive serum βhCG levels suggest ectopic pregnancy.
- *Multiple pregnancy (Figs. 15 and 16)*: Sometimes, two or more gestational sacs are visible suggestive of twins or higher-order pregnancies. In the first trimester scan, it is advisable to clarify the chorionicity of the high-order pregnancy.

PROGNOSTICATION OF PREGNANCY

Nowadays, there is possibility of prognostication of pregnancy or to detect possible maldevelopment of the embryo by evaluating some early pregnancy ultrasound signs. These signs are as follows:
- Decreased values of gestational sac (Fig. 17) diameter or its abnormal growth and/or its irregular shape

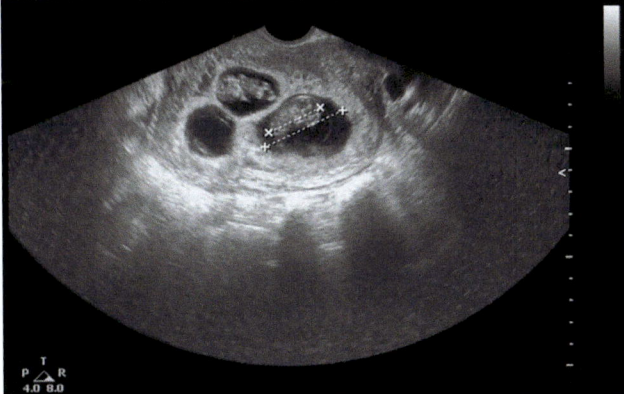

Fig. 16: Triamniotic trichorionic triplet pregnancy.

(Figs. 18A and B) can suggest upcoming incident and may be used as a marker for chromosomopathies.
- Lack of double decidual sign or thin decidual reaction.

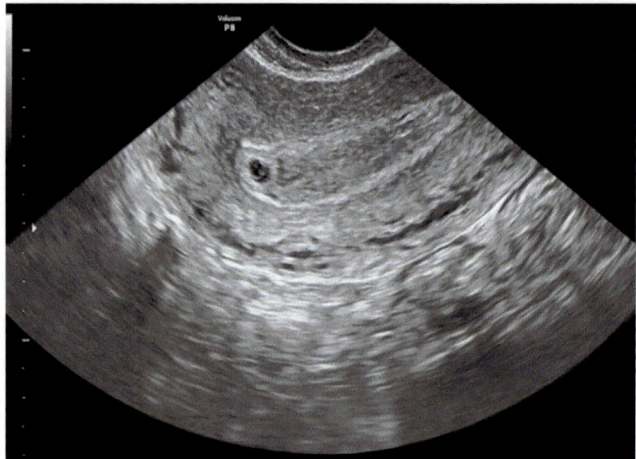

Fig. 17: Too tight fitting yolk sac is poor prognostic factor for continuation of pregnancy (review sac showed missed miscarriage).

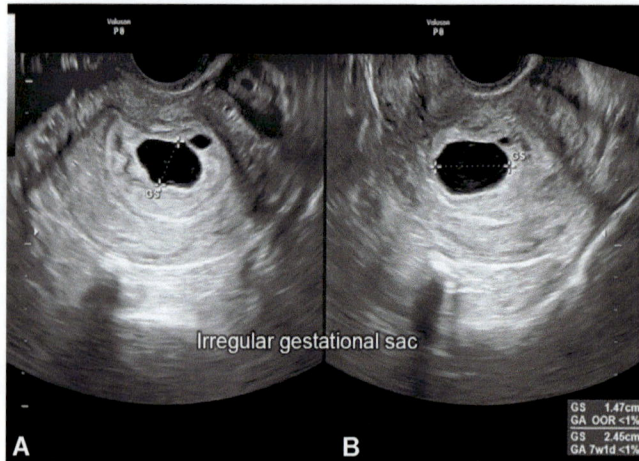

Figs. 18A and B: Irregular gestational sac which resulted in miscarriage in subsequent scan.

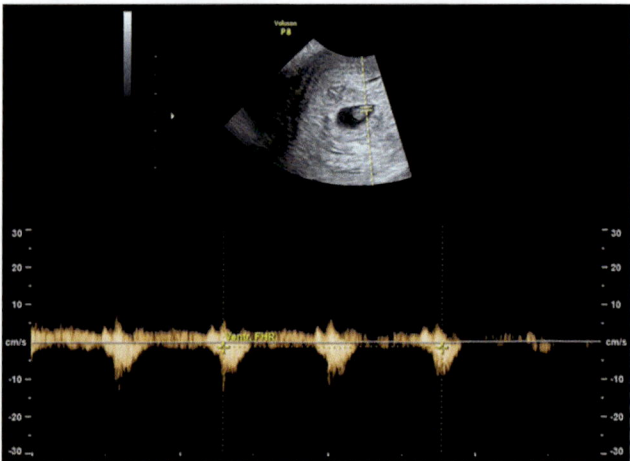

Fig. 19: Cardiac activity of 80 bpm (poor prognostication of pregnancy) which resulted in missed miscarriage in review scan after 1 week.

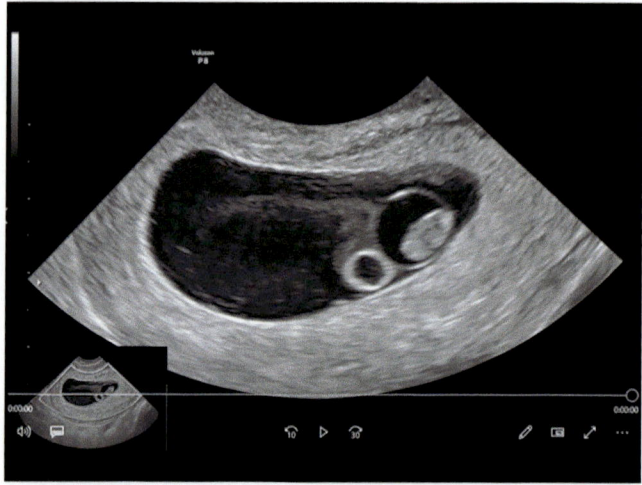

Fig. 20: Cardiac activity is not appreciated (follow-up scan of Fig. 19).

- Absence of the yolk sac.
- Too large—more than 6 mm or too small—less than 3 mm diameter of yolk sac.
- Irregular-shaped yolk sac—mainly wrinkled with indented walls.
- Degenerative changes—abundant calcifications with decreased translucency of the yolk sac.
- Number of yolk sacs—has to be equal to the number of the embryos.
- An embryonic heart rate less than expected at that CRL has been reported to result in risk of fetal demise (Figs. 19 and 20).
- When the amniotic membrane is clearly visualized or its thickness and echogenicity approach that of yolk sac, abnormal amnion development should always be suspected.
- Mean amniotic sac diameter is approximately equal to the CRL in normal early pregnancy. Enlarged amniotic cavity in relation to CRL measurement suggests early pregnancy abnormality.

Thus, first trimester scan gives enormous amount of information regarding ongoing pregnancy including predictors of chromosomal abnormalities (soft markers), major and minor fetal defects affecting fetal outcome and fetal growth. The detailed timely first trimester scan in high-risk cases along with biochemical markers increases the aneuploidy detection rate to almost 96%. Major fetal defects such as holoprosencephaly, acrania, anencephaly, megacystis, hypoplastic heart syndrome, omphalocele, etc. should never be missed in first trimester scan. Definitely, the expertise in ultrasound is key to conquer. Although all the pathological conditions are not covered in detail in the chapter, but the commonly encountered situations are tried to explain well.

CONCLUSION

In a nutshell, first trimester ultrasound is nowadays not at all limited to just localize the position of sac and look for viability of embryo but a detailed ultrasound in hands of skilled practitioner is a good guide for prognostication, prediction and prevention of untoward obstetric accidents.[8]

REFERENCES

1. Economides DL, Braithwaite JM. First trimester ultrasonographic diagnosis of fetal structural abnormalities in a low risk population. Br J Obstet Gynaecol. 1998;105:53-7.
2. Saltvedt S, Almström H, Kublickas M, et al. Ultrasound dating at 12–14 or 15–20 weeks of gestation? A prospective cross-validation of established dating formulae in a population of in-vitro fertilized pregnancies randomized to early or late dating scan. Ultrasound Obstet Gynecol. 2004;24:42-50.
3. Whitworth M, Bricker L, Neilson JP, et al. Ultrasound for fetal assessment in early pregnancy. Cochrane Database Syst Rev. 2010;(4):CD007058.
4. Nicolaides KH, Brizot ML, Snidjers RJ. Fetal nuchal translucency: ultrasound screening for fetal trisomy in the first trimester of pregnancy. Br J Obstet Gynaecol. 1994;101:782-6.
5. Borrell A. The ductus venosus in early pregnancy and congenital anomalies. Prenat Diagn. 2004;24:688-92.
6. Martinez JM, Comas M, Borrell A, et al. Abnormal first-trimester ductus venosus blood flow: a marker of cardiac defects in fetuses with normal karyotype and nuchal translucency. Ultrasound Obstet Gynecol. 2010;35:267-72.
7. Papatheodorou S, Evangelou E, Makrydimas G, et al. First-trimester ductus venosus screening for cardiac defects: a meta-analysis. BJOG. 2011;118:1438-45.
8. Baser A, Dhingra H, Zaidi AK (Eds). Obstetrics and Gynaecological Ultrasound for Beginners. New Delhi: Jaypee Brothers Medical Publishers; 2019.

12
Ultrasound and Doppler in Multiple Pregnancy

Parth Shah, Jayprakash Shah

INTRODUCTION

Multiple pregnancies may result from two or more fertilization events, from a single fertilization followed by splitting of the zygote, or from a combination of both. Fueled largely by infertility therapy, both the rate and the number of twins and high-order multifetal births are growing dramatically. Increasing multiple pregnancies rates have direct effect on preterm birth rates, its comorbidities, and infant death rates. The mother may also experience higher obstetric morbidity and mortality rates. Here, we will be mainly discussing twin pregnancy, its diagnosis, complications, and how to manage them.

MECHANISM OF MULTIFETAL GESTATION

Dizygotic or Fraternal Twins

These twin fetuses usually result from fertilization of two separate ova. They are almost always dichorionic-diamniotic (Figs. 1A and B).

Monozygotic or Identical Twins

A single fertilized ovum divides to create monozygotic twins. These can be dichorionic-diamniotic, monochorionic-diamniotic (MCDA) (Figs. 1A and B), or monochorionic monoamniotic (MCMA). Figure 2 shows the process of formation of different types of monozygotic twins.

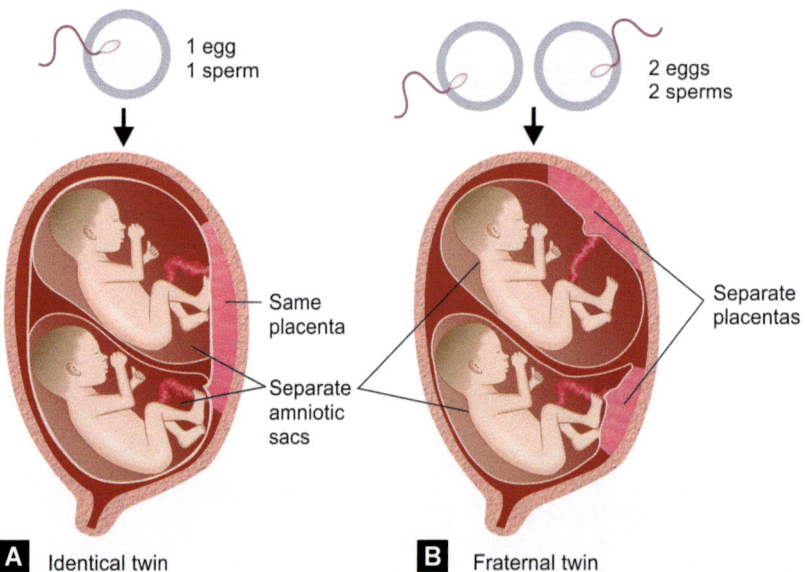

Figs. 1A and B: (A) Identical or monozygotic twins are shown, resulting from single fertilized ovum. Monozygotic twins can be dichorionic or monochorionic, this figure shows monochorionic twins; (B) Twins resulting from fertilization of two separate eggs and two separate ova are shown, forming dizygotic or fraternal twins. Dizygotic twins are always dichorionic diamniotic with two separate placentas.

Ultrasound and Doppler in Multiple Pregnancy

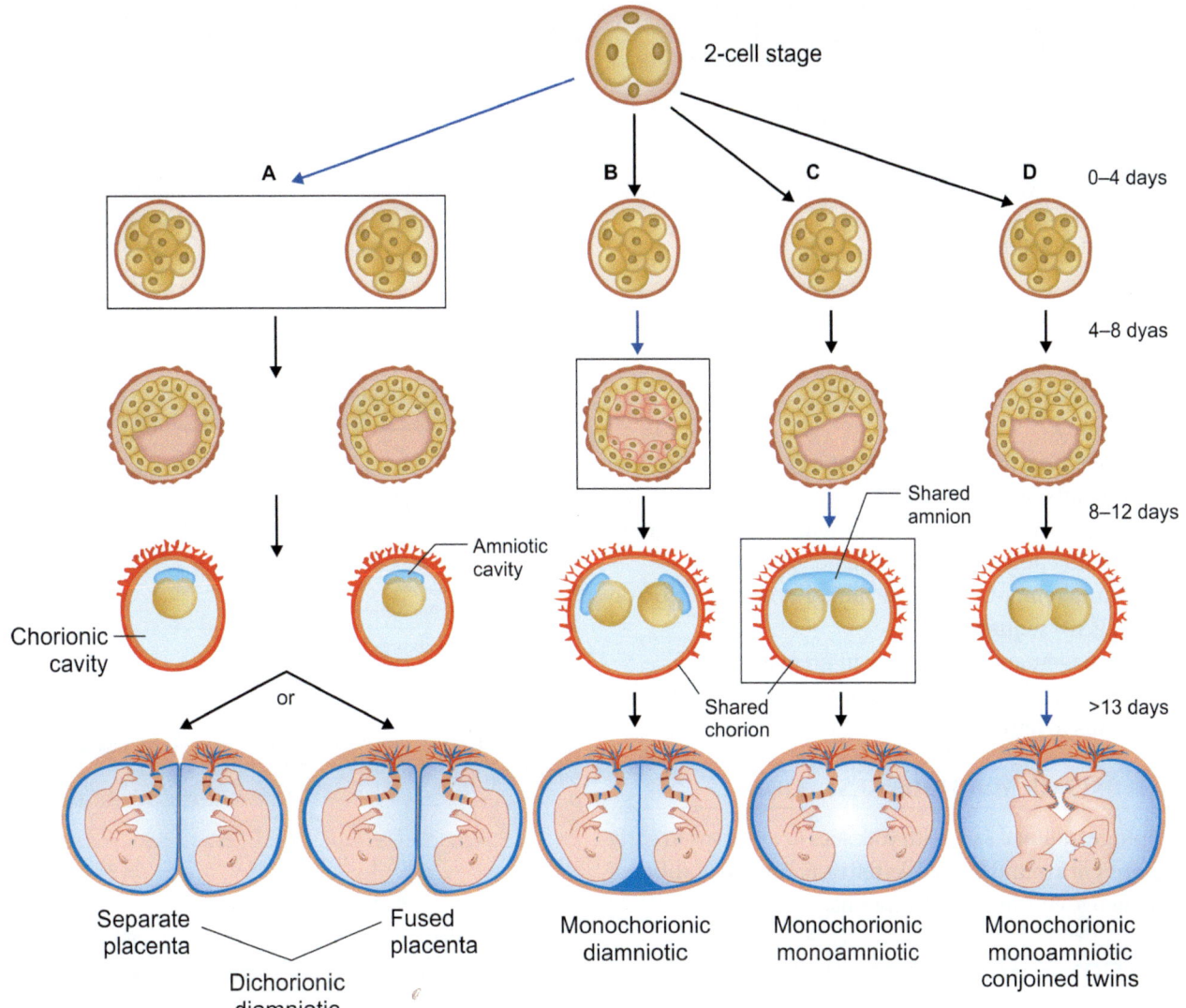

Fig. 2: Mechanism of monozygotic twinning. Black boxing and blue arrows in columns A, B, and C indicate timing of the division. (A) At 0–4 days postfertilization, an early conceptus may divide into two. Division at this early stage creates two chorions and two amnions (dichorionic and diamniotic). Placentas may be separate or fused; (B) Division between 4 and 8 days leads to the formation of a blastocyst with two separate embryoblasts (inner cell masses). Each embryoblast will form its own amnion within a shared chorion (monochorionic and diamniotic); (C) Between 8 and 12 days, the amnion and amniotic cavity form above the germinal disc. Embryonic division leads to two embryos with a shared amnion and shared chorion (monochorionic and monoamniotic); (D) Differing theories explain conjoined twin development. One describes an incomplete splitting of one embryo into two. The other describes fusion of a portion of one embryo from a monozygotic pair onto the other.

Either or both the processes may be involved in the formation of higher numbers.

GENESIS OF MONOZYGOTIC TWINS (FIG. 2)

The risk for twin-specific complications varies in relation to both zygosity and chorionicity—the number of chorions; the latter is the more important determinant as depicted in Table 1.

ROLE OF PRENATAL ULTRASOUND IN MULTIFETAL GESTATION

- Diagnosis of multiple gestation
- Dating of the pregnancy (determining gestational age)
- Determining chorionicity and amnionicity
- Twin labeling
- Timing, frequency, and content of ultrasound assessment
- Screening for aneuploidy
- Prenatal diagnosis of aneuploidy
- Screening for structural abnormalities
- Diagnosis and management of discordant twin pregnancy
- Fetal reduction/selective termination
- Screening for preterm birth
- Screening, diagnosis, and management of fetal growth restriction (FGR)
- Management of multiple pregnancy complicated by single intrauterine device (IUD)

Table 1: Overview of the incidence of twin pregnancy, zygosity, and corresponding twin-specific complications.[1]

Type of twinning	Twins (%)	Fetal growth restriction (%)	Preterm delivery[a] (%)	Placental vascular anastomoses (%)	Perinatal mortality (%)
Dizygotic	80	25	40	0	10–12
Monozygotic	20	40	50		15–18
Diamniotic/dichorionic	6–7	30	40	0	18–20
Diamniotic/monochorionic	13–14	40	60	100	30–40
Monoamniotic/monochorionic	<1	50	60–70	80–90	58–60
Conjoined	0.002–0.008	–	70–80	100	70–90

[a]Delivery before 37 weeks.

- Complications unique to monochorionic twin pregnancy:
  - Screening, diagnosis, and management of twin-twin transfusion syndrome (TTTS)
  - Screening, diagnosis, and management of twin anemia polycythemia sequence (TAPS)
  - Management of twin reversed arterial perfusion (TRAP) sequence
  - Management of MCMA twin pregnancy
  - Diagnosis and management of conjoined twins
  - Fetus in fetu

DIAGNOSIS OF MULTIPLE GESTATION

Multiple gestational sacs with yolk sacs or embryos in early pregnancy at around 5–6 weeks tell us about the number of pregnancies, chorions, and amnions.

GESTATIONAL AGE ASSESSMENT IN MULTIFETAL PREGNANCY

Gestational age assessment in twin pregnancy should ideally be done when crown-rump length (CRL) measures between 45 mm and 84 mm, as is done between 11+0 weeks and 13+6 weeks:
- In pregnancy spontaneously conceived, the larger of two CRLs should be used to date the pregnancy.
- In IVF (in vitro fertilization) pregnancy, oocyte retrieval date or the embryonic age from fertilization should be used to date the pregnancy.

Note: If the women present after 14 weeks of gestation in spontaneously conceived pregnancy, the larger head circumference should be used to date the pregnancy.

DETERMINING CHORIONICITY AND AMNIONICITY IN MULTIFETAL PREGNANCY

- *Early pregnancy*: In early pregnancy, presence of separate gestational sacs each with echogenic ring (trophoblast) surrounding it tells us about the chorionicity while the number of yolk sacs tells about the amnionicity.

Table 2: Ultrasound signs of chorionicity.

Sign	Dichorionic pregnancy	Monochorionic diamniotic pregnancy
T-sign or Lambda sign	Lambda sign	T-sign
Placental mass	Double/fused placenta	Single
No. of intertwin membranes	4	2
Thickness of membrane	≥2 mm	<2 mm
Fetal gender	Different/same	Same

Table 3: Statistical accuracy of antenatal prediction of monochorionicity by ultrasound.[2]

	Sensitivity (%)	Specificity (%)	PPV (%)	NPV (%)
Overall	88.9	97.7	92.6	96.5
First trimester	89.8	99.5	97.8	97.5
Second trimester	88.0	94.7	88.0	94.7

(PPV: positive predictive values; NPV: negative predictive values)

- *In first trimester*: Chorionicity should be determined between 11+0 weeks and 13+6 weeks using the membrane thickness at the point of insertion of amniotic membrane into the placenta, identifying the "T-sign" or the "lambda sign," number of placental masses, number of membranes, and thickness of membranes. Table 2 shows various ultrasound signs of monochorionic and dichorionic pregnancy. The sensitivity, specificity, positive predictive values (PPV) as well as negative predictive values (NPV) of ultrasound diagnosis of chorionicity are all higher in the first trimester as compared to the second trimester (Table 3):
  - *T-sign*: T-sign is defined as the right-angle relationship between the membranes and placenta with no apparent extension of placenta between the dividing membranes.
  - *Lambda sign*: It is a triangular projection of placental tissue extending a short distance between the layers of the dividing membrane.

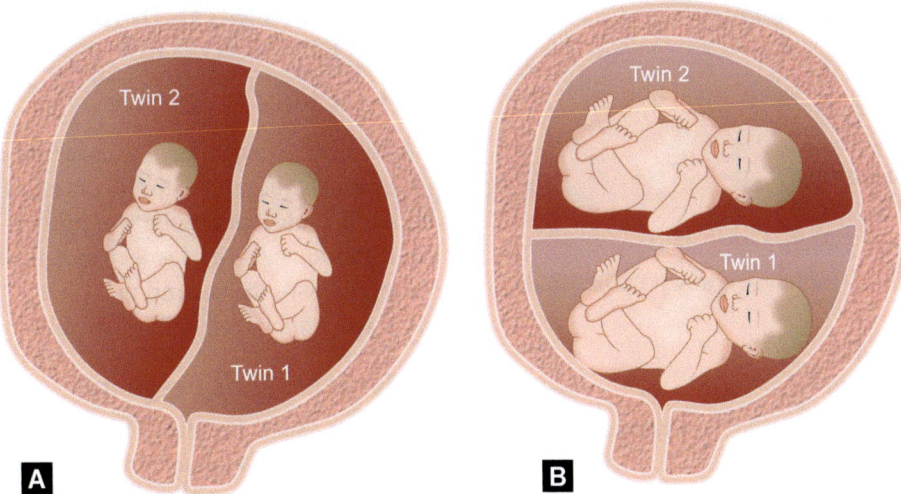

Figs. 3A and B: The fetuses are labeled according to site. (A) The fetus is labeled as twin 1 on right side and twin 2 on left side; (B) Fetuses are divided according proximity to the cervix, fetus 1 is closer to the cervical canal and fetus 2 is the upper one.

- *After 14 weeks*: Chorionicity is determined by using the same ultrasound signs, in particular by counting the membrane layers and noting the discordant or concordant fetal sex:
  - Both a bipartite placenta and discordant sex have been reported in monochorionic pregnancies.[3]
  - If there is an uncertainty about placenta, it is safe to consider it as monochorionic.
- The time at which chorionicity is identified, amnionicity, i.e., whether or not the twins share the same amniotic sac, should be determined and documented.

LABELING OF THE FETUSES

The labeling once done should be consistent and mentioned nicely in the pregnant women's ultrasound report. The labeling options include:

- Labeling as fetus 1 and fetus 2 according to site—as either right and left, or lower and upper (Figs. 3A and B).
- Fetus near internal os to be labeled as fetus 1 and other as fetus 2. If more than two fetuses, then they shall be labeled in clockwise direction starting the fetus near internal os as fetus 1.
- Mapping in the first trimester according to the insertion of their cords relative to the placental edges and membrane insertion.

MONITORING OF THE MULTIFETAL PREGNANCY

Women with uncomplicated dichorionic twin pregnancy should have:

- A first trimester scan between 11+0 weeks and 13+6 weeks
- A detailed second trimester anomaly scan at around 20 weeks
- And then follow-up scans every 4 weeks
- Complicated dichorionic pregnancy should be monitored more frequently, depending on the condition and its severity.

Women with uncomplicated monochorionic twin pregnancy should have:

- A first trimester scan between 11+0 weeks and 13+6 weeks
- And then scanning should be done every 2 weeks after 16 weeks in order to detect TTTS and TAPS earlier
- Complicated monochorionic pregnancy should be monitored more frequently, depending on the condition and its severity.

At each ultrasound assessment, the parameters that are to be looked in for both twins are described below.

Dichorionic Twin Pregnancy

- *11–14 weeks*:
  - Dating and labeling
  - Chorionicity
  - Screening for trisomy 21
  - Early malformation screening
- *20–22 weeks*:
  - Detailed anatomy
  - Biometry
  - Deepest vertical pocket (DVP)
  - Cervical length
- *24–26 weeks*:

28–30 weeks	Assessment of fetal growth,
32–34 weeks	amniotic fluid volume, and
36–37 weeks	fetal Doppler

Monochorionic Twin Pregnancy

- *11–14 weeks*:
  - Dating and labeling
  - Chorionicity
  - Screening for trisomy 21
  - Early malformation screening
- 16 weeks } Fetal growth and DVP
- 18 weeks } UA-PI (umbilical artery pulsatility index)
- *20 weeks*:
  - Detailed anatomy
  - Biometry and DVP
  - UA-PI and MCA-PSV (middle cerebral arterial peak systolic velocity)
  - Cervical length
- 22 weeks
  24 weeks
  26 weeks } Fetal growth DVP,
  28 weeks } UA-PI, and MCA-PSV
  30 weeks
  32 weeks
  34 weeks
  36 weeks

SCREENING FOR ANEUPLOIDY IN MULTIFETAL GESTATION

In twin gestation, the detection rate (DR) for Down syndrome may be lower compared to singleton pregnancy.[4] Also screening and diagnostic testing for trisomy are more complex in twins compared with singleton pregnancy.

Screening for trisomy 21 can be performed in the first trimester using the combined test [nuchal translucency (NT) thickness] and double marker test [free beta-human chorionic gonadotropin (βhCG) level and pregnancy-associated plasma protein-A (PAPP-A) level]. An alternative is the combination of maternal age and NT only.

But while using combined test, there is an increased likelihood of being offered invasive testing on the basis of a combined screening result compared with singleton pregnancy. Moreover, invasive testing carries greater risks in twins. A meta-analysis showed that the overall pregnancy loss rate following chorionic villus sampling (CVS) in twin pregnancy was 3.8% and following amniocentesis was 3.1%. So, a thorough counseling is required prior to testing by the healthcare providers.

Cell-free deoxyribonucleic acid (cfDNA) analysis of maternal blood for risk assessment for fetal trisomy 21 is used increasingly in clinical practice. In a recent meta-analysis, the weighted pooled DR for trisomy 21 in twin pregnancy was 94.4% for a false-positive rate (FPR) of 0%.[5]

INVASIVE PRENATAL DIAGNOSIS IN MULTIFETAL GESTATION

In Dichorionic Pregnancy

In dichorionic pregnancy, CVS is preferred because it can be performed earlier than amniocentesis. Earlier diagnosis of any aneuploidy is particularly important in twin pregnancy, given the lower risk of selective termination in the first compared with the second trimester (*7% risk of loss of the entire pregnancy and 14% risk of delivery before 32 weeks*).

In Monochorionic Pregnancy

Amniocentesis is preferred in monochorionic pregnancy as we sample single placenta in CVS and we may miss the rare discordant chromosomal anomalies in monochorionic pregnancy (Figs. 4A and B).

During amniocentesis, if the fetuses appear concordant for growth and anatomy, it is acceptable to sample only one amniotic sac. Otherwise, both amniotic sacs should be sampled because of the rare discordant chromosomal anomalies in monochorionic pregnancy.

In case of heterokaryotypic monochorionic pregnancy, selective reduction by umbilical cord occlusion can be offered from 16 weeks onward, with *a survival rate of more than 80%* for the healthy twin.[6,7]

ULTRASOUND SCREENING FOR STRUCTURAL ANOMALIES

The risk of fetal anomaly is greater in multifetal gestation compared to singleton pregnancy. The risk of anomalies is probably the same as that in singleton pregnancy, for each fetus in dizygotic twins, but it is two to three times higher in monozygotic twins. In around 1 in 25 dichorionic, 1 in 15 MCDA, and 1 in 6 monoamniotic twin pregnancies, there is a major congenital anomaly that typically affects only one twin.[8,9] A list of congenital anomalies showing increased incidence are mentioned in Table 4.

- Twin fetuses should be assessed for any major anomalies at the first trimester scan, and a routine anomaly scan at around 20 weeks of gestation.
- Fetal cardiac screening should also be performed in monochorionic twins.

MANAGEMENT OF TWIN PREGNANCY DISCORDANT FOR FETAL ANOMALY

In such a case, invasive fetal chromosomal or genetic testing is indicated, and a discussion of the likely prognosis of both the affected and the normal twin should be done.

If the condition is lethal and carry a high risk of intrauterine demise, conservative management is preferred in dichorionic twins, whereas in monochorionic twin

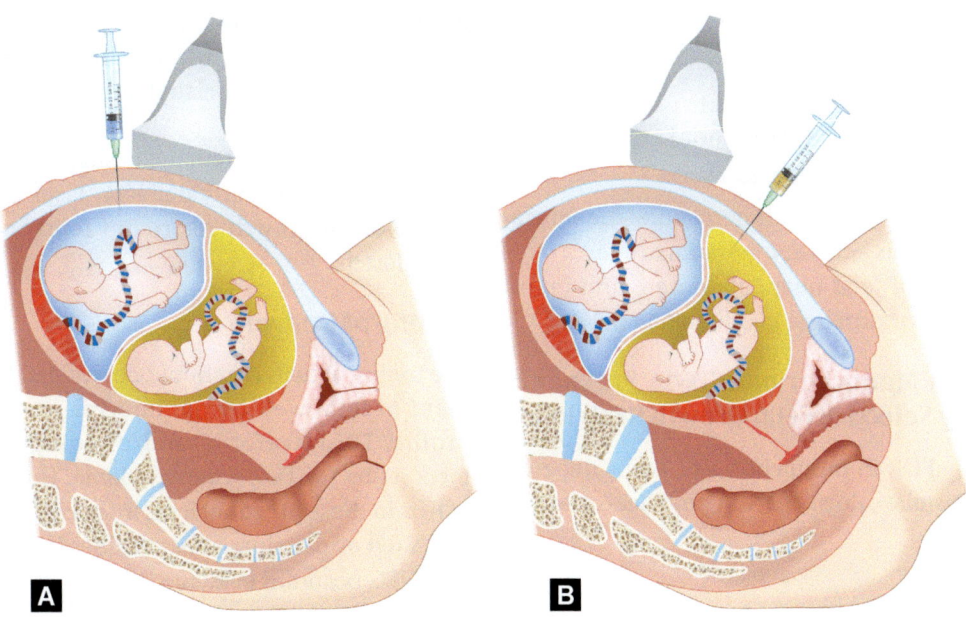

Figs. 4A and B: A dichorionic diamniotic pregnancy with two separate placental masses and two amniotic cavities. After amniocentesis from fetus A, methylene blue is injected in sac of fetus A. Then sonographically-guided needle inserted in amniotic sac of fetus B. Amniotic fluid will not be having methylene blue color, confirming tapping of fetus B sac.

Table 4: Congenital anomalies showing an increased incidence in monochorionic twins.[10]

CNS	Facial	Heart	Gastrointestinal	Genitourinary
• Neural tube defect • Holoprosencephaly • Cerebellar anomalies • Agenesis of corpus callosum	• Ocular • Cleft palate and/or cleft lip	• ASD • Common arterial trunk • Pulmonary stenosis • TOF • Univentricular heart	• GI atresia • Wall defects • Diaphragmatic hernia	• Hypospadias • Epispadias • UPJ and urethral obstruction • Cloacal or bladder exstrophy

(CNS: central nervous system; ASD: atrial septal defect; TOF: tetralogy of Fallot; GI: gastrointestinal; UPJ: ureteropelvic junction)

pregnancy, this would warrant intervention, by occluding the cord or radiofrequency ablation (RFA) of the cord, to protect the healthy co-twin against the adverse effects of spontaneous demise of the other.

FETAL REDUCTION/SELECTIVE TERMINATION IN MULTIFETAL GESTATION

In Dichorionic Pregnancy

In dichorionic pregnancy, selective feticide is performed using ultrasound-guided intracardiac injection of KCL (potassium chloride) or lignocaine, using a 23 gauge needle, under aseptic precautions, preferably at 11–13 weeks.

In Monochorionic Pregnancy

Using intracardiac KCL is not an option here because of risk to the healthy co-twin. Selective feticide in monochorionic pregnancy is performed by cord occlusion, intrafetal laser ablation, or RFA after 18 weeks. By this method, demise of one fetus does not lead to hypotension in the surviving twin. The survival rate of co-twin is 80% and the risk of premature rupture of membranes and preterm birth prior to 32 weeks is 20%.

SCREENING FOR RISK OF PRETERM BIRTH IN MULTIFETAL GESTATION

The preferred method for screening preterm birth in multifetal gestation is cervical length measurement. The cut-off value is 25 mm in the second trimester.

Cervical length of <25 mm between 18 weeks and 24 weeks is a moderator predictor of preterm birth before 34 weeks, but not before 37 weeks.

FETAL GROWTH RESTRICTION

- *Selective fetal growth restriction (sFGR)*, conventionally, is defined as one fetus with estimated fetal weight (EFW) <10th percentile and the intertwin EFW discordance

>25%. Formula for calculating fetal weight discordance is as follows:

$$\text{EFW discordance} = \frac{(\text{Weight of larger twin} - \text{Weight of smaller twin})}{\text{Weight of larger twin}} \times 100$$

- If both twins have EFW <10th percentile, the fetuses should be termed as small-for-gestational age.
- A combination of fetal head, abdomen, and femur measurements perform best in calculating EFW.

Classification of Monochorionic Twin Pregnancy Complicated by Selective Fetal Growth Restriction

Classification of sFGR in monochorionic twins depends upon the end-diastolic velocity flow in umbilical artery.

Type I

In type I, the umbilical artery waveform has positive end-diastolic flow. The survival rate is >90%.

Type II

In type II, there is absence or reversal of end diastolic-flow. The risk of IUD in either twin is 29% and risk of neurological sequelae is 15% in cases born prior to 30 weeks.

Type III

In type III, there is cyclical/intermittent pattern of absent or reversed end-diastolic flow. There is 10–20% risk of sudden death of the growth-restricted fetus, which is unpredictable. Also, there is a high (up to 20%) risk of neurological morbidity in surviving larger twin.

Management of Twin Pregnancy Complicated by Selective Fetal Growth Restriction

Dichorionic Pregnancy

In dichorionic pregnancy affected by sFGR, follow-up is done with fetal Doppler approximately every 2 weeks, depending on the severity. As these twins have separate circulations, the pregnancy can be followed as in growth-restricted singleton pregnancy, monitoring for progressive deterioration of umbilical artery, of MCA (middle cerebral artery) and ductus venosus (DV) Doppler, and of biophysical profile scores.

Monochorionic Pregnancy

In monochorionic pregnancy affected by sFGR, fetal growth should be assessed at least every 2 weeks and fetal Doppler should be assessed at least weekly with umbilical artery and MCA Doppler. If umbilical artery Doppler is abnormal, DV Doppler should be done. The aim in managing these pregnancies is to prolong the pregnancy at least until viability is achieved, while at the same time avoiding single IUD with its associated serious consequences for the surviving co-twin.

Options for treatment including conservative management followed by early delivery, laser ablation, or cord occlusion of growth-restricted fetus in twins may be considered.

Timing of Delivery

The timing of delivery should be decided based on assessment of fetal well-being, interval growth, biophysical profile, DV waveform, and/or computerized cardiotocography (cCTG), when available. However, as the risk of IUD in these pregnancies is increased, delivery might be indicated even before abnormalities in the DV Doppler or the cCTG becomes evident.

MANAGING THE SURVIVING TWIN AFTER DEMISE OF ITS CO-TWIN

Following single IUD, many complications occur in monochorionic and dichorionic pregnancies.[11-13] Table 5 shows complications that occur after single fetus demise.

Mechanism of Injury in Co-twin in Monochorionic Twin Pregnancy

In monochorionic pregnancy, when one twin dies in utero, the surviving twin may then lose part of its circulating volume to the dead twin, leading to potentially severe hypotension in the survivor. This can lead to hypoperfusion of the brain and other organs, which can cause brain damage or death.

Vanishing Twin

It is the "disappearance" or "vanishing" of one of the twins in the second trimester, which was visualized in the first trimester. This occurs in 10–40% of all twin pregnancies.

Fetus Papyraceus

When fetal death occurs in slightly more advanced gestation, it may go undetected until delivery of a normal-appearing live infant along with a dead fetus that is barely identifiable.

Table 5: Complications after single fetal demise in the co-twin (%).

Complication	Monochorionic	Dichorionic
Death of the co-twin	15%	3%
Preterm delivery	68%	54%
Abnormal postnatal cranial imaging of the surviving twin	34%	16%
Neurodevelopmental impairment of surviving twin	26%	2%

It may be compressed appreciably—fetus compressus—or it may be flattened remarkably through desiccation—fetus papyraceus.

Management of Pregnancy after Death of One Twin in Monochorionic Pregnancy

After the death of one twin, pregnancy should be monitored with relevant expertise. Conservative management is followed, because the neurological harm has often already happened in the surviving co-twin by the time the demise of the twin has been diagnosed.

If the pregnancy is at term, then it makes sense to deliver without delay, but if it is preterm, prolonging the pregnancy for the benefit of the surviving twin (in terms of increased maturity) is usually recommended.

Parents should be counseled in detail about the risk that there might be significant long-term morbidity (neurological or otherwise) to the surviving twin, but that this damage may have taken place already and urgent delivery may be too late to prevent such harm.

If conservative management is being followed then fetal biometry and assessment of umbilical and MCA Doppler to rule out anemia should be scheduled every 2–4 weeks or earlier if abnormal Doppler, and delivery should be considered at 34–36 weeks after a course of maternal steroids and magnesium sulfate.

The fetal brain should be imaged around 4–6 weeks after the death of the co-twin to search for evidence of cerebral morbidity. In cases where there is a strong evidence that the surviving co-twin may have suffered serious neurological harm, late termination of pregnancy should be considered as an option, where it is legal. Neurodevelopmental assessment of the surviving twin at the age of 2 years should be done.

COMPLICATIONS SPECIFIC TO MONOCHORIONIC TWIN PREGNANCIES

These complications specific to monochorionic pregnancy include conjoined twins, TRAP sequence, TAPS, TTTS, and complications in monoamniotic pregnancy such as cord entanglement.

CONJOINED TWINS

Incidence

The incidence is from 1 in 50,000 to 1 in 100,000.[14]

Pathogenesis

For conjoined twins, the following two theories have been postulated:
1. *Fission theory*: It states that conjoined twins originate from an incomplete split of the embryonic axis after the 12th day of fertilization. Most conjoined twins are symmetrical.
2. *Fusion theory*: Fusion theory states that a fertilized egg completely separates, but stem cells (which search for similar cells) find like-stem cells on the other twin and fuse the twins together.

Ultrasound Diagnosis

Ultrasound diagnosis is possible as early as the ninth week of pregnancy, with most cases being detected usually before the midtrimester anomaly scan.

When scanning a MCMA pregnancy, it is always mandatory to check that fetal bodies and head are well apart and are moving independently.

Various types of conjoined twins, their incidence, extent, and separability during surgery have been mentioned in Table 6. Most conjoined twins are symmetrical. The most common variety is parapagus followed by thoracopagus and omphalopagus.

Conjoined twins explained above are symmetric conjoined twins. Asymmetric conjoined twins include parasitic twin and fetus in fetu (Fig. 6).

Parasitic Twin

This is a grossly defective fetus or merely fetal parts, attached externally to a relatively normal twin. A parasitic twin usually consists of externally attached supernumerary limbs, often with some viscera. Classically, however, a functional heart or brain is absent. Parasites are believed to result from demise of the defective twin, with its surviving tissues attached to and vascularized by its normal twin.

Table 6: Classification of conjoined twins.[15]

Type	Incidence	Extent	Separability
Cephalopagus	11%	Top of head to umbilicus (Fig. 5)	None
Thoracopagus	19%	Thorax, upper abdomen, and conjoined heart	Rare
Omphalopagus	18%	Thorax, upper abdomen, and separate heart	Likely 82% success
Ischiopagus	11%	Lower abdomen and genitourinary tract	Likely 63% success
Parapagus	28%	Pelvis, variable trunk, diprosopus-2 faces, and dicephalus-2 heads	Rare
Craniopagus	5%	Cranial vault	Unlikely without sequelae
Rachipagus	2%	Vertebra column	None reported
Pygopagus	6%	Sacrum	Likely; 68% success

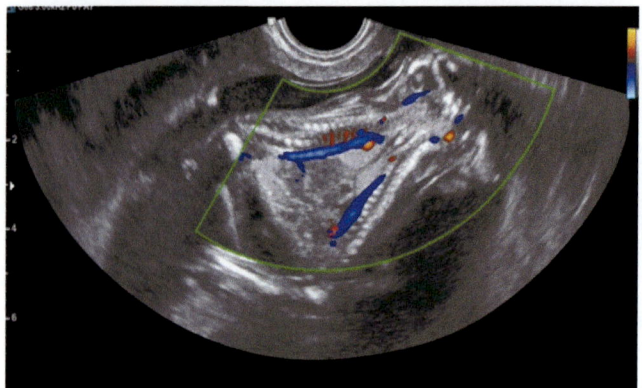

Fig. 5: Cephalopagus conjoined twins where the two fetuses are joined from head to umbilicus.

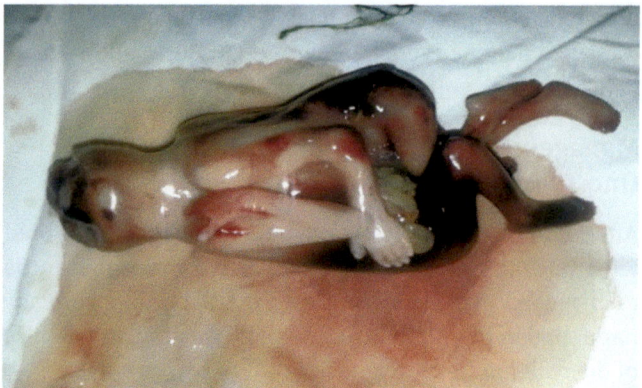

Fig. 6: Postabortion picture of the same cephalopagus conjoined twins.

Fetus in Fetu

Early in development, one embryo may be enfolded within its twin. Normal development of this rare parasitic twin usually arrests in the first trimester. Classically, vertebral or axial bones are found in these fetiform masses, whereas the heart and brain are lacking. These masses are typically supported by their host by a few large parasitic vessels.

Management

- Patient should be counseled regarding the outcome of the fetus and complexity of situation and the problems with surgery of the conjoined twins.
- As most cases of conjoined twins are being detected usually before the mid-trimester anomaly scan, termination of pregnancy can be considered.
- Surgical separation of an almost completely joined twin pair may be successful if essential organs are not shared.
- Viable conjoined twins should be delivered by cesarean. For the purpose of pregnancy termination, however, vaginal delivery is possible because the union is most often pliable.
- Still, dystocia is common, and if the fetuses are mature, vaginal delivery may be traumatic to the uterus or cervix.

TWIN REVERSED ARTERIAL PERFUSION SEQUENCE

It is also known as an *acardiac twin*. In the TRAP sequence, there is usually a normally formed donor twin that has features of heart failure and a recipient twin that lacks a heart (acardius) and other structures.

Incidence

The incidence is 1 in 35,000.

Pathophysiology

Twin reversed arterial perfusion sequence is caused by a large artery-to-artery placental shunt, often also accompanied by a vein-to-vein shunt. Within the single, shared placenta, arterial perfusion pressure of the donor twin exceeds that in the recipient twin, who thus receives reverse blood flow of deoxygenated arterial blood from its co-twin. This "used" arterial blood reaches the recipient twin through its umbilical arteries and preferentially goes to its iliac vessels. Thus, only the lower body is perfused, and disrupted growth and development of the upper body result. Because of this vascular connection, the normal donor twin must not only support its own circulation but also pump its blood through the underdeveloped acardiac recipient. This may lead to cardiomegaly and high-output heart failure in the normal twin.

Ultrasound Diagnosis

It is feasible from the first trimester itself:
- First, we should make a diagnosis of monochorionic pregnancy, and then the absence of heartbeat in acardiac twin is demonstrated, with other vascularity in acardiac fetus visible.
- Care should be taken not to mistake it for monochorionic pregnancy with demise of one twin.
- The parasitic twin may appear amorphous, edematous mass or as a partially formed fetus, or as a fetus with almost normal body, usually with abnormalities of the cephalic pole.
- Rarely fetus may show some active limb movements.
- Color Doppler is very helpful in establishing the diagnosis as it demonstrates the presence of blood vessels inside the TRAP fetus despite the absence of heartbeat, located alongside a bladder-like structure in the pelvis of the acardiac fetus that sometimes continues

with an aorta toward the upper part of the body, if the latter is present.
- Directional color or power Doppler tells the reverse perfusion of the cord and the cord pattern.

Classification

- *Acardius acephalus*: Failure of head growth
- *Acardius myelacephalus*: A partially developed head with identifiable limbs
- *Acardius amorphous*: Failure of any recognizable structure.

Differential Diagnosis

The only differential diagnosis is twin monochorionic pregnancy with single fetal demise; however, the abnormal body of the acardiac twin rules out single fetal demise in a monochorionic pregnancy.

Management

- Once the diagnosis of TRAP sequence is established, the pump twin should be assessed thoroughly for any anomalies as 10% of the pump twins are associated with major malformations.
- Echocardiography should be done to rule out any impending cardiac failure; if that is the case, cord occlusion of the acardiac twin should be considered.
- If cord occlusion is done after 18 weeks, survival rate of the pump twin is around 94%.[16] The reason for high success of cord occlusion is because it blocks the growth of acardiac twin and at the same time prevents overload and heart failure in the pump twin.
- Karyotyping should also be considered in the pump twin.

TWIN ANEMIA POLYCYTHEMIA SEQUENCE

This form of chronic fetofetal transfusion is characterized by significant hemoglobin differences between the donor and the recipient twins without the discrepancies in amniotic fluid volumes typical of TTTS.

Incidence

The incidence of TAPS occurring spontaneously in MCDA twins is up to 5%. However, it may complicate up to 13% of cases of TTTS following laser ablation.[17]

Pathophysiology

Twin anemia polycythemia sequence is believed to be due to the presence of miniscule arteriovenous anastomoses

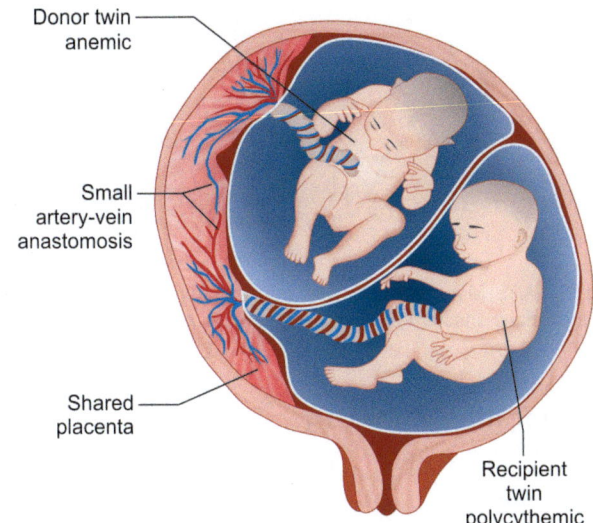

Fig. 7: Monochorionic diamniotic twins with twin anemia polycythemia sequence (TAPS), small arteriovenous anastomoses leading to slow transfusion of blood from one twin to another. The donor twin has become pale and the recipient twin has become plethoric.

(<1 mm) which allows slow transfusion of blood from the donor to the recipient, leading to highly discordant hemoglobin concentrations at birth (Fig. 7).

Spontaneous TAPS usually occurs after 26 weeks and iatrogenic TAPS develops within 5 weeks of a procedure.

Ultrasound Diagnosis

It is diagnosed antenatally by MCA-PSV >1.5 multiples of the median (MoM) in the donor and <1.0 MoM in the recipient twin, indicating anemia in the donor and polycythemia in the recipient.

Additional ultrasound findings in TAPS include differences in placental echogenicity and thickness, with a bright, thickened section associated with the donor and an echolucent thin section associated with the recipient.

The polycythemic twin might have a "starry sky" appearance of the liver pattern due to diminished echogenicity of the liver parenchyma and increased brightness of the portal venule walls.

Postnatal Diagnosis

The criteria for diagnosis of TAPS include the following:[18,19]
- A difference in hemoglobin concentration between the twins of more than 8 g/dL and at least one of either reticulocyte count ratio greater than 1.[7]
- Small vascular anastomoses (<1 mm in diameter) in the placenta (Fig. 8).

Screening

For the screening for TAPS, the MCA-PSV should be measured from 20 weeks onward in both fetuses and during the follow-up of cases treated for TTTS.

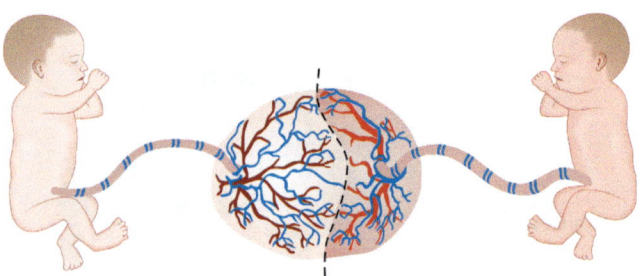

Fig. 8: TAPS: Monochorionic twins with shared placenta and the small arteriovenous anastomoses, showing plethora of one twin and anemia of the other twin.

Classification of Severity

Antenatal and postnatal staging of TAPS is shown in Table 7.[18,19]

Management and Counseling

- In monochorionic twins complicated by TAPS, the risk of neurodevelopmental delay is increased (20%). Therefore, brain imaging during the third trimester and neurodevelopmental assessment at the age of 2 years are recommended.
- The line of treatment in TAPS depends on the gestational age at diagnosis, parental choice, severity of the disease, and technical feasibility of intrauterine therapy. Therefore, the management of twin pregnancies complicated by TAPS should be individualized.
- The various options include the following:
  - Conservative management
  - Early delivery
  - Laser ablation
  - Intrauterine blood transfusion (IUT) for the anemic twin
  - Combined IUT for the anemic twin and partial exchange transfusion to dilute the blood of the polycythemic twin.

TWIN-TWIN TRANSFUSION SYNDROME

In TTTS, blood is transfused from a donor twin to its recipient sibling such that the donor may eventually become anemic and its growth may be restricted. In contrast, the recipient becomes polycythemic and may develop circulatory overload which menifest as hydrops. The donor twin is pale and its recipient sibling is plethoric. Similarly, one portion of the placenta often appears pale compared with the remainder. The recipient neonate may have circulatory overload from heart failure and severe hypervolemia and hyperviscosity. Occlusive thrombosis is another concern. Finally, polycythemia in the recipient twin may lead to severe hyperbilirubinemia and kernicterus.

Table 7: Antenatal and postnatal staging of TAPS.

Stage	Antenatal staging	Postnatal staging: Intertwin Hb difference (g/dL)
1	Donor MCA-PSV>1.5 MoM and recipient MCA-PSV<1.0 MoM, without other signs of fetal compromise	>8.0
2	Donor MCA-PSV>1.7 MoM and recipient MCA-PSV<0.8 MoM, without other signs of fetal compromise	>11.0
3	Stage 1 or 2 and cardiac compromise in donor (UA-AREDF, UV pulsatile flow, or DV increased or reversed flow)	>14.0
4	Hydrops of donor twin	>17.0
5	Death of both fetuses, preceded by TAPS	>20.0

(TAPS: twin anemia polycythemia sequence; MCA-PSV: middle cerebral arterial peak systolic velocity; MoM: multiples of the median; Hb: hemoglobin; UA-AREDF: umbilical artery-absent or reversed end diastolic flow; UV: umbilical vein; DV: ductus venosus)

Twin-twin transfusion syndrome affects 10–15% of monochorionic twin pregnancies and is associated with increased perinatal mortality and morbidity; if untreated, it leads to fetal demise in up to 90% of cases, with morbidity rates in survivors of over 50%.

Incidence

The incidence is 1–3 per 100,000 live births.

Pathophysiology

Chronic TTTS is the result of unidirectional flow through arteriovenous anastomoses between the monochorionic twins. Deoxygenated blood from a donor placental artery is pumped into a cotyledon shared by the recipient. Once the oxygen exchange is completed in the chorionic villus, the oxygenated blood leaves the cotyledon via a placental vein of the recipient twin. If this flow is not compensated by arterioarterial anastomoses, this unidirectional flow leads to an imbalance in blood volumes.

Ultrasound Diagnosis and Staging

- Early prediction of TTTS:
  - *Increased NT*: Increase in the NT in one or both of the fetuses is predictive of TTTS.
  - *Abnormal DV*: Another early marker of TTTS is abnormal Doppler flow velocity waveform in the ductus of the recipient twin.
  - *Intertwin membrane folding*: It is an early manifestation of amniotic fluid discrepancy, the folding points toward the recipient amniotic sac.

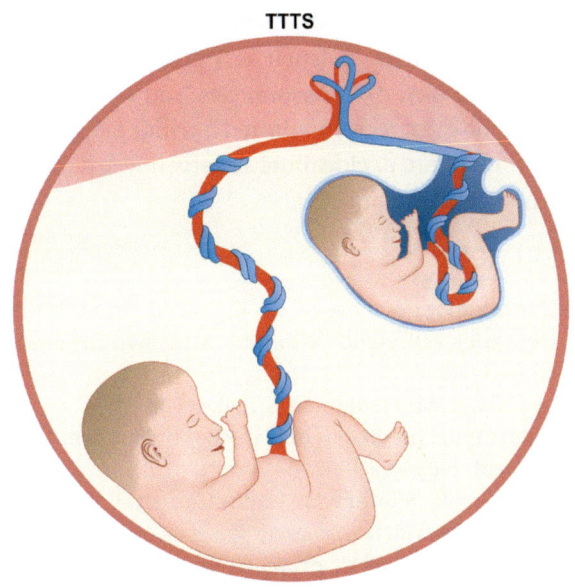

Fig. 9: Monochorionic diamniotic twins with twin-to-twin transfusion syndrome (TTTS) showing oligohydramnios in the donor twin, and polyhydramnios in the recipient twin due to unidirectional blood flow from donor to recipient twin. TTTS has large A-A anastomoses.

Table 8: Quintero classification of TTTS.	
Stage	Classification
I	Polyhydramnios-oligohydramnios sequence: DVP > 8 cm in recipient twin and DVP <2 cm in donor twin
II	Bladder in donor twin not visible on ultrasound
III	Absent or reversed umbilical artery diastolic flow, reversed ductus venosus a-wave flow, and pulsatile umbilical venous flow in either twin
IV	Hydrops in one or both twins
V	Death of one or both twins

(TTTS: twin-twin transfusion syndrome; DVP: deepest vertical pocket)

- The diagnosis of TTTS requires the presence of significant amniotic fluid discordance between the donor and the recipient twin. The "donor" twin has a DVP of <2 cm (oligohydramnios) and the "recipient" twin has a DVP >8 cm (polyhydramnios) (Fig. 9). The most widely used classification system is the one given by Quintero (Table 8). But the problem with this classification system is that Stage 1 does not always mean good prognosis and, also it does not represent a chronological order of deterioration, e.g., Stage 1 can become Stage 5 without passing through Stages 2, 3, and 4, and it does not predict survival well after treatment. But, still this is the most widely used classification system.

Screening

In monochorionic twin pregnancy, the screening for TTTS should start at 16 weeks, with scans repeated every 2 weeks thereafter.

Screening plays an important role in the management of TTTS as early diagnosis and may allow intervention with fetoscopic laser ablation, which significantly improves the prognosis in TTTS. Laser treatment in these pregnancies results in 60–70% survival of both twins and 80–90% survival of at least one twin.

Management

- Monochorionic twin pregnancies with uncomplicated amniotic fluid discordance (the discordance is not the typical 8 cm/2 cm, which we use in the diagnosis of TTTS) and normal umbilical artery Doppler generally have a good outcome and a low risk of progression to severe TTTS and can be followed up on a weekly basis to exclude progression to TTTS.
- For *Quintero Stage II* and above, laser ablation is the treatment of choice. Following laser treatment, the recurrence rate of TTTS is up to 14%, which is likely to be due to anastomoses missed at the time of the initial laser treatment. The risk of recurrence of TTTS and occurrence of TAPS is reduced by use of the Solomon technique (equatorial laser dichorionization) compared with the highly-selective technique.
- Conservative management with close surveillance or laser ablation can be considered for Quintero Stage I. Both conservative and laser ablation have similar results in Stage I. If conservative management is chosen for Quintero Stage I, worsening polyhydramnios, maternal discomfort, and shortening of the cervical length are considered "rescue" criteria signaling a need to proceed with fetoscopic laser treatment.
- *Follow-up after laser treatment*:
  - After laser treatment, normalization of amniotic fluid occurs in 14 days[20] and the normalization of cardiac function in recipient occurs in 1 month.[21]
  - A common practice is weekly ultrasound assessment for the first 2 weeks after treatment, reducing to alternate weeks following clinical evidence of resolution.
  - At each ultrasound scan we should assess the DVP, biometry (every 2 weeks), and umbilical artery, MCA, MCA-PSV and DV Doppler in both fetuses. There should be a detailed assessment of the brain, heart, and limbs (risk of amputation secondary to thrombi or amniotic bands) during these follow-up scans.
- When laser treatment is not available, serial amnioreduction is an acceptable alternative after 26 weeks' gestation.
- Another option for the management of severe TTTS is selective termination of pregnancy using bipolar diathermy, laser coagulation, or RFA of one of the

umbilical cords. This means that this fetus is sacrificed in the hope of protecting the other twin from death or cerebral damage.

Timing of Delivery

For monochorionic pregnancy previously treated for TTTS, delivery should be done at 34 weeks after a course of steroids.

Similarly this criteria can be applied in all monochorionic twins, with delivery at 34 weeks of gestation for persisting abnormalities and up to 37 weeks where there is complete resolution.

MONOCHORIONIC MONOAMNIOTIC TWINS

Only about 1% of all monozygotic twins will share an amniotic sac. Said another way, approximately 1 in 20 monochorionic twins are monoamniotic. Perinatal loss rate before 16 weeks' gestation is as high as 50% and most of these losses are attributable to fetal abnormalities and spontaneous miscarriages.

Ultrasound Diagnosis

The presence of monochorionic pregnancy with both the fetuses in a single amniotic sac is best seen at 11–14 weeks.

Umbilical cord entanglement is present in almost all monoamniotic twins evaluated systematically by ultrasound and color Doppler, and cord entanglement does not contribute to prenatal morbidity and mortality in monoamniotic twin pregnancy.[22]

Management

In MCMA twin pregnancy with discordant anomaly, TRAP sequence, severe TTTS, or sFGR, selective reduction by cord occlusion and transaction are recommended to prevent fetal demise of the other twin due to cord accidents.

Timing of Delivery

Monochorionic-monoamniotic twin pregnancies are at increased risk of IUD compared with other types of twin pregnancy and should be delivered by cesarean section between 32 weeks and 34 weeks of gestation. This is based on the finding that after 32+4 weeks gestation, the risk of IUD is greater in ongoing MCMA pregnancy compared with the risk of nonrespiratory neonatal complications when the twins are delivered.[23]

CONCLUSION

Multiple pregnancy is high-risk pregnancy. Dichorionic twin sIUGR and FGR require follow-up with color Doppler. Monochorionic twins share placenta and placental circulation. In situations such as TTTS, TAPS or TRAPS, large or small A-A, A-V anastomoses lead to in utero risk which can be effectively monitored by color Doppler twice month or earlier to decide timely intervention/delivery for better neonatal outcome.

REFERENCES

1. Cunningham G, Leveno KJ, Bloom SL, et al. Williams Obstetrics, 24th edition. New York: McGraw-Hill Education; 2014. p. 896.
2. Lee YM, Cleary-Goldman J, Thaker HM, et al. Antenatal sonographic prediction of twin chorionicity. Am J Obstet Gynecol. 2006;195:863-7.
3. Lopriore E, Sueters M, Middeldorp JM, et al. Twin pregnancies with two separate placental masses can still be monochorionic and have vascular anastomoses. Am J Obstet Gynecol. 2006;194:804-8.
4. National Collaborating Center for Women's and Children's Health (UK). Multiple Pregnancy: The Management of Twin and Triplet Pregnancies in the Antenatal Period. RCOG Press: London; 2011.
5. Gil MM, Quezada MS, Revello R, et al. Analysis of cell-free DNA in maternal blood in screening for fetal aneuploidies: updated meta-analysis. Ultrasound Obstet Gynecol. 2015;45:249-66.
6. Lewi L, Blickstein I, Van Schoubroeck D, et al. Diagnosis and management of heterokaryotypic monochorionic twins. Am J Med Genet A. 2006;140:272-5.
7. Lewi L, Gratacos E, Ortibus E, et al. Pregnancy and infant outcome of 80 consecutive cord coagulations in complicated monochorionic multiple pregnancies. Am J Obstet Gynecol. 2006;194:782-9.
8. Lewi L, Jani J, Blickstein I, et al. The outcome of monochorionic diamniotic twin gestations in the era of invasive fetal therapy: a prospective cohort study. Am J Obstet Gynecol. 2008;199:514.e1-8.
9. Baxi LV, Walsh CA. Monoamniotic twins in contemporary practice: a single-center study of perinatal outcomes. J Matern Fetal Neonatal Med. 2010;23:506-10.
10. Paladini D, Volpe P. Ultrasound of Congenital Fetal Anomalies: Differential Diagnosis and Prognostic Indicators. Florida: CRC Press; 2014. p. 455.
11. Ong SSC, Zamora J, Khan KS, et al. Prognosis for the co-twin following single-twin death: a systematic review. BJOG. 2006;113:992-8.
12. Hillman SC, Morris RK, Kilby MD. Co-twin prognosis after single fetal death: a systematic review and meta-analysis. Obstet Gynecol. 2011;118:928-40.
13. Shek NW, Hillman SC, Kilby MD. Single-twin demise: pregnancy outcome. Best Pract Res Clin Obstet Gynaecol. 2014;28:249-63.
14. Rees AE, Vujanic GM, Williams WM. Epidemic of conjoined twins in Cardiff. Br J Obstet Gynaecol. 1993;100(4):388-91.

15. Osmanağaoğlu MA, Aran T, Güven S, et al. Thoracopagus conjoined twins: a case report. ISRN Obstet Gynecol. 2011;2011:238360.
16. Rossi AC, D'addario V. Umbilical cord occlusion for selective feticide in complicated monochorionic twins: a systematic review of literature. Am J Obstet Gynecol. 2009;200:123-9.
17. Robyr R, Lewi L, Salomon LJ, et al. Prevalence and management of late fetal complications following successful selective laser coagulation of chorionic plate anastomoses in twin-to-twin transfusion syndrome. Am J Obstet Gynecol. 2006;194:796-803.
18. Slaghekke F, Kist WJ, Oepkes D, et al. Twin anemia-polycythemia sequence: diagnostic criteria, classification, perinatal management and outcome. Fetal Diagn Ther. 2010;27:181-90.
19. Lopriore E, Slaghekke F, Oepkes D, et al. Hematological characteristics in neonates with twin anemia-polycythemia sequence (TAPS). Prenat Diagn. 2010;30:251-5.
20. Assaf SA, Korst LM, Chmait RH. Normalization of amniotic fluid levels after fetoscopic laser surgery for twin-twin transfusion syndrome. J Ultrasound Med. 2010;29:1431-6.
21. Mieghem TV, Lewi L, Gucciardo L, et al. The fetal heart in twin-to-twin transfusion syndrome. Int J Pediatr. 2010; 2010:379792.
22. Rossi AC, Prefumo F. Impact of cord entanglement on perinatal outcome of monoamniotic twins: a systematic review of the literature. Ultrasound Obstet Gynecol. 2013; 41:131-5.
23. Van Mieghem T, De Heus R, Lewi L, et al. Prenatal management of monoamniotic twin pregnancies. Obstet Gynecol. 2014;124:498-506.

13

Ultrasound in Second Trimester
Chinmayee Ratha

INTRODUCTION

Ultrasound has become an extremely important method of monitoring fetal growth and development in pregnancy. It helps not only in reassuring parents about the well-being of the fetus, but also in vital procedures such as diagnosing fetal anomalies and growth disorders, and in the screening for fetal aneuploidies and maternal complications in pregnancy. In contemporary obstetrics, starting from establishment of viability and dating in early pregnancy till decisions for delivery are taken near term or preterm in special cases, the role of ultrasound cannot be undermined. It is therefore important that all practitioners understand and update themselves about how best to use this powerful tool in pregnancy care.

This chapter will focus specifically on the role of ultrasound in the second trimester of pregnancy. To achieve the best possible results of the second trimester scan, use of optimal equipment is of paramount importance. The ISUOG (International Society of Ultrasound in Obstetrics and Gynecology) has recommended some criteria in its practice guidelines (2010) which include the following features:
- Real-time, grayscale ultrasound capabilities
- Transabdominal transducers (3–5 MHz range)
- Adjustable acoustic power output controls with output display standards
- Freeze frame capabilities
- Electronic calipers
- Capacity to print/store images
- Regular maintenance and servicing for optimum performance of equipment

SCOPE OF THE SECOND TRIMESTER SCAN

In the second trimester of pregnancy, ultrasound can be used for the following indications:
- Fetal biometry
- Targeted imaging for fetal anomalies (TIFFA) scan
- Placental localization
- Uterine artery Doppler studies
- Cervical length assessment

FETAL BIOMETRY IN THE SECOND TRIMESTER

The standard fetal biometric measurements reported on the second trimester ultrasound are as follows (Table 1):
- Biparietal diameter (BPD)
- Occipitofrontal diameter (OFD)
- Head circumference (HC)
- Transabdominal diameter (TAD)
- Anteroposterior abdominal diameter (APAD)
- Abdominal circumference (AC)
- Femur length (FL)

These measurements when calculated together based on formulas give the estimated fetal weight. The measurements can be taken in millimeter or centimeter and then plotted on graphs depicting centiles for that stage of gestation. It is reiterated here that the second-trimester biometry should be corroborated as per the dating established in the first trimester ideally. Once the dates have been allotted in the first trimester, they should not be changed in the second trimester, rather the growth pattern can be evaluated by analyzing

Table 1: Standard fetal biometric measurements.	
Biparietal diameter (BPD)	This is measured on the transventricular plane perpendicular to falx cerebri at the broadest part of the skull, from the outer margin of proximal parietal bone to inner margin of distal parietal bone
Occipitofrontal diameter (OFD)	This is measured on the transventricular plane along the falx cerebri, perpendicular to the BPD between the outer edges of the calvarium
Head circumference (HC)	It is measured at the outer edges of calvarium—in many cases when both BPD and OFD are measured, the machine automatically calculates the HC using formula
Transverse abdominal diameter	This is measured on the transverse section of the abdomen, where the stomach bubble is seen and the entry of umbilical vein to DV is seen as a J shape curving toward right with a single rib on each side. It is the measurement of the transverse diameter between the outer edges of the abdomen
Anteroposterior abdominal diameter	This is measured on the transverse section of the abdomen. It is the anteroposterior diameter of the abdomen
Abdominal circumference	This is measured on the transverse section of the abdomen as the outer margin of this section. It is the first measurement that is altered in IUGR. The smallest measurement is most accurate
Femur length	In the second trimester, it can be used to estimate the gestational age of the fetus. All long bones must be measured from end to end excluding the epiphysis. When measuring the femur length, the long axis of the femur should be aligned with the transducer and the tip to tip should be measured

(DV: ductus venosus; IUGR: intrauterine growth restriction)

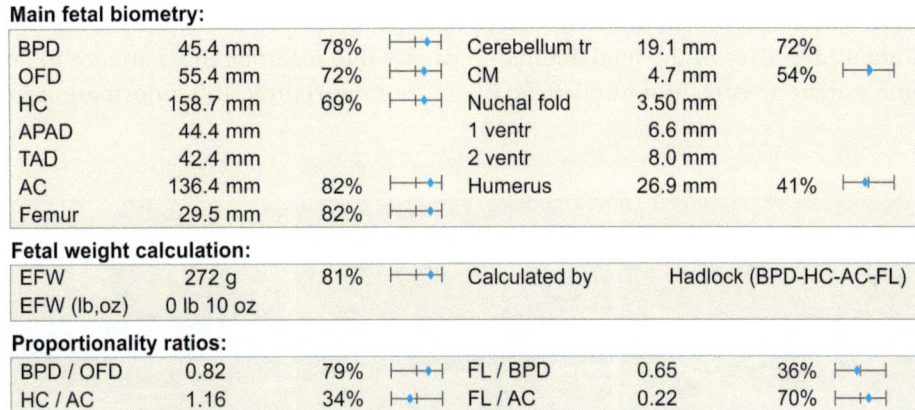

Main fetal biometry:

BPD	45.4 mm	78%		Cerebellum tr	19.1 mm	72%	
OFD	55.4 mm	72%		CM	4.7 mm	54%	
HC	158.7 mm	69%		Nuchal fold	3.50 mm		
APAD	44.4 mm			1 ventr	6.6 mm		
TAD	42.4 mm			2 ventr	8.0 mm		
AC	136.4 mm	82%		Humerus	26.9 mm	41%	
Femur	29.5 mm	82%					

Fetal weight calculation:

EFW	272 g	81%		Calculated by	Hadlock (BPD-HC-AC-FL)
EFW (lb,oz)	0 lb 10 oz				

Proportionality ratios:

BPD / OFD	0.82	79%		FL / BPD	0.65	36%	
HC / AC	1.16	34%		FL / AC	0.22	70%	

Fig. 1: Second trimester biometry—appropriate for gestational age.

Main fetal biometry:

BPD	40.4 mm	1%		Cerebellum tr	18.6 mm	28%	
OFD	52.7 mm	5%		CM	4.0 mm	24%	
HC	146.9 mm	1%		Nuchal fold	2.90 mm		
APAD	36.3 mm			1st ventr	5.1 mm		
TAD	31.8 mm			2nd ventr	5.1 mm		
AC	107.1 mm	<1%		Humerus	23.1 mm	<1%	
Femur	22.1 mm	<1%					

Fetal weight calculation:

EFW	169 g	<1%		Calculated by	Hadlock (BPD-HC-AC-FL)
EFW (lb,oz)	0 lb 6 oz				

Proportionality ratios:

BPD / OFD	0.77	26%		FL / BPD	0.55	<1%	
HC / AC	1.37	>99%		FL / AC	0.21	28%	

Fig. 2: Second trimester biometry showing fetal growth restriction.

the centiles of various biometry parameters at this stage. In these examples of biometry documentation, Figure 1 shows an appropriately growing fetus while Figure 2 shows a fetus with growth restriction where biometry parameters are lagging behind the gestational age in the second trimester.

TARGETED IMAGING FOR FETAL ANOMALIES

The midtrimester anomaly scan for routine screening of fetal anatomy in the second trimester must be offered to all pregnant women. This helps to reassure most parents about normal anatomy of the fetus and also helps in detection of fetal structural abnormalities in 2–3% of pregnancies where they are expected in an apparently "low-risk" population. Detection of congenital anomalies is vital in planning reasonable obstetric care for any pregnant woman. Hence, every pregnant woman should be offered the second-trimester ultrasound screening—the "midtrimester anomaly scan." This scan must also be conducted in a systematic manner so as to detect any fetal abnormalities that may be amenable to in-utero treatment or as in lethal cases, early termination may be offered, saving the parents the agony of giving birth to a child with a serious debilitating condition due to either a physical or a mental subnormality as a result of detectable structural abnormalities.

As per the ISUOG guideline on the midtrimester anomaly scan, the main objectives of the fetal anomaly scan are to determine cardiac activity, fetal number, fetal age and size, basic fetal anatomy, placental appearance, and location.

After making a general survey of the uterine cavity to establish the number and lie of fetus/fetuses, it is important to document fetal cardiac activity. Then, a detailed evaluation of fetal structure from "head-to-toe" is performed at this scan. There are recommended "standard views" of each part of the body, some examples are shown in Figures 3 and 4. This helps to ensure uniformity of evaluation and minimizes the possibility of interoperator differences with optimal detection rate of relevant structural anomalies.

The Fetal Medicine Foundation (FMF), UK, and the ISUOG have recommended standard criteria to complete the checklist of evaluation of fetal anatomy (Table 2). The points to be noted on fetal structural assessment are given in Table 2.

Despite the fact that the second trimester anomaly scan is an important checkpoint for almost 90–95% of major structural anomalies, the fact remains that "all" fetal anomalies cannot be determined by ultrasound scan. We are used to inserting this sentence in our disclaimers but more importantly, this information must be conveyed

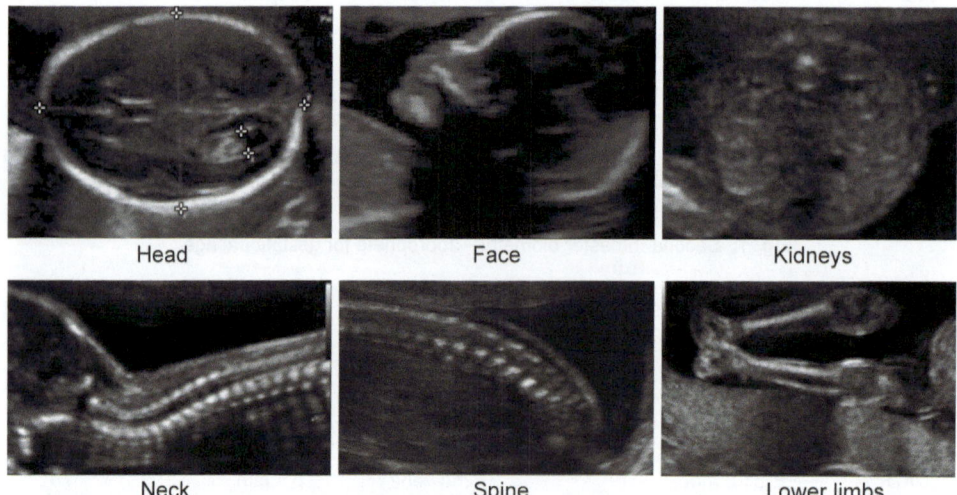

Fig. 3: Standard views for some important fetal structural evaluation at the midtrimester scan.

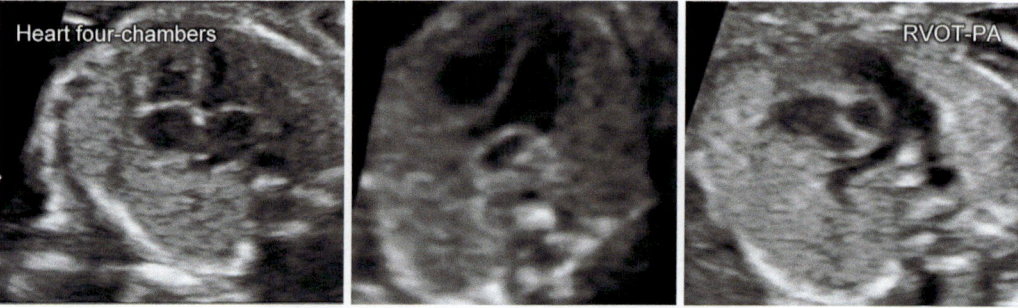

Fig. 4: Cardiac structure evaluation at an anomaly scan.

sensitively to the parents so as to allow them to have realistic expectations from the scan. Some fetal anomalies cannot be seen on ultrasound and some structural issues such as late-onset microcephaly, intestinal obstructive pathologies, nonlethal skeletal dysplasias, cerebral ventriculomegaly, and congenital heart blocks may become apparent only later in pregnancy.

Detection of problems in the third trimester after an apparently normal second-trimester evaluation is a cause of a lot of anguish to both parents and doctors. It is imperative, therefore, to include parents in an appropriate "pretest" counseling explaining to them that although a detailed anatomy check is undertaken, detection of structural anomalies will never be 100%. Detection rates will be different depending on the type of anomaly, the gestational age at scanning, the skill of the operator, the quality of the equipment used, and the time allocated for the scan. It is therefore also suggestive that all these parameters need to be optimized to obtain the best results from an anomaly scan.

Table 3 is based on the NHS, UK, patient information leaflet for anomaly scans and it shows the expected detection rate of various fetal anomalies at this scan.

Table 3 can be used to explain the limitations of the scan to the parents. It may be useful to provide a "pretest" information leaflet to them so that they are well informed about the scope and limitations of the scan.

Every operator must make an attempt of obtaining the standard views and completing the checklist for fetal anatomy survey. If the standard views are unattainable despite correct position and machine settings, an anomaly is suspected. Based on the operator's knowledge of fetal anatomy, the anomaly is identified and defined. Presence of any anomaly must alert the operator to look for any other issue as isolated abnormalities and multisystem anomalies are different in terms of their cause, effect, and recurrence risk.

Some common fetal anomalies are depicted in Figures 5 to 8.

In case, a fetal anomaly is detected on the second trimester anomaly scan, a detailed evaluation of the fetus must be done using advanced methods of evaluation available in contemporary medicine to firmly establish the anomaly and its severity. Fetal anomalies detected maybe "lethal" or "not lethal" but associated with significant postnatal morbidity and long-term disability. Some fetal

Table 2: Checklist of fetal anatomy evaluation in the second trimester scan.

Part examined	Points to be noted at the "anomaly scan"
Skull	Examination of the integrity and normal shape and measurement of the biparietal diameter and the head circumference
Brain	Examination of the cerebral ventricles, choroids plexuses, mid-brain, and posterior fossa (cerebellum and cisterna magna), and measurement of the posterior horn of the lateral ventricle
Face	Examination of the median profile, presence of both orbits, intact upper lip, presence of the mouth, and the evaluation of the nasal bone in the midsagittal view
Neck	Measurement of the nuchal fold thickness and absence of neck masses
Abdomen	Examination of the stomach, liver, kidneys, bladder, abdominal wall, and umbilicus, and measurement of the abdominal circumference
Spine	Examination in longitudinal, coronal, and transverse views. No spinal defects or masses
Limbs	Examination of the femur, tibia, fibula, humerus, radius, ulna, hands, and feet (including shape and echogenicity of the long bones and mobility at the joints), and measurement of the femur length
Thorax	Examination of the shape of the thorax, the lungs and diaphragm
Heart	Presence of cardiac activity, examination of the rate and rhythm, four-chamber view, and outflow tracts (Fig. 4)

Table 3: Detection rates of common anomalies on targeted imaging for fetal anomalies.

Condition	Predicted detection rate
Anencephaly	98%
Open spina bifida	90%
Cleft lip	75%
Diaphragmatic hernia	60%
Gastroschisis	98%
Exomphalos	80%
Serious cardiac abnormalities	50%

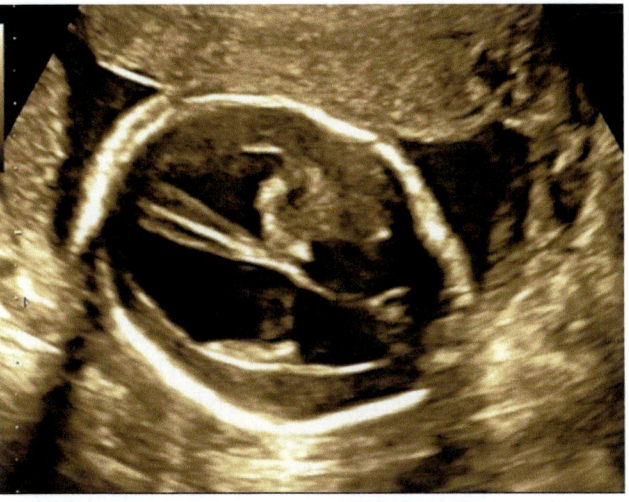

Fig. 5: Bilateral cerebral ventriculomegaly.

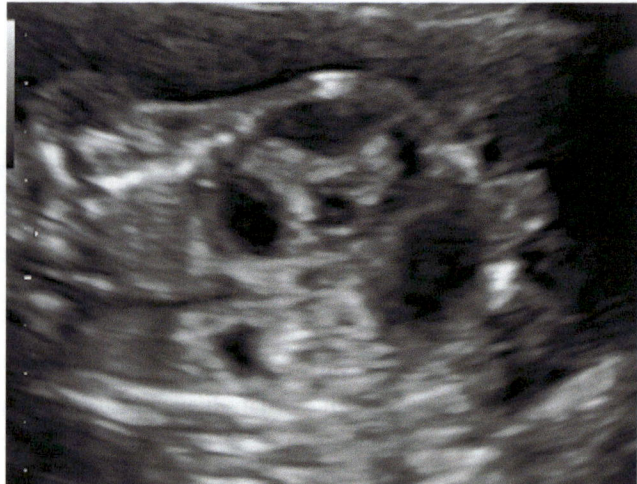

Fig. 6: Multicystic dysplastic kidneys.

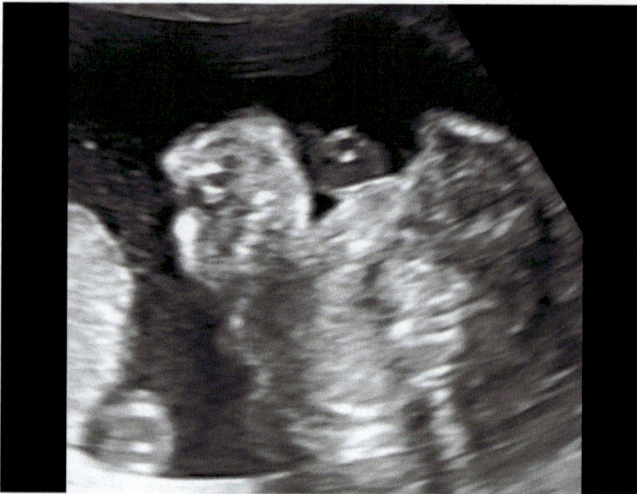

Fig. 7: Unilateral cleft lip.

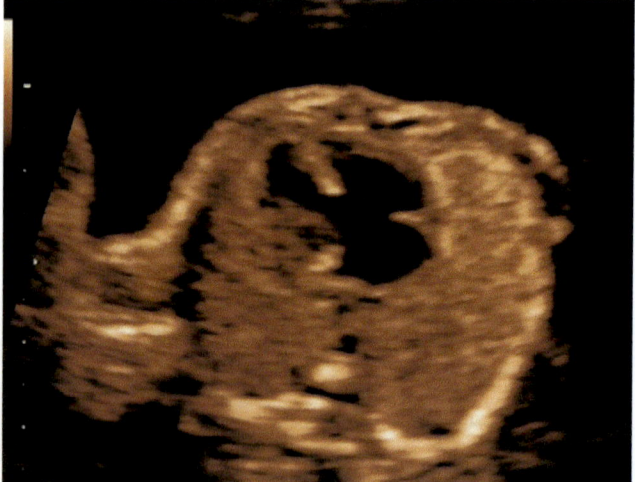

Fig. 8: Atrioventricular septal defect.

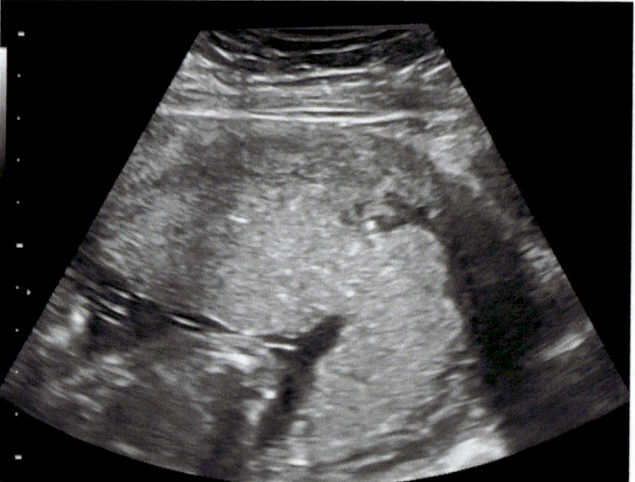

Fig. 9: Placenta previa.

conditions can be offered potential intrauterine therapy to prevent morbidity and mortality, while others will require postnatal investigation or treatment and lead to a reasonably good outcome. Thus, timely diagnosis of fetal anomalies allows for institution of a relevant multidisciplinary care team for counseling the parents, allowing them to clarify all their doubts, and apprehensions summarily, and planning further care.

PLACENTAL LOCALIZATION IN THE SECOND TRIMESTER

The placenta is an important organ mediating nutrient and oxygen transfer from the mother to the fetus. It is a very vascular organ and can be a cause of life-threatening obstetric hemorrhage. If the placenta is in the lower uterine segment or covering the internal os (complete placenta previa in Fig. 9), the categorization of the pregnancy and further care protocol is significantly changed. Therefore, localization of placenta is important in the second trimester scans. If the placental lower edge is 3 cm or more away from the internal os, it is classified as "high" and that is reassuring (Fig. 10). If the placenta is not covering the internal os but within 3 cm of the same, it is a "low lying" placenta (Fig. 11) but has the tendency to "move" away from the os further as the pregnancy progresses and lower segment develops. These cases should be kept on follow up and reassessed in the third trimester. The second trimester scan thus helps in triaging cases based on placental location.

UTERINE ARTERY DOPPLER STUDIES IN THE SECOND TRIMESTER

Blood flow patterns through the uterine arteries are indicative of the distal resistance in the uteroplacental bed. In case of high resistance, the spectral flow pattern of the uterine artery shows impeded flow in diastole with

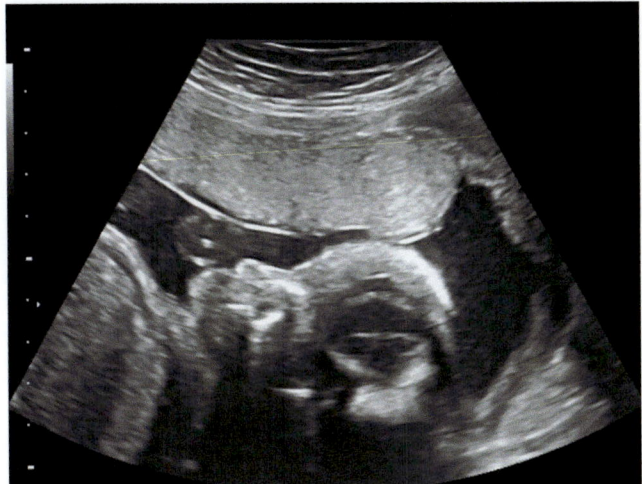

Fig. 10: Placenta—anterior high.

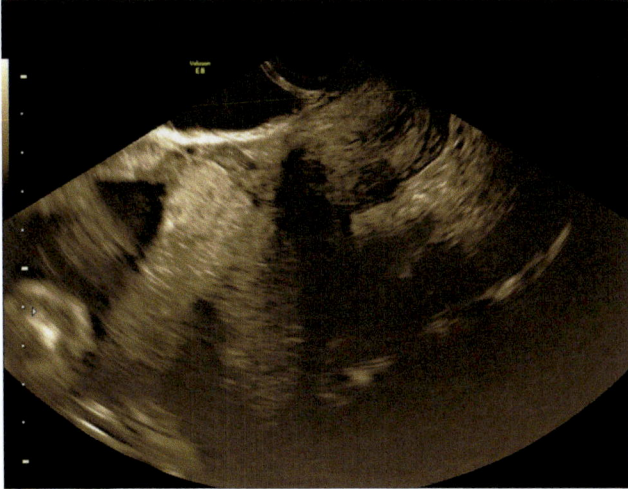

Fig. 11: Placenta—posterior low lying.

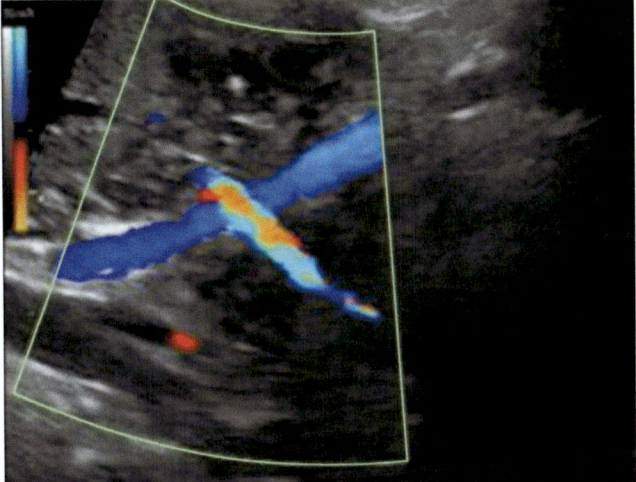

Fig. 12: Identifying the uterine artery with color Doppler.

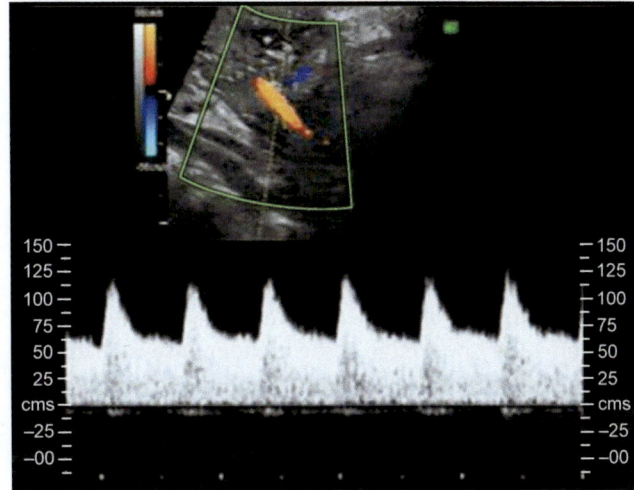

Fig. 13: Normal uterine artery flows.

high pulsatility indices. This is reflective of suboptimal placentation and in the second trimester, it is highly predictive of the risk of pre-eclampsia in the mother in that pregnancy.

Uterine artery Doppler in the second trimester is usually done transabdominally. The ultrasound probe is moved laterally in the lower segment and color Doppler is used to identify the uterine artery at the apparent crossover with the external iliac arteries (Fig. 12). Then, the pulsed wave (PW) Doppler is used to get a waveform which may be representative of good diastolic flow (Fig. 13) or high-resistance flow (Fig. 14).

CERVICAL LENGTH ASSESSMENT IN THE SECOND TRIMESTER

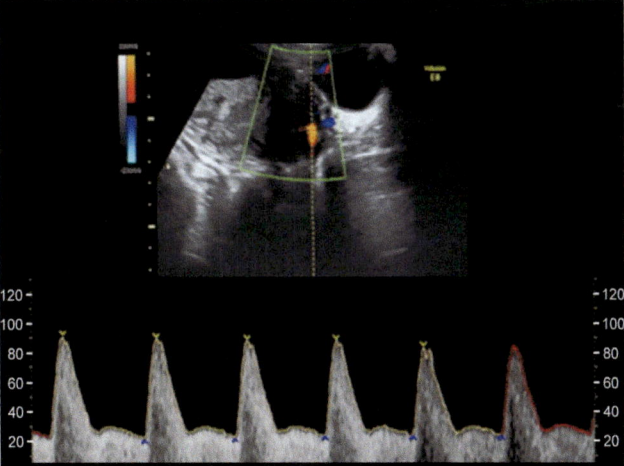

Fig. 14: High-resistance flows in uterine artery.

Assessment of the length of the cervical canal in mid pregnancy as well as detecting any signs of "funneling" of membranes has been known to be of use in predicting the risk of preterm birth. There is still a controversy about whether cervical length assessment should be done as part of "routine" assessment or only when there are known risk

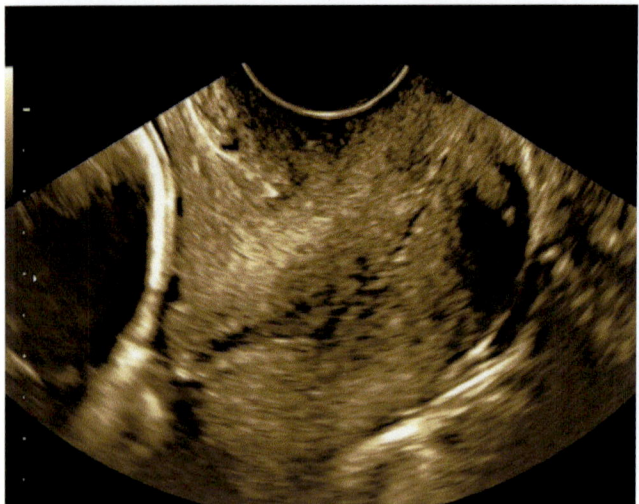

Fig. 15: Assessment of cervix in the second trimester.

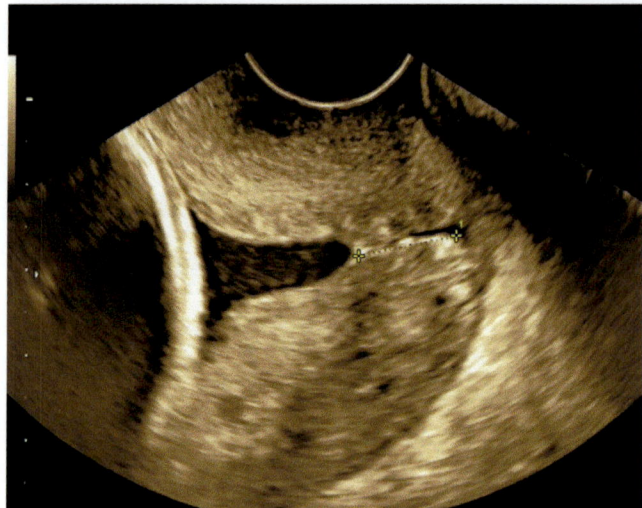

Fig. 16: Short cervix with funneling of membranes.

factors for preterm birth. Nevertheless, the importance of this measurement is accepted and when done using a correct technique, cervical assessment can provide vital information to guide obstetric care.

The most accurate method of cervical length measurement in the second trimester is by transvaginal sonography (TVS). It is preferably done with the patient in the dorsal lithotomy position and an empty bladder. The anterior and posterior lips of the cervix are seen with the canal in between—the lower edge of the bladder base is taken as a reference point for the internal os and the canal length is measured. It may be normal as shown in Figure 15 or may show funneling as shown in Figure 16.

The TVS probe is introduced in the vagina and directed in the anterior fornix avoiding undue pressure on the cervix, which may artificially increase the length. The cervical length is measured on a sagittal view of the cervical canal. It is recommended not to hurry with this assessment as there may be dynamic changes at times and detecting these are important.

The best approach for measurement of cervical length is by TVS, although transabdominal and transperineal approaches have been described. Detection of a short cervix helps in modifying obstetric care and instituting measures to prevent preterm birth. Even though measures of preventing preterm birth may not always be successful, awareness of the possibility of such an event helps prepare the family and healthcare professionals so that they can optimize the circumstances around the delivery, thus improving perinatal outcome.

CONCLUSION

The second trimester ultrasound scan is an important landmark in obstetric care which provides a timely opportunity for a comprehensive evaluation of the fetus and maternal structures in a manner that can help in planning pregnancy care meaningfully. Undetected congenital anomalies have been a major cause of neonatal morbidity and mortality, so timely detection of such problems prevents such adverse outcomes. The diagnostic potential of antenatal ultrasound varies significantly depending on many factors, the most important of which are operator experience and machine resolution. Maternal complications such as pre-eclampsia and preterm labor pose a major challenge to perinatal healthcare delivery and again while most of these are not completely preventable, being forewarned helps in optimizing care delivery.

Every passing year is witness to advent of new technology and better understanding of fetal physiology and development. Also the sociolegal parameters of fetal evaluation may change in different times with varying cultural pressures. Hence, the nature and scope of the second trimester ultrasound may undergo subtle modifications from time to time. It is imperative on practitioners to keep themselves abreast such developments and update their protocols from time to time.

SUGGESTED READING

1. Pilu G, Nicolaides K, Ximenes R, et al. Diagnosis of fetal abnormalities—the 18–23 weeks scan; 2002. [online] Available from https://fetalmedicine.org/var/uploads/18-23_Weeks_Scan.pdf.
2. Salomon LJ, Alfirevic Z, Berghella V, ISUOG Clinical Standards Committee, et al. Practice guidelines for performance of the routine mid-trimester fetal ultrasound scan. Ultrasound Obstet Gynecol. 2011;37(1):116-26.

14

Placental Abnormalities

Shreyasi Sharma

INTRODUCTION

Pregnancy is an organic whole comprising of fetus, placenta, and umbilical cord, where the placenta is its signature. Often ignored, it is home to important clues about the pregnancy. Alternatively, it is a reflection of the health of the fetus. Thus, any prenatal/postnatal examination is incomplete without detailed evaluation of the placenta and umbilical cord. The importance of prenatal ultrasound cannot be undermined as it differentiates between anatomic variations and lesions of clinical significance. This chapter aims to review the normal placenta, the commonly encountered abnormalities, their ultrasound detection, and clinical relevance.

NORMAL PLACENTA

Understanding a normal placenta can provide better insights into placental abnormalities. A "typical" placenta at term, weighs 470 g, is round to oval with 22 cm in diameter and has a central thickness of 2.5 cm.[1] Its three components include placental disk, extraplacental membranes, and umbilical cord. It is composed of two surfaces, i.e., the maternal and fetal, termed as basal and chorionic plate, respectively. The former is divided by clefts into small portions, known as cotyledons. These clefts coincide with internal septae, which extend into the intervillous space. The latter (chorionic plate) is the site for umbilical cord insertion. It is spanned by large fetal vessels, which originate from the cord vessels and enter into the placental parenchyma (Fig. 1). A thin layer of amnion covers the chorionic plate, which is loosely adherent and can be easily peeled away. The details of placental implantation and development are beyond the scope of this chapter.

On ultrasound, the placenta appears as a 2–4 cm thick homogeneous structure lying against the myometrium and indenting into the amniotic sac. It is separated from the myometrium by a hypoechoic area measuring around 1–2 cm called as retroplacental area (Figs. 2A and B).

SIZE AND SHAPE ABNORMALITIES

When there is an occurrence of multiple seemingly-equal placental lobes, the abnormality is termed as a multilobate/bilobate placenta. Bilobate placenta, also referred to as bipartite placenta and placenta duplex, is the condition where placentas may infrequently form as separate disks. The usual anatomical location of the cord insertion in such placentas is between the two lobes which are connected either through an intervening membrane or a chorionic bridge (Fig. 3). Multilobate placenta describes a placenta with three or more equally sized lobes.

Succenturiate (accessory) lobe, as depicted in Figure 3, is a separate mass positioned distinctly away from the placenta. This gains clinical importance as fatal hemorrhage might result if there is shearing of umbilical vessels that supply the succenturiate lobe and traverse the internal os (vasa previa—to be discussed in a later section). A succenturiate lobe can also cause postpartum hemorrhage if it gets retained in uterus postdelivery.

Thickness Abnormalities

Routinely, the thickness of the placenta increases by 1 mm/week of gestation.[2,3] Thus, the placenta at term is roughly 40 mm, barring a few exceptions.[2] Although not measured routinely, it is mostly the subjective assessment which triggers the sonographer to obtain this measurement.

Placentomegaly (thickened placenta) may occur due to several causes including diabetes mellitus, anemia, fetal hydrops, and fetal infection (Fig. 4). Multiple hypoechoic spaces (cystic areas) with placentomegaly may be seen

Placental Abnormalities

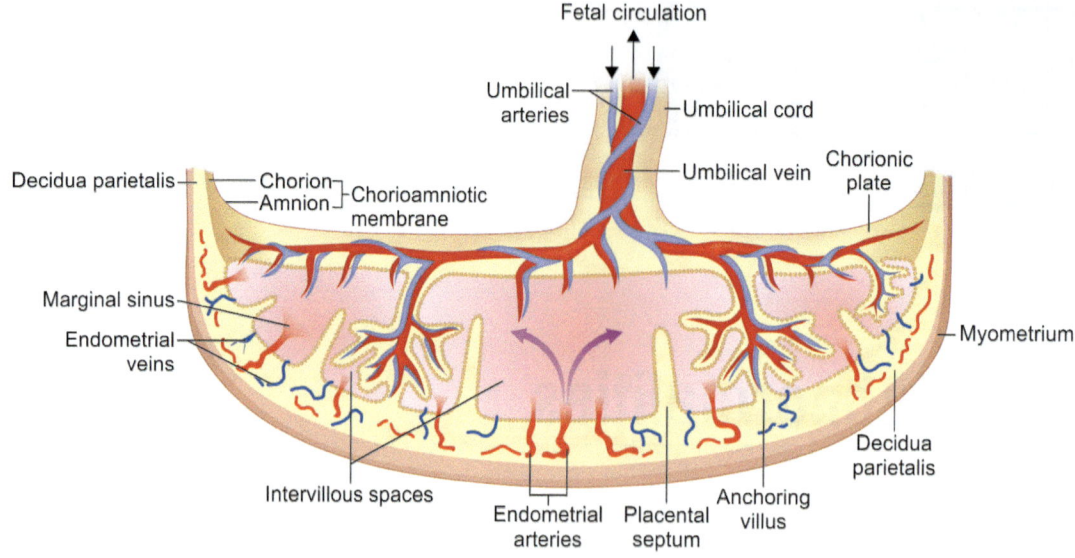

Fig. 1: Anatomy of placenta.

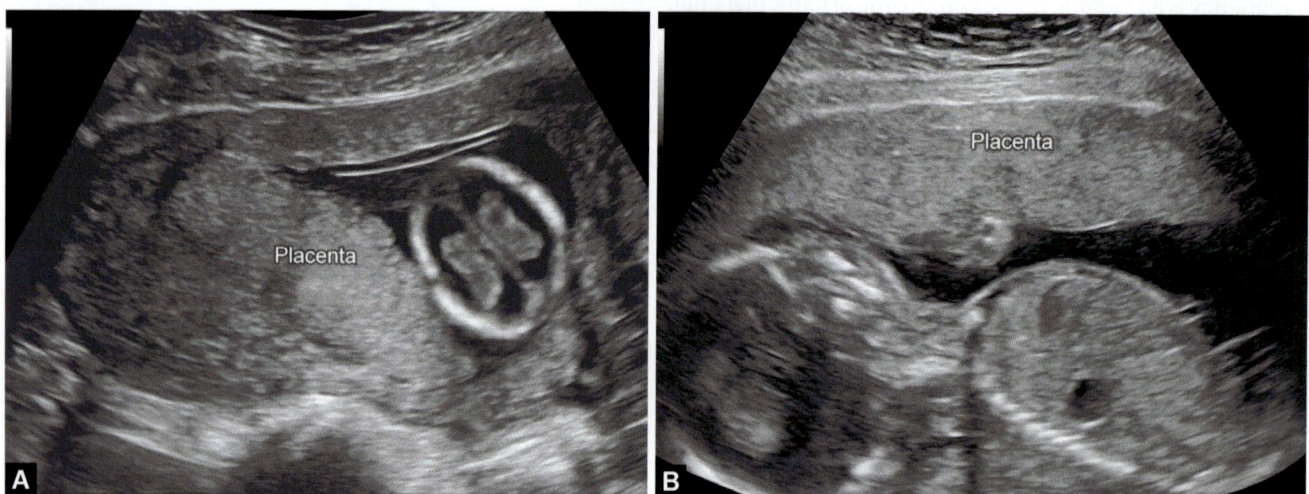

Figs. 2A and B: (A) Image of a normal first trimester placenta; and (B) Image of a normal second trimester placenta.

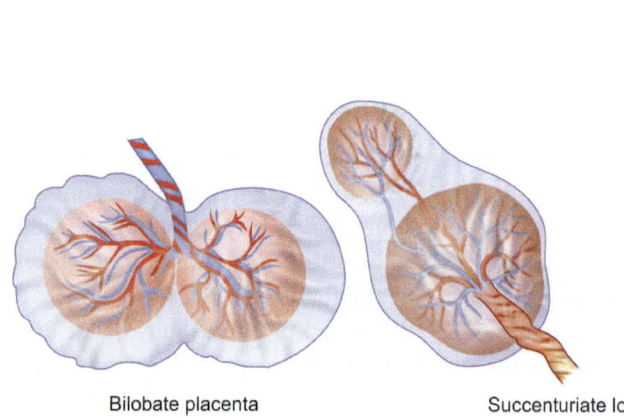

Fig. 3: Bilobate placenta and succenturiate lobe.

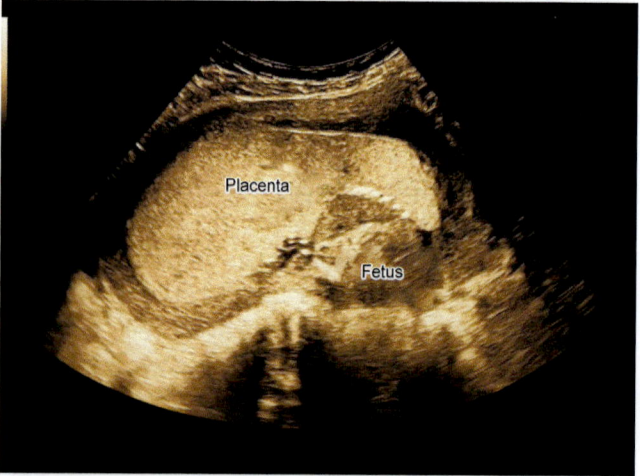

Fig. 4: A case of placentomegaly with oligohydramnios where the fetus is pushed toward one side. A cord blood sampling confirmed the diagnosis of cytomegalovirus (CMV) infection.

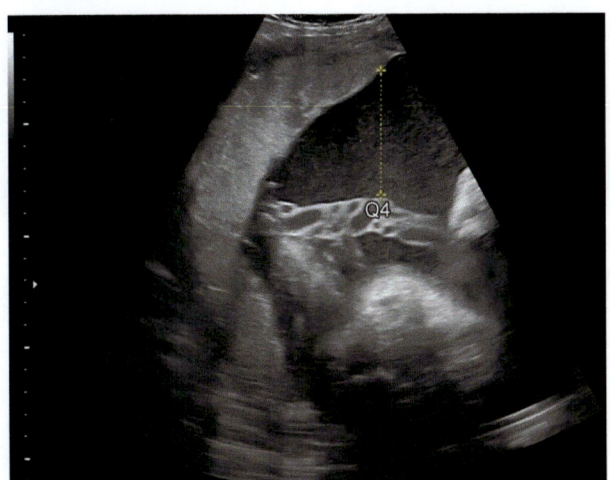

Fig. 5: Apparent placental thinning on ultrasound due to polyhydramnios.

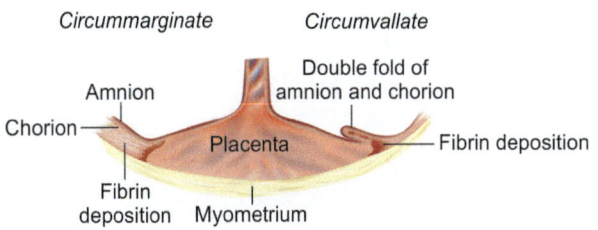

Fig. 6: Circummarginate placenta versus circumvallate placenta.

in placental mesenchymal dysplasia, villitis, placental hemorrhage, triploidy, partial mole, or a complete mole with a coexisting fetus.[4] An intraplacental hemorrhage may also make the placenta appear heterogeneously thickened. A thin placenta may occur in a growth-restricted fetus. Sometimes, polyhydramnios causing distension of uterus may also make the placenta appear thin as depicted in Figure 5.

Since the alteration in placental size may have multiple underlying reasons, it is imperative for the sonographer to look beyond what meets the eye. The sonographer should attempt to look for associated signs which may help in triangulating the exact cause.

EXTRACHORIAL PLACENTATION

Usually, the basal and chorionic plates of the placenta are equal in size and meet at the placental margins. In the event of failure of the chorionic plates to reach the placental periphery, there is inequality of size and the chorionic plate is much smaller than the basal plate. Thus, there is a complete/partial inward rolling of the placental margins. This condition of chorioamnion folding upon itself is termed as circumvallate placenta (Fig. 6). The same is apparent as a shelf on ultrasound, in a cross-sectional view. Care should be taken to differentiate this finding from uterine synechiae.

A circummarginate placenta (Fig. 6), on the other hand, occurs when there is fibrin deposition between the placenta and the chorioamnion with no infolding of the membranes.

Clinically, the outcomes of such placentation are usually normal. Although Taniguchi et al. reported a high incidence of preterm delivery, placental abruption, small for gestational age (SGA), and neonatal death associated with extrachorial placentation,[5] most of the studies including a recent one by Temming et al. suggest no increase in adverse obstetric and neonatal outcomes reaffirming that these are benign findings.[6]

ABNORMALITIES OF LOCATION

Placenta Previa

Placenta previa is defined as a condition where the placental tissue extends over the internal os. It is one of the important causes of antepartum hemorrhage. Although reported variably, it occurs in approximately 0.4% of live births.[7,8] Since most placenta previas (~90%) resolve prior to delivery, its prevalence in earlier gestations is higher.[9]

There are two possible theories explaining the higher occurrence of placenta previa in early gestations as compared to term pregnancies. The first theory hypothesizes that lengthening of the lower uterine segment with advancing gestation results in the displacement of lower end of placenta away from the internal os.[10] According to the second theory, as the pregnancy advances, trophotropism induces the trophoblastic tissue to preferentially grow toward the uterine fundus, resulting in placental migration away from internal os.

The diagnosis of placenta previa is established by ultrasound determination of placenta tissue extending over the internal os during the second or third trimester (Fig. 7). It is referred to as low lying when the distance between the lower edge of the placenta and the internal os is less than 2 cm, and it does not overlie the os. It is imperative that an ultrasound report makes a clear mention of the distance between the lower edge of the placenta from the internal os.[11] Figure 8 illustrates the method of measuring this distance. Previously used terminologies like marginal and partial are obsolete and should not be used as they do not add value to the accuracy of reporting.

Although transabdominal ultrasound is the standard initial modality for placental localization (Fig. 9), transvaginal or translabial sonography can be used for better visualization. The transabdominal ultrasonography (USG) performs fairly well as a screening tool. The sensitivity ranges from 86.7% to 93.3% depending upon

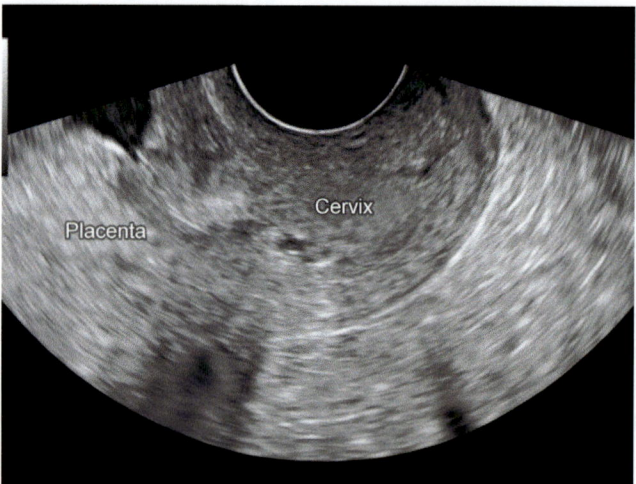

Fig. 7: Placenta previa as demonstrated on a transvaginal ultrasound where the lower edge of the placental tissue is seen extending over the internal os.

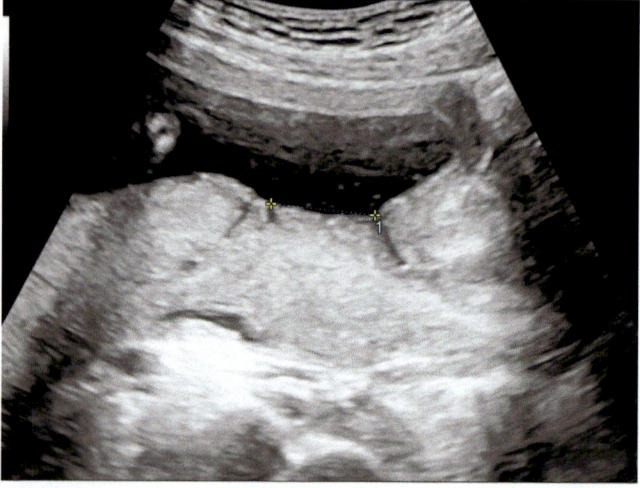

Fig. 8: Measuring distance between placental lower edge and internal os on a transabdominal ultrasound.

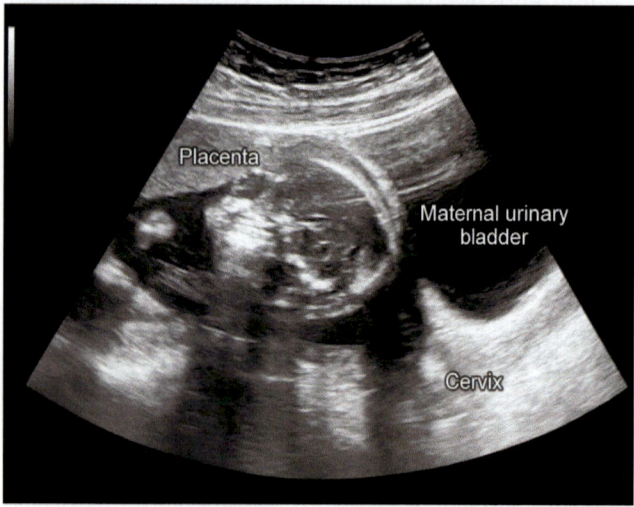

Fig. 9: Placental localization on a transabdominal ultrasound.

the cutoff used[12] with a false-positive rate which may go up to 25%.[13,14]

Few practical considerations to avoid pitfalls of transabdominal sonography (TAS) include:
- An overdistended urinary bladder causes the apposition of the uterine walls thereby increasing false positives. Care should be taken that the bladder is emptied and there is no lower uterine segment contraction while the placental localization is being noted (Figs. 10A and B).
- Placental location may be difficult to ascertain at term due to the fetal head, especially in the case of a posterior placenta. A transvaginal scan serves as a better modality in such instances.
- In case of an hematoma near the leading edge of the placenta, the true relation between the internal os and placenta might be obscured, resulting in false-positive reporting (Fig. 11).

A transvaginal USG is safe and provides better visualization of the relationship between the placental edge and internal os. Figures 12A and B provide a comparison of TAS and transvaginal sonography (TVS) for localization of the placenta. Diagnostic superiority of transvaginal scan over transabdominal scan has been proven beyond doubt by prospective studies and randomized trials.[15-17] In a study by Leerentveld et al., the specificity and negative predictive value were as high as 98.8% and 97.6%, respectively.[18] Color Doppler finds its use where there is a suspicion of the placenta accreta spectrum (PAS) (to be discussed in later sections). Also, its use during transvaginal scan serves to rule out vasa previa, especially when the umbilical cord insertion is in the lower segment.

PLACENTA ACCRETA SPECTRUM/MORBIDLY ADHERENT PLACENTA

Placenta accreta spectrum, formerly referred to as morbidly adherent placenta, is a placental implantation defect, which occurs as a result of the invasion of the trophoblastic tissue into the myometrium in the absence of decidua basalis (Fig. 13). The depth of invasion determines the type of PAS. The attachment and invasion of the trophoblastic tissue to the myometrium are termed as placenta accreta and increta, respectively. Placenta percreta occurs where the integrity of serosa is breached (Fig. 14). The rise in the frequency of PAS is primarily attributable to an increased cesarean delivery rate. The incidence of PAS increases from 3% after one cesarean section to 67% after five or more cesarean sections.[19] Its associations with grave complications such as

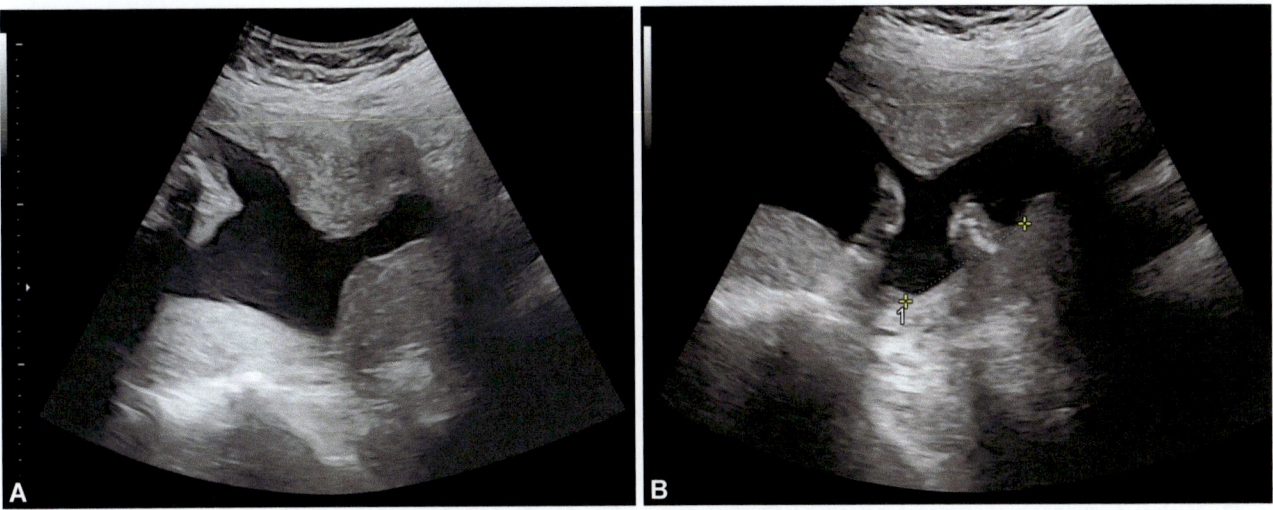

Figs. 10A and B: (A) Lower segment uterine contraction giving a false impression of low-lying placenta; and (B) Postuterine contraction view portrays that placenta is not low lying.

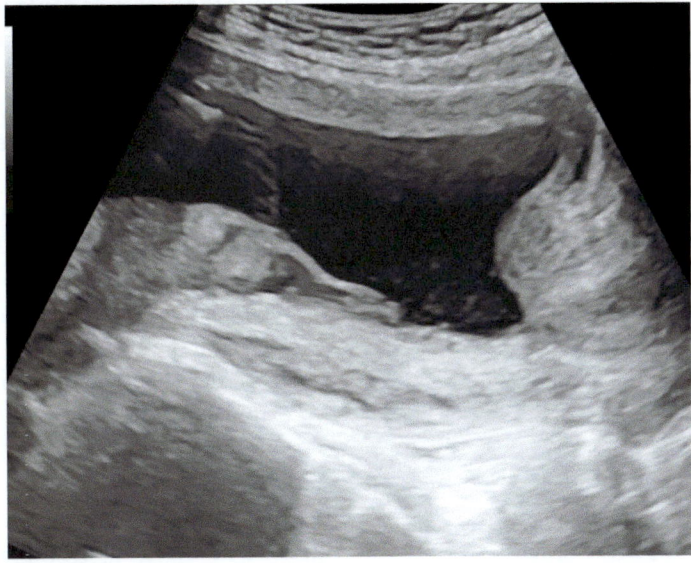

Fig. 11: Hematoma at the leading edge of placenta obscuring the relationship between the placenta and internal os.

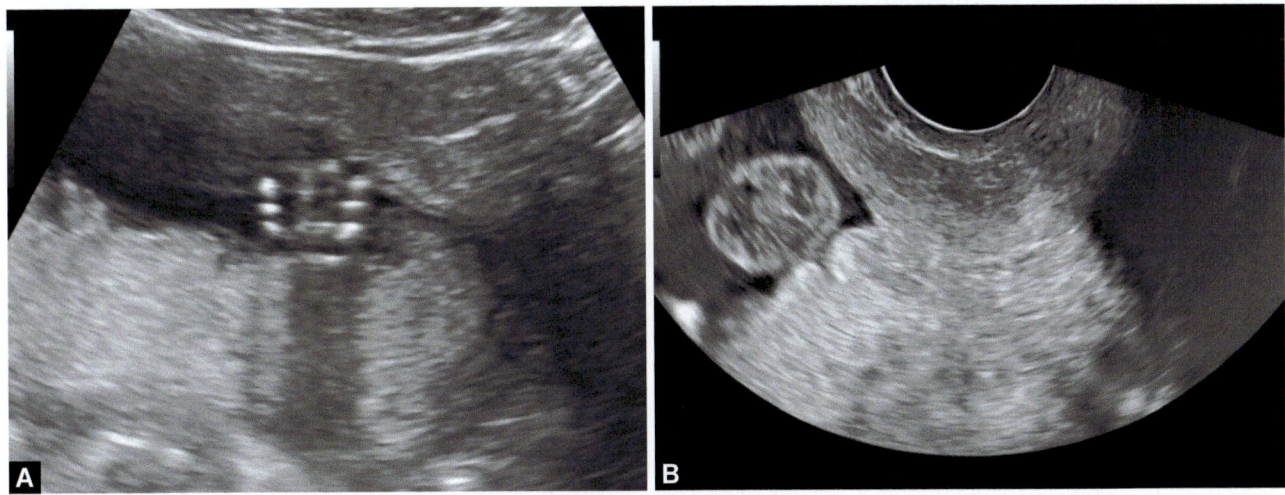

Figs. 12A and B: (A) Transabdominal ultrasound where the relationship between placenta and internal os cannot be clearly established; and (B) The same is clearly visualized on a transvaginal scan.

Placental Abnormalities

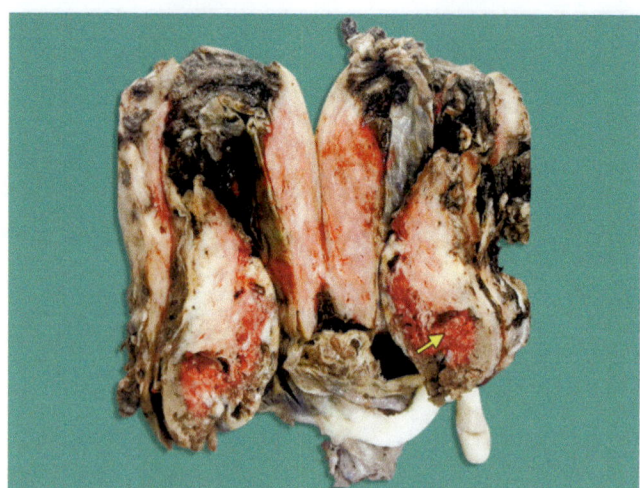

Fig. 13: Hysterectomy specimen where the indication for hysterectomy was placenta accreta. The yellow arrow depicts placental tissue invasion into the myometrium.

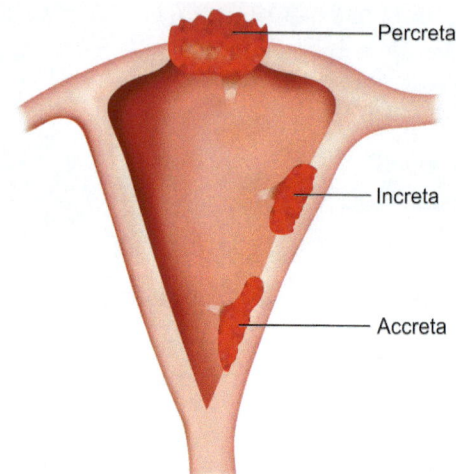

Fig. 14: Classification of placenta accreta spectrum.

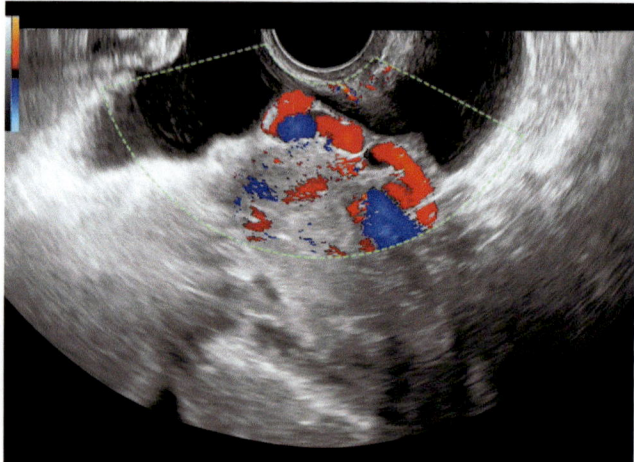

Fig. 15: Ultrasound image showing disruption of the clear zone and neovascularization at the bladder wall-serosa interface.

postpartum hemorrhage, consumption coagulopathy, renal failure, acute respiratory failure, and maternal mortality make the prenatal diagnosis of this condition essential.[19]

Ultrasound provides important clues for diagnosis and in the presence of a normal USG, PAS may be reasonably excluded. Ultrasound features associated with PAS that may be present in isolation or with each other are described below.

- Presence of placental lacunae which are large, irregular hypoechoic areas present along with thinning of the underlying myometrium. Placental lacunae are distinct from vascular lakes which are small and relatively regular in shape.[20]
- Loss in the continuity of the normal interface of the bladder wall—uterine serosa—by either neovascularity or the placental tissue itself in the case of placenta percreta (Fig. 15).

While the presence of placental lacunae and disruption of the bladder line are the most reliable ultrasound features, other associated ultrasound features include:

- Loss or irregularity of the normal retroplacental hypoechoic area otherwise called the clear space or the clear zone (Fig. 15)
- Thinning of the myometrium
- Abnormal vascularity extending from the placenta through the myometrium
- Ballooning of the uterus into the bladder, apparent as a placental bulge
- Presence of a focal mass breaching uterine serosa and extending into the bladder, hinting toward placenta percreta.

Color Doppler serves as a helpful adjunct for reaffirming the diagnosis of PAS. Features on color Doppler include lacunae blood flow turbulence, intraparenchymal blood flow, and increased vascularity of the serosa-bladder junction (Fig. 15). The overall diagnostic accuracy of ultrasound (including color Doppler) is reasonably good in identifying the depth of placental invasion with a sensitivity greater than 80% and a specificity greater than 94%.[20,21]

CIRCULATORY DISTURBANCES

Circulatory disturbances can be functionally classified into disturbances of maternal blood flow and those of fetal blood flow through the villi. These lesions are often noted as sonolucent areas within the placenta. They are considered incidental findings unless associated with fetal or maternal complications.

Disruption of Maternal Blood Flow

Disruption of maternal blood flow can result in various conditions which can be correctly differentiated histopathologically. Blood stasis occurring in the subchorionic area causes subchorionic fibrin deposition. The lesions so formed are commonly encountered as white or yellow plaques on the fetal surface. On the other hand, fibrin deposition around an individual villus is known as perivillous fibrin deposition, which is a benign finding. In its extreme form, perivillous fibrin deposition is referred to as maternal floor infarction. In the latter, the maternal blood flow into the intervillous space gets restricted by the deposition of a dense fibrinoid layer within the basal plate of the placenta. The adverse pregnancy outcomes associated with this condition include miscarriage, preterm delivery, and stillbirths.[21] Apart from a thickened basal plate, there are no definitive ultrasound signs for diagnosing this condition.

A break in villus might result in the collection of coagulated maternal and fetal blood occasionally. Such lesions can occur at any placental depth and are not associated with any adverse obstetric outcomes. An individual villus might get infarcted when its blood supply is reduced due to any uteroplacental disease. Although mostly benign, extensive infarction can result in placental insufficiency.

Hematoma

Placental hematoma is classified into retroplacental, marginal, subchorial, and subamnionic based on the location of occurrence (Fig. 16). A retroplacental hematoma occurs between the placenta and the decidua (Fig. 17). Marginal hematomas, commonly known as subchorionic hematomas (Fig. 18), are located at the placental periphery between the chorion and decidua. The subchorial hematoma is located underneath the chorionic plate along the periphery of the intervillous space. Subamnionic hematoma is sandwiched between the amnion and the chorionic plate.

On ultrasound, hematomas initially appear as hyperechoic to isoechoic areas in the first week. Over 2 weeks, they morph to become hypoechoic and settle as anechoic. Usually, the small hematomas bear no clinical significance. However, higher rates of miscarriage, placental abruption, fetal growth restriction, and preterm delivery are associated with extensive retroplacental, marginal, and subchorial hematomas.[22,23]

Disruption of Fetal Blood Flow

A fetal thrombotic vasculopathy occurs due to thrombosis of stem villi thereby obstructing the fetal blood flow as it renders the distal portion of the villi nonfunctional. This condition gains clinical significance only when multiple villi are infarcted.

As described earlier, a subamnionic hematoma is sandwiched between the amnion and the chorionic plate. It is important to differentiate it from other placental masses

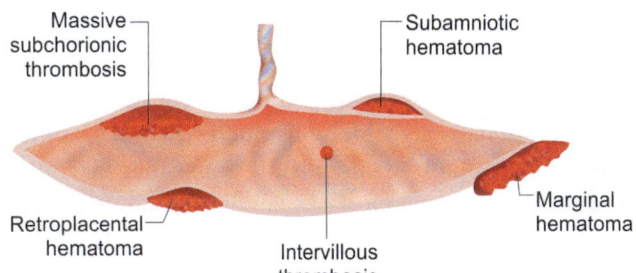

Fig. 16: Types of placental hematoma.

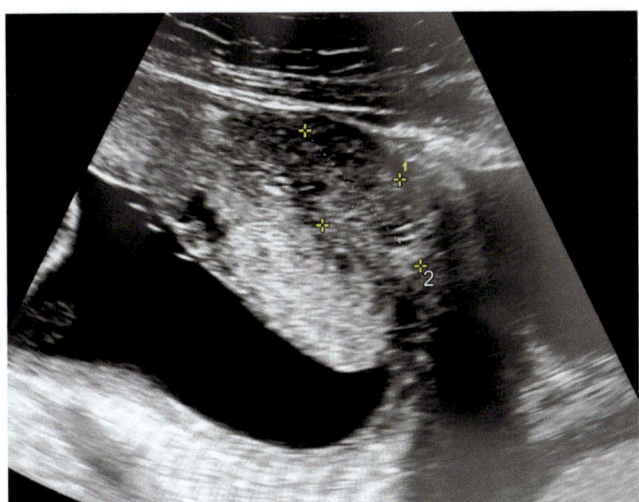

Fig. 17: Two-dimensional ultrasound image of a retroplacental hematoma.

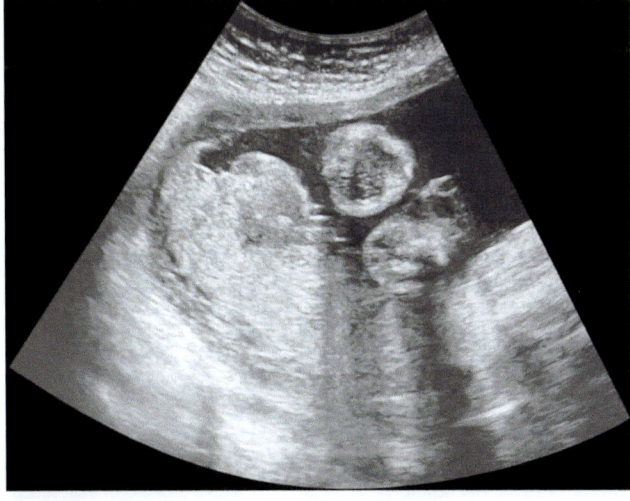

Fig. 18: Two-dimensional ultrasound image of a subchorionic hematoma.

such as chorioangioma. A color Doppler evaluation aids this differentiation as hematomas are devoid of any vascularity. Occasionally, chronic lesions may be associated with preterm delivery and fetal growth restriction.[24]

PLACENTAL CALCIFICATION

Deposition of calcium salts in the placenta occurs as a universal phenomenon associated with placental aging (Fig. 19). The deposition most commonly occurs at the basal plate (Fig. 20). Other conditions causing calcium deposition in the placenta include smoking, maternal hypertension, pre-eclampsia, and fetal growth restriction.[25] Grannum et al. developed a grading scale based upon placental calcification to indicate placental maturity.[26] Despite being widely used, it is pertinent to note that it neither correlates with fetal lung maturity nor predicts neonatal outcomes.[27-29]

PLACENTAL TUMORS

Placental tumors can be trophoblastic or nontrophoblastic in origin. Chorioangiomas are the most common nontrophoblastic tumors. These are found in approximately 1% of pregnancies.[30] On ultrasound, they appear as well-circumscribed, rounded masses which are hypoechoic or have mixed echogenicity. They are mostly located near the umbilical cord insertion, on the chorionic surface of the placenta, and protruding into the amniotic cavity. Increased vascularity is demonstrated by color Doppler which is essential to distinguish it from other placental masses like hematoma, partial hydatidiform mole, teratoma, etc.[31] Small lesions usually have a benign course. However, chorioangiomas more than 5 cm may lead to fetal anemia and hydrops owing to placental arteriovenous shunting. To abate complications associated with large tumors, laser coagulation of the feeding vessel has been described in literature.[32,33]

Figures 21A and B detail two-dimensional (2D) and color Doppler imagery of placental chorioangioma detected at 19 weeks of gestation. The gross specimen of the same case viewed from the fetal surface obtained postnatally is represented in Figure 21C. This chorioangioma did not lead to any fetal complications and only a close prenatal follow-up sufficed.

Placental trophoblastic tumors are distinct from non-trophoblastic placental tumors. In this section, we have limited the discussion to nontrophoblastic placental tumors as gestational trophoblastic disease is beyond the scope of the chapter.

ABNORMALITIES OF THE UMBILICAL CORD

Placental evaluation is incomplete without examination of the umbilical cord. Much of the umbilical cord abnormalities having clinical significance can be detected on an ultrasound examination.

Single Umbilical Artery

The usual umbilical cord comprises of two umbilical arteries and one umbilical vein. Documenting the number of vessels of the umbilical cord forms an essential component of the second-trimester reporting. A single umbilical artery (SUA) is the most common abnormality of the umbilical cord and is noted in approximately 0.48% of pregnancies when scanned between 16 weeks and 23 weeks of gestation.[34] The evaluation of the number of vessels of the cord is done at the level of the fetal urinary bladder, wherein the urinary bladder is flanked by the two umbilical arteries normally (Fig. 22). Alternatively, a cross-sectional view may also

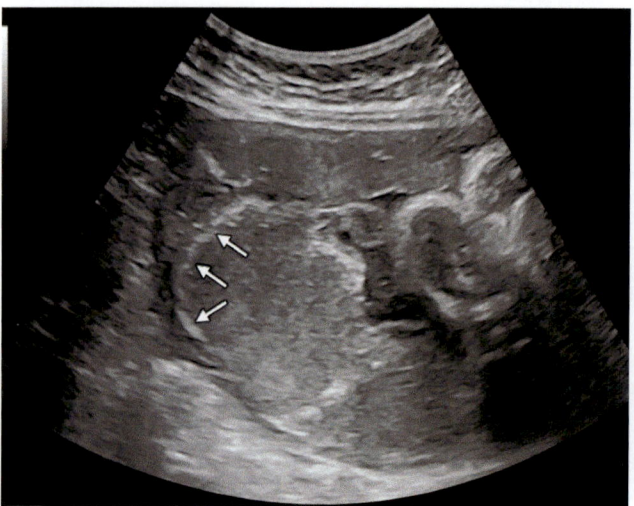

Fig. 19: Placental calcification on ultrasound. Hyperechoic areas depicting calcification are highlighted (arrows).

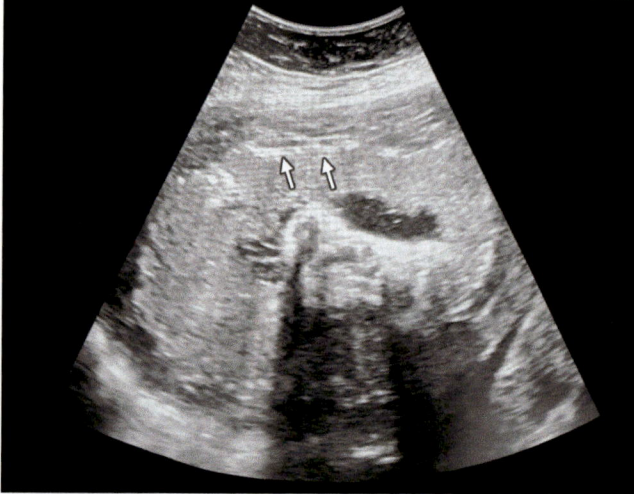

Fig. 20: Ultrasound image of calcification located primarily at the basal plate (arrows).

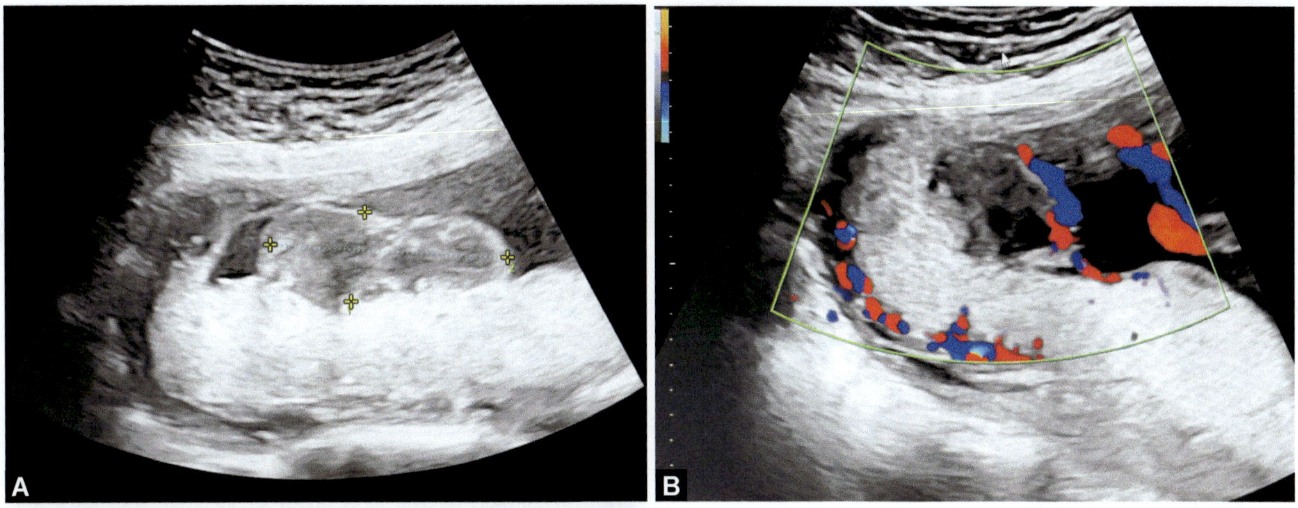

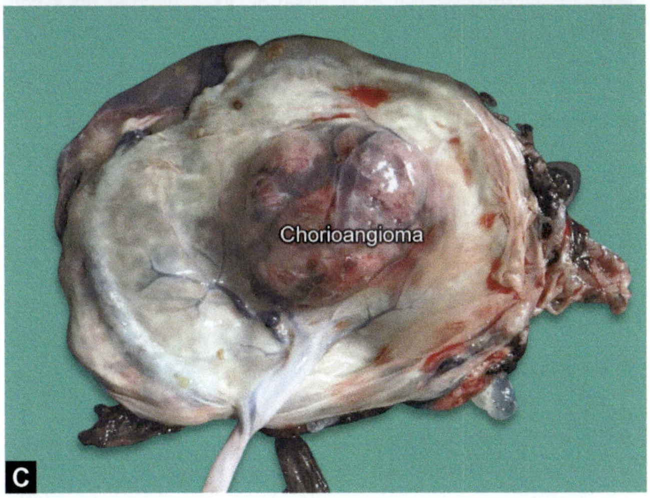

Figs. 21A to C: (A) Placental chorioangioma at 19 weeks of gestation; (B) Vascularity of chorioangioma as seen on color Doppler; and (C) Gross specimen of chorioangioma.

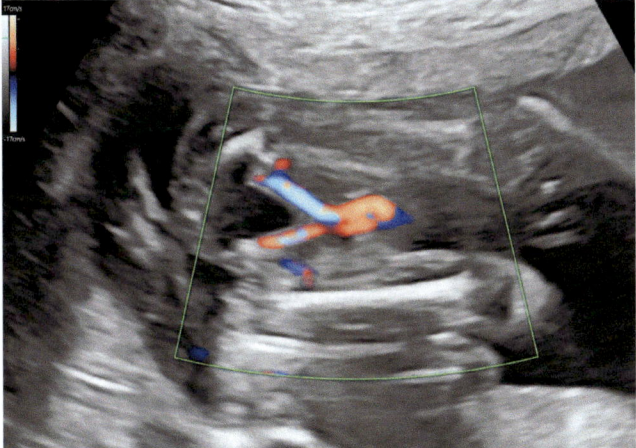

Fig. 22: Ultrasound evaluation of three-vessel umbilical cord—normal view.

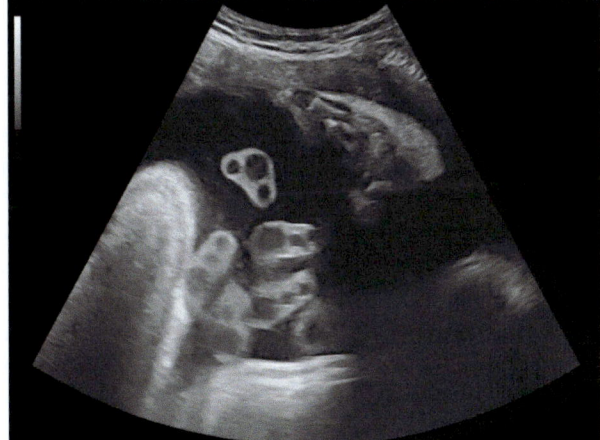

Fig. 23: Cross-sectional view of three-vessel umbilical cord.

reveal the number of blood vessels in the umbilical cord (Fig. 23).

In the case of a SUA, only one vessel is visible which runs along the fetal urinary bladder before it joins the umbilical vein (Fig. 24). Once noted, it warrants a detailed evaluation of the fetal anatomy with special emphasis on the cardiovascular and the genitourinary system. Even though there exists an increased risk of fetal growth restriction,[35,36]

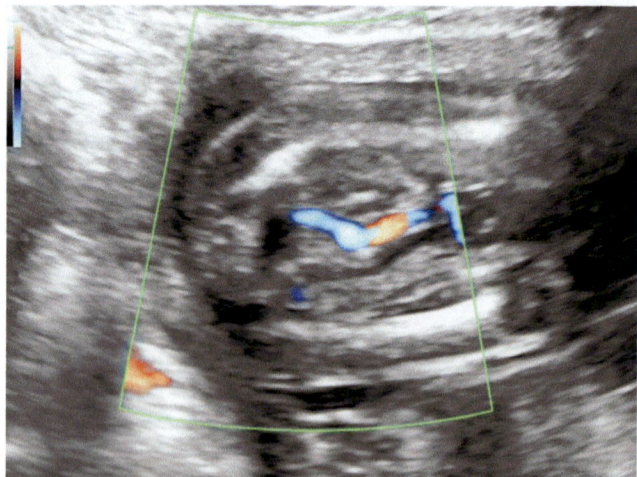

Fig. 24: Single umbilical artery.

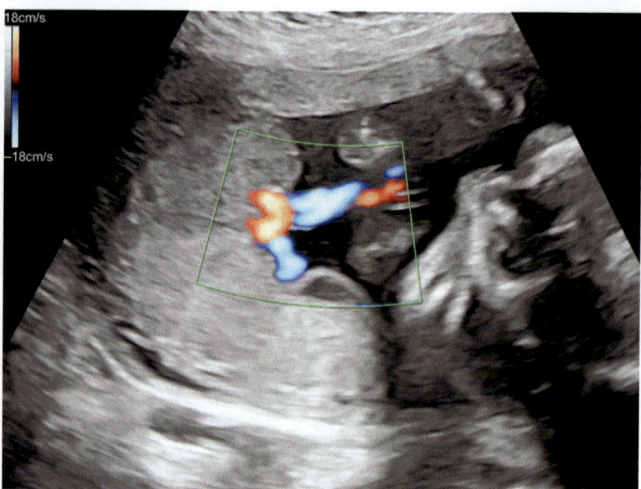

Fig. 25: Normal central cord insertion as evaluated on a color Doppler.

it should be remembered that there is no increased risk of aneuploidies if SUA is present as an isolated finding in an otherwise low-risk pregnancy. However, if it is associated with any major malformation, the risk of aneuploidies is increased.[37] Thus, in cases of SUA, follow-up ultrasounds to check for interval fetal growth is a prudent approach.

Length Abnormalities

The usual length of the umbilical cord is 40–70 cm. Although there is no specific method of measurement and cutoff, clinical associations with short umbilical cord include fetal growth restriction, congenital malformations, intrapartum fetal distress, and risk of fetal death.[38] Long cords, on the other hand, are associated with cord entanglement, prolapse, fetal malformations, etc.

Coiling Abnormalities

Although not part of a routine examination, umbilical cord coiling can be expressed in terms of the umbilical coiling index (UCI) which is calculated as the ratio of the number of complete coils to the length of the coil in centimetres.[39] An ultrasound computed UCI of 0.4 is usually considered normal.[40] Adverse fetal outcomes associated with hypercoiling include fetal growth restriction and intrapartum fetal acidosis while hypocoiling has been associated with fetal demise.[41]

Insertion Abnormalities

The cord usually gets inserted centrally on the placenta (Fig. 25); however, variants include eccentric, marginal, and velamentous insertion of cord (Fig. 26). The cord gets attached to the edge of the placenta in the marginal variant/ battledore placenta. Such insertion may sometimes cause the cord to snap while delivering the placenta.

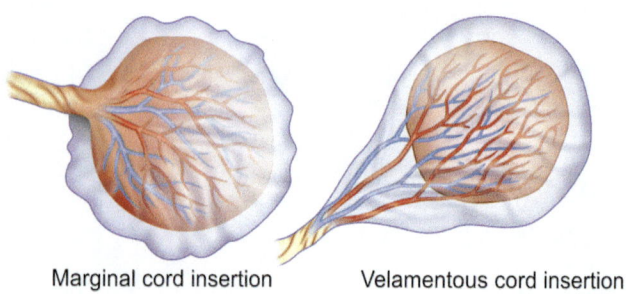

Marginal cord insertion   Velamentous cord insertion

Fig. 26: Illustration of marginal and velamentous cord insertion.

When the umbilical vessels, surrounded only by a layer of the amnion, traverse a considerable distance along the uterine wall before getting inserted in the placenta, it is termed as velamentous insertion. This renders the umbilical vessels amenable to compression which might lead to adverse fetal events. In prenatal sonography, color Doppler reveals the umbilical cord vessels against the uterine wall before they get inserted in the placenta.

Lastly, in furcate insertion, there is loss of the Wharton's jelly of the cord vessels, just before placental insertion. Covered only by the amnion, the cord vessels become susceptible to compression and thrombosis.

Vasa Previa

A variant of velamentous cord insertion that occurs in <0.02% of pregnancies (1 in 5,200 pregnancies),[42] vasa previa is associated with catastrophic implications. In this condition, the umbilical vessels cross the internal os while surrounded by a thin layer of amnion. Thus, they are prone to compression and avulsion, which might lead to rapid exsanguination of the fetus. A bilobate or succenturiate placenta acts as important predisposing factors.

A prenatal diagnosis is cardinal for preventing fetal complications resulting from vasa previa. A transvaginal scan may reveal umbilical cord vessels overlying the internal os before they get inserted into the placenta. Thus, a prudent approach would be to routinely examine the cord insertion by color Doppler, especially in low lying placentas thereby improving detection of vasa previa. Once detected, a planned cesarean delivery is suggested at 34–35 weeks to balance prematurity and fetal exsanguination.[43] Care should also be taken to hasten the delivery in case the laceration of a vessel is suggested during uterine entry. In the event of an unexplained antepartum/intrapartum hemorrhage, the differential of vasa previa should be considered. Therefore, efforts should be directed toward ruling out this condition to prevent fatal complications.

Cord Cysts

Figures 27A and B depict 2D and Doppler ultrasound images of a cord cyst detected at 12 weeks of gestation which did not lead to any fetal complications. Although similar in sonographic appearance, cord cysts can be classified into true and false cysts. The former are remnants of the vitelline duct and are located closer to the fetus, whereas the latter are a resultant of Wharton's jelly degeneration occurring anywhere along the length of the cord. First-trimester identification of a single cyst is usually inconsequential; however, multiple cysts may be associated with miscarriage or aneuploidies.[44]

Knots, Strictures, and Loops

True knots may occur due to fetal movements and are associated with an increased risk of stillbirths.[45] In contrast, false knots carry no clinical significance. An umbilical cord knot on ultrasound is portrayed in Figure 28A. This knot was confirmed to be a true knot postnatally (Fig. 28B).

A stricture implies a focal narrowing of the cord, which usually occurs near the fetal end. Owing to stenosis of the cord vessels, it may be associated with stillbirths.[46]

Cord loop, especially a nuchal cord (cord around the neck), is a frequently encountered sonographic finding (Fig. 29). These might act as a cause for intrapartum variable fetal heart decelerations due to cord compression and bear an associa-tion with a lower cord pH;[47] however, they are not associated with any significant adverse perinatal outcomes.[48]

Vascular Abnormalities

Cord vessel thromboses are mostly venous; however, it is the arterial thromboses that are associated with higher rates of perinatal mortality and morbidity, fetal growth restriction, fetal acidosis, and stillbirths.[49]

Focal dilatation of the umbilical vein (intra-abdominal/intra-amniotic) is referred to as an umbilical vein varix. It is seen as a vascular cystic dilatation on the ultrasound with a normal caliber of the umbilical vein proximal and distal to it. If isolated, the pregnancy outcome is usually favorable; however once detected, close fetal monitoring should be performed to reduce untoward perinatal events such as stillbirth.[50]

Umbilical vein aneurysm results from thinning of the vessel wall. These are most commonly located near the placental end, as the support from Wharton's jelly is compromised. They appear as cystic structures with a hyperechoic rim and low-velocity turbulent blood flows on color Doppler.[51] Associations include single umbilical artery, aneuploidies, fetal growth restriction, and stillbirth.[52,53]

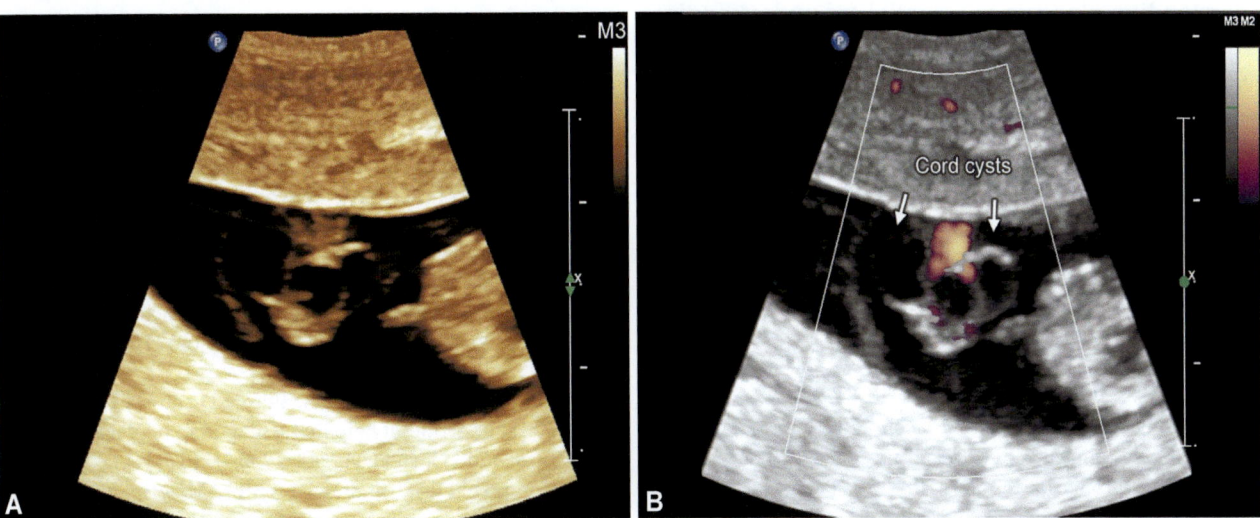

Figs. 27A and B: (A) Two-dimensional (2D) ultrasound image of a cord cyst; and (B) Cord cyst appearing avascular on Doppler.

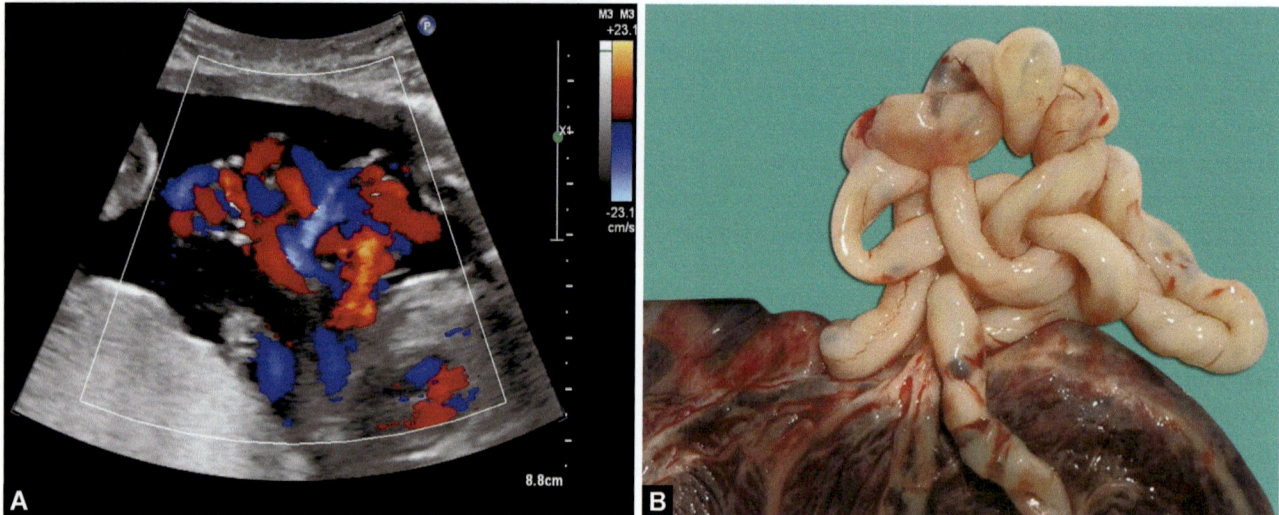

Figs. 28A and B: (A) Ultrasound image of umbilical cord knot; and (B) Gross specimen of the umbilical cord knot that confirms prenatal findings.

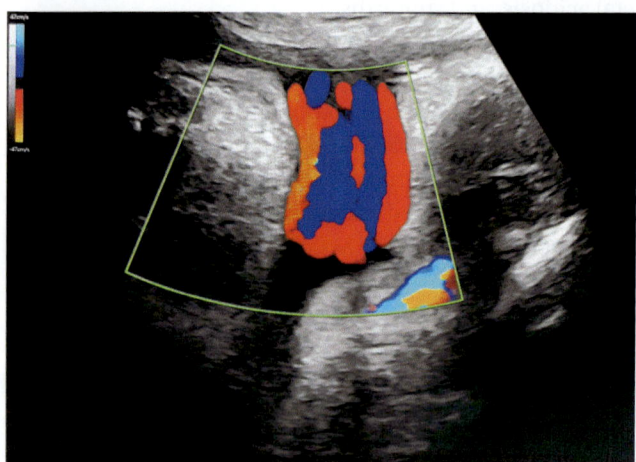

Fig. 29: Ultrasound image of two loops around the fetal neck.

CONCLUSION

Understanding placenta is essential for understanding the health of mother and unborn child. While this chapter attempted to explain important placental signatures, much yet remains to be uncovered. Hence, it is not surprising that placenta continues to attract medical research for improving pregnancy outcomes.

REFERENCES

1. Yetter JF. Examination of the placenta. Am Fam Physician. 1998;57(5):1045-54.
2. Hoddick WK, Mahony BS, Callen PW, et al. Placental thickness. J Ultrasound Med. 1985;4(9):479-82.
3. Tongsong T, Boonyanurak P. Placental thickness in the first half of pregnancy. J Clin Ultrasound. 2004;32(5):231-4.
4. Jauniaux E, Nicolaides KH, Hustin J. Perinatal features associated with placental mesenchymal dysplasia. Placenta. 1997;18(8):701-6.
5. Taniguchi H, Aoki S, Sakamaki K, et al. Circumvallate placenta: associated clinical manifestations and complications—a retrospective study. Obstet Gynecol Int. 2014;2014:986230.
6. Temming LA, Raghuraman N, Woolfolk C, et al. 432: Clinical significance of circumvallate placenta. Am J Obstet Gynecol. 2018;218(1):S262-3.
7. Faiz AS, Ananth CV. Etiology and risk factors for placenta previa: an overview and meta-analysis of observational studies. J Matern Fetal Neonatal Med. 2003;13(3):175-90.
8. Cresswell JA, Ronsmans C, Calvert C, et al. Prevalence of placenta praevia by world region: a systematic review and meta-analysis. Trop Med Int Health. 2013;18(6):712-24.
9. Oyelese Y, Smulian JC. Placenta previa, placenta accreta, and vasa previa. Obstet Gynecol. 2006;107(4):927-41.
10. Lavery JP. Placenta previa. Clin Obstet Gynecol. 1990;33(3): 414-21.
11. Thurmond A, Mendelson E, Böhm-Vélez M, et al. Role of imaging in second and third trimester bleeding. American College of Radiology. ACR Appropriateness Criteria. Radiology. 2000;215 Suppl:895-7.
12. Quant HS, Friedman AM, Wang E, et al. Transabdominal ultrasonography as a screening test for second-trimester placenta previa. Obstet Gynecol. 2014;123(3):628-33.
13. McClure N, Dornal JC. Early identification of placenta praevia. Br J Obstet Gynaecol. 1990;97(10):959-61.
14. Oppenheimer L. Diagnosis and management of placenta previa. J Obstet Gynaecol Can. 2007;29(3):261-6.
15. Sunna E, Ziadeh S. Transvaginal and transabdominal ultrasound for the diagnosis of placenta praevia. J Obstet Gynaecol. 1999;19(2):152-4.
16. Smith RS, Lauria MR, Comstock CH, et al. Transvaginal ultrasonography for all placentas that appear to be low-lying or over the internal cervical os. Ultrasound Obstet Gynecol. 1997;9(1):22-4.
17. Sherman SJ, Carlson DE, Platt LD, et al. Transvaginal ultrasound: does it help in the diagnosis of placenta previa? Ultrasound Obstet Gynecol. 1992;2(4):256-60.
18. Leerentveld RA, Gilberts EC, Arnold MJ, et al. Accuracy and safety of transvaginal sonographic placental localization. Obstet Gynecol. 1990;76(5 Pt 1):759-62.

19. Silver RM, Landon MB, Rouse DJ, et al. Maternal morbidity associated with multiple repeat cesarean deliveries. Obstet Gynecol. 2006;107(6):1226-32.
20. Pagani G, Cali G, Acharya G, et al. Diagnostic accuracy of ultrasound in detecting the severity of abnormally invasive placentation: a systematic review and meta-analysis. Acta Obstet Gynecol Scand. 2018;97(1):25-37.
21. Andres RL, Kuyper W, Resnik R, et al. The association of maternal floor infarction of the placenta with adverse perinatal outcome. Am J Obstet Gynecol. 1990;163(3):935-8.
22. Madu AE. Breus' mole in pregnancy. J Obstet Gynaecol. 2006;26(8):815-6.
23. Nagy S, Bush M, Stone J, et al. Clinical significance of subchorionic and retroplacental hematomas detected in the first trimester of pregnancy. Obstet Gynecol. 2003;102(1):94-100.
24. Owada M, Shibata Y, Suzuki S. Case Series of Intrauterine Subamniotic Hemorrhage. Case Rep Obstet Gynecol. 2019;2019:1828457.
25. Pinette MG, Loftus-Brault K, Nardi DA, et al. Maternal smoking and accelerated placental maturation. Obstet Gynecol. 1989;73(3 Pt 1):379-82.
26. Grannum PA, Berkowitz RL, Hobbins JC. The ultrasonic changes in the maturing placenta and their relation to fetal pulmonic maturity. Am J Obstet Gynecol. 1979;133(8):915-22.
27. McKenna D, Tharmaratnam S, Mahsud S, et al. Ultrasonic evidence of placental calcification at 36 weeks' gestation: maternal and fetal outcomes. Acta Obstet Gynecol Scand. 2005;84(1):7-10.
28. Montan S, Jorgensen C, Svalenius E, et al. Placental grading with ultrasound in hypertensive and normotensive pregnancies. A prospective, consecutive study. Acta Obstet Gynecol Scand. 1986;65(5):477-80.
29. Sau A, Seed P, Langford K. Intraobserver and interobserver variation in the sonographic grading of placental maturity. Ultrasound Obstet Gynecol. 2004;23(4):374-7.
30. Guschmann M, Henrich W, Entezami M, et al. Chorioangioma—new insights into a well-known problem. I. Results of a clinical and morphological study of 136 cases. J Perinat Med. 2003;31(2):163-9.
31. Prapas N, Liang RI, Hunter D, et al. Color Doppler imaging of placental masses: differential diagnosis and fetal outcome. Ultrasound Obstet Gynecol. 2000;16(6):559-63.
32. Sepulveda W, Alcalde JL, Schnapp C, et al. Perinatal outcome after prenatal diagnosis of placental chorioangioma. Obstet Gynecol. 2003;102(5 Pt 1):1028-33.
33. Quintero RA, Reich H, Romero R, et al. In utero endoscopic devascularization of a large chorioangioma. Ultrasound Obstet Gynecol. 1996;8(1):48-52.
34. Granese R, Coco C, Jeanty P. The value of single umbilical artery in the prediction of fetal aneuploidy: findings in 12,672 pregnant women. Ultrasound Q. 2007;23(2):117-21.
35. Murphy-Kaulbeck L, Dodds L, Joseph KS, et al. Single umbilical artery risk factors and pregnancy outcomes. Obstet Gynecol. 2010;116(4):843-50.
36. Hua M, Odibo AO, Macones GA, et al. Single umbilical artery and its associated findings. Obstet Gynecol. 2010;115(5):930-4.
37. Dagklis T, Defigueiredo D, Staboulidou I, et al. Isolated single umbilical artery and fetal karyotype. Ultrasound Obstet Gynecol. 2010;36(3):291-5.
38. Krakowiak P, Smith EN, de Bruyn G, et al. Risk factors and outcomes associated with a short umbilical cord. Obstet Gynecol. 2004;103(1):119-27.
39. Strong TH, Jarles DL, Vega JS, et al. The umbilical coiling index. Am J Obstet Gynecol. 1994;170(1 Pt 1):29-32.
40. Sebire NJ. Pathophysiological significance of abnormal umbilical cord coiling index. Ultrasound Obstet Gynecol. 2007;30(6):804-6.
41. de Laat MW, Franx A, Bots ML, et al. Umbilical coiling index in normal and complicated pregnancies. Obstet Gynecol. 2006;107(5):1049-55.
42. Lee W, Lee VL, Kirk JS, et al. Vasa previa: prenatal diagnosis, natural evolution, and clinical outcome. Obstet Gynecol. 2000;95(4):572-6.
43. Robinson BK, Grobman WA. Effectiveness of timing strategies for delivery of individuals with vasa previa. Obstet Gynecol. 2011;117(3):542-9.
44. Gilboa Y, Kivilevitch Z, Katorza E, et al. Outcomes of fetuses with umbilical cord cysts diagnosed during nuchal translucency examination. J Ultrasound Med. 2011;30(11):1547-51.
45. Airas U, Heinonen S. Clinical significance of true umbilical knots: a population-based analysis. Am J Perinatol. 2002;19(3):127-32.
46. French AE, Gregg VH, Newberry Y, et al. Umbilical cord stricture: a cause of recurrent fetal death. Obstet Gynecol. 2005;105(5 Pt 2):1235-9.
47. Hankins GD, Snyder RR, Hauth JC, et al. Nuchal cords and neonatal outcome. Obstet Gynecol. 1987;70(5):687-91.
48. Mastrobattista JM, Hollier LM, Yeomans ER, et al. Effects of nuchal cord on birthweight and immediate neonatal outcomes. Am J Perinatol. 2005;22(2):83-5.
49. Sato Y, Benirschke K. Umbilical arterial thrombosis with vascular wall necrosis: clinicopathologic findings of 11 cases. Placenta. 2006;27(6-7):715-8.
50. Lee SW, Kim MY, Kim JE, et al. Clinical characteristics and outcomes of antenatal fetal intra-abdominal umbilical vein varix detection. Obstet Gynecol Sci. 2014;57(3):181-6.
51. Olog A, Thomas JT, Petersen S, et al. Large umbilical artery aneurysm with a live healthy baby delivered at 31 weeks. Fetal Diagn Ther. 2011;29(4):331-3.
52. Hill AJ, Strong TH, Elliott JP, et al. Umbilical artery aneurysm. Obstet Gynecol. 2010;116 Suppl 2:559-62.
53. Weber MA, Sau A, Maxwell DJ, et al. Third trimester intrauterine fetal death caused by arterial aneurysm of the umbilical cord. Pediatr Dev Pathol. 2007;10(4):305-8.

15
Amniotic Fluid Assessment

Seetha Ramamurthy Pal, Kanchan Mukherjee

INTRODUCTION

Amniotic fluid is vital for the well-being of the fetus and evaluation of amniotic fluid is a very important and integral part of assessment of the fetus. Throughout the pregnancy, amniotic fluid has several functions in the development of the embryo and the fetus. It allows the fetus to grow and move, cushions the fetus from injury, provides a thermally stable environment, and protects the fetus from infections due to its bacteriostatic action.[1] Abnormalities in the fetus and placenta can cause alterations in the amount of fluid which can affect the well-being of the fetus and increase perinatal morbidity and mortality (Fig. 1).

The amniotic fluid volume (AFV) is a complex balance of fluid between the maternal and fetal structures that produce or allow passage of fluid into the amniotic cavity (Fig. 2). Several pathways like fetal swallowing, urination, pulmonary secretions, intramembranous, and transmembranous routes help to maintain the dynamic equilibrium (Fig. 3).[2-5]

Amniotic fluid essentially contains 98–99% water, but its solute composition keeps changing. It contains proteins, electrolytes, immunoglobulins, and vitamins from the mother. Occasionally, echogenic particles can be seen in the amniotic fluid. This was initially thought to be "vernix", but later termed as "amniotic fluid sludge".[6] Their significance is unknown, but one study found that in term patients, their presence was not associated with any adverse pregnancy outcome.[7]

In early pregnancy, the production of amniotic fluid is poorly understood. Multiple sources operate in the first

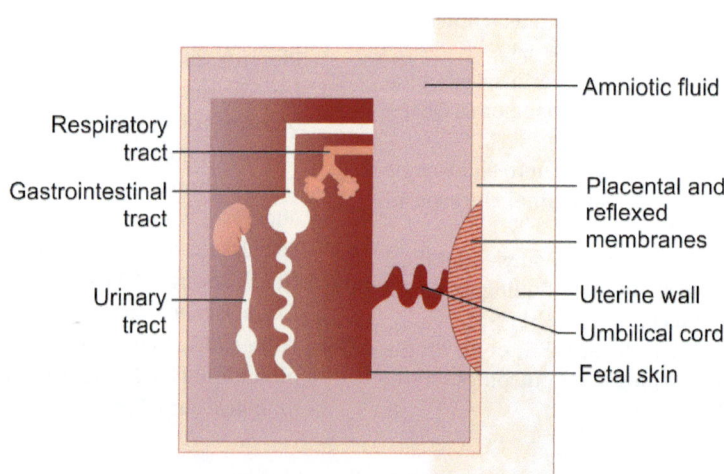

Fig. 1: The major fetal and maternal amniotic structures involved in the formation and reabsorption of amniotic fluid.
Source: Adapted from Wallenburg HC. The amniotic fluid I. Water and electrolyte homeostasis. J Perinat Med. 1977;5:193-205.

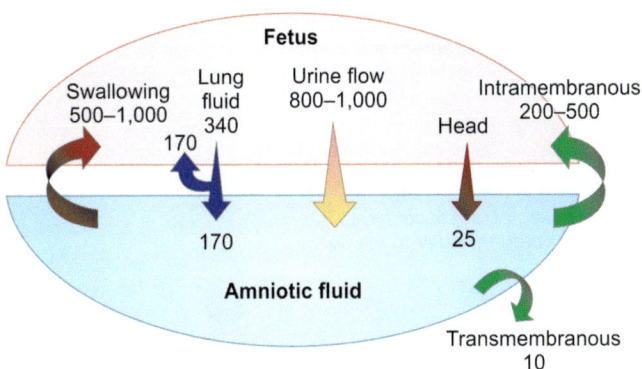

Fig. 2: Summary of water flow into and out of the amniotic space in late gestation.
Source: Adapted from Brace RA. Physiology of amniotic fluid volume regulation. Clin Obstet Gynecol. 1997;40:280-9.

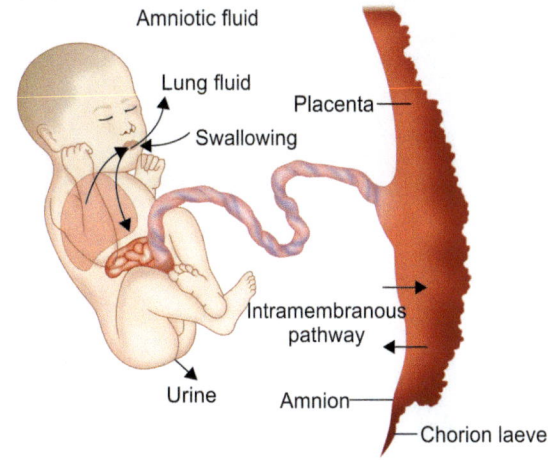

Fig. 3: Amniotic fluid dynamics.
Source: Seeds AE. Amniotic fluid physiology. In: Sciarra JJ (Ed). Gynecology and Obstetrics. New York: Harper & Row; 1989.

trimester but given the fact that the osmolality of amniotic fluid and maternal plasma is similar, amniotic fluid is basically a transudate of maternal plasma from the placenta and minimal from the fetus.[8] In the second trimester, the fetal urine is a major contributor and once the fetal skin gets keratinized (22-24 weeks), the fetal kidneys and lungs take over. However, confirmation of functioning renal system can be seen by the presence of urine in the fetal bladder at 8-10 weeks.[9] It has also been found that maternal disease status and hydration can affect AFV.[10]

Amniotic fluid is mainly removed by fetal swallowing[11] and the fetal pulmonary system, though a small amount is removed by the placenta and bulk flow.

NORMAL AMNIOTIC FLUID VOLUME (FIG. 4)

The amniotic fluid gradually increases in the first trimester, stabilizes in the second trimester, and decreases late in the third trimester. At 12 weeks, it measures 60 mL which increases to 175 mL by 16 weeks (time of genetic amniocentesis). It then increases steadily to 400–1,200 mL by 34–38 weeks and then declines after 38 weeks to measure an average of around 800 mL by 40 weeks.[12]

In the case of multifetal gestation, one study evaluated amniotic fluid between 27 weeks and 38 weeks in dichorionic diamniotic (DCDA) twins and found that the volumes per sac were similar to singletons.[13]

Measurement of Amniotic Fluid Volume

There are numerous methods to evaluate AFV during pregnancy, but the most accurate noninvasive method is yet to be determined. The most accurate, but most invasive and impractical method is obtaining direct measurements with the use of dye-dilution techniques. The disadvantage is that it is invasive, time-consuming, requires laboratory support, and cannot be used throughout pregnancy.[14]

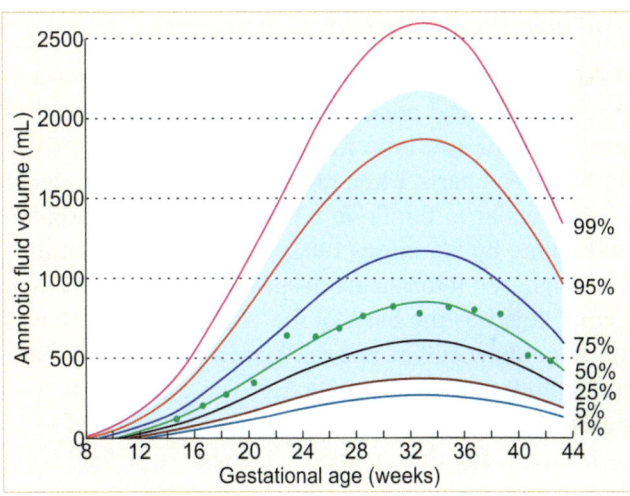

Fig. 4: Amniotic fluid volume as a function of gestational age. Shaded area covers 95% confidence interval.
Source: Brace RA, Wolf EJ. Normal amniotic fluid volume changes throughout pregnancy. Am J Obstet Gynecol. 1989;161:382-8.

Another limitation is that the dye-dilution technique reflects the AFV only at the time of cesarean delivery. Due to these limitations, ultrasound is used to measure AFV at any given point in pregnancy.

Sonographic techniques include subjective (qualitative) estimation and semi-quantitative methods to measure AFV. The advantages of using ultrasound are that it is noninvasive, easy to use, and reproducible. The disadvantage relates to the tomographic nature, where it is a two-dimensional representation of a complex three-dimensional (3D) structure.

Subjective evaluation is based on the overall impression of amniotic fluid by a sonographer by looking at anechoic spaces between fetal parts and placenta. Many studies have demonstrated good correlation between subjective and objective evaluations of amniotic fluid.

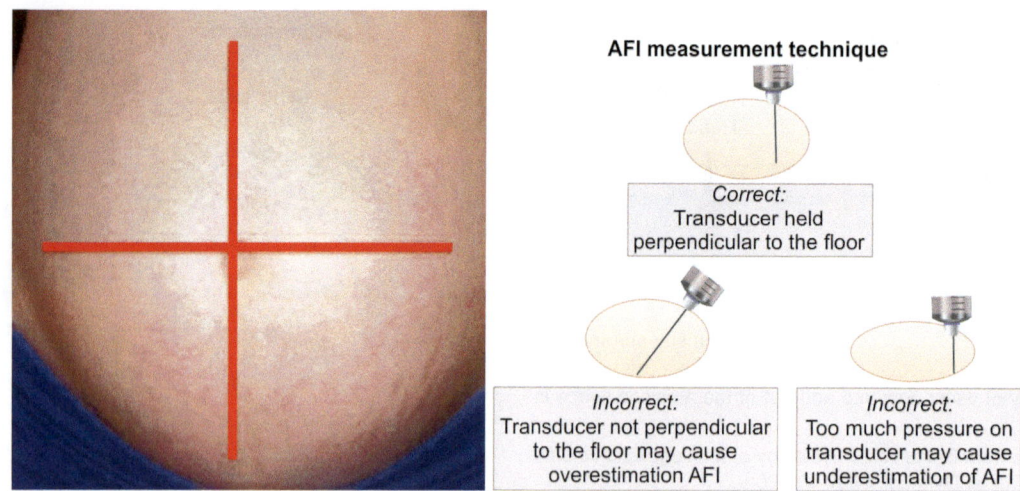

Fig. 5: Technique for amniotic fluid index (AFI).
Source: Adapted from Moore TR. Clinical assessment of amniotic fluid. Clin Obstet Gynecol. 1997;40:303-13.

Semi-quantitative Methods

Maximum vertical pocket or deepest vertical pocket: Maximum vertical pocket (MVP) is the greatest vertical dimension of amniotic fluid pocket free of umbilical cord and fetal parts, when measured with the transducer perpendicular to the floor. It dates back to the original study done by Manning (1980) where oligohydramnios was diagnosed if the single deepest pocket was less than 1 cm.[15] This was the basis of the "1 cm rule" which was subsequently modified to 2 cm, 3 cm, and 0.5 cm. By 1990, the definition of an adequate AFV was a pocket of fluid measuring 2 cm minimum in the vertical axis and 1 cm horizontally. This threshold of 2 × 1 cm pocket of fluid is the current measurement used when using the MVP method.

As of now, oligohydramnios is diagnosed when the MVP is <2 cm and polyhydramnios when MVP >8 cm. MVP between 2 cm and 8 cm is considered normal.

Amniotic fluid index: First introduced by Phelan et al. (1987),[16] this measurement involves the division of the uterus into four quadrants and measuring the deepest vertical pocket in each quadrant. The measurements are then added to give the sum which is the amniotic fluid index (AFI) (Fig. 5).

Technique: Position the patient supine. A linear, curvilinear, or sector transducer can be used. Divide the uterus into four quadrants using the maternal sagittal midline vertically and an arbitrary transverse line approximately halfway between the symphysis pubis and the upper edge of the uterine fundus. The transducer should be kept parallel to the maternal sagittal plane and perpendicular to the maternal coronal plane. The deepest unobstructed and clear pocket of amniotic fluid is visualized and the image frozen. The ultrasound calipers are used to measure the pocket in a strictly vertical direction. The process is repeated in each of the four quadrants and the pockets measurements are added.

If the AFI is <8 cm, perform the four-quadrant evaluation three times and average the values.

The International Society of Ultrasound in Obstetrics and Gynecology recommends that AFI can be measured after 16 weeks (though ideally after 25 weeks) and minimum pressure can be used to measure a pocket free of cord or fetal parts.

A normal AFI measures between 5 cm and 24 cm, but ideally the values are plotted on a graph to assess the percentile values. AFI less than or equal to 5 cm is oligohydramnios and polyhydramnios if AFI >24 cm.

In cases of twins, AFV is stable in normal monochorionic (MC) and dichorionic (DC) twins between 17 and 37 weeks. Definitions for oligohydramnios and polyhydramnios for twins are the same as for singletons. Various techniques have been described to measure AFV by using AFI, but they are very cumbersome and ideally. Deepest vertical pocket should be used rather than AFI to measure the amniotic fluid in twins. The criteria are the same as for singletons to diagnose oligo-/polyhydramnios. Assesment of amniotic fluid in twins should start from 18 weeks onward and done every 4 weeks in cases of DCDA twins and from 16 weeks onward and every 2 weeks in cases of monochorionic diamniotic (MCDA) twins (Table 1).[17]

Earlier studies by Moore[18] has compared the AFI with the MVP technique in 1,168 patients had concluded that AFI method was superior as it identified more women with low AFV. Subsequently, Magann et al.[19] found that both techniques were unreliable in the detection of abnormal AFV and neither technique was superior to the other. A Cochrane review in 2007[14] concluded that MVP measurement seems

Table 1: Amniotic fluid index percentile values.

Weeks	2.5th	5th	50th	95th	97.5th	n
16	73	79	121	185	201	32
17	77	83	127	194	211	26
18	80	87	133	202	220	17
19	83	90	137	207	225	14
20	86	93	141	212	230	25
21	88	95	143	214	233	14
22	89	97	145	216	235	14
23	90	98	146	218	237	14
24	90	98	147	219	238	23
25	89	97	147	221	240	12
26	89	97	147	223	242	11
27	85	95	146	226	245	17
28	86	94	146	228	249	25
29	84	92	145	231	254	12
30	82	90	145	234	258	17
31	79	88	144	238	263	26
32	77	86	144	242	269	25
33	74	83	143	245	274	30
34	72	81	142	248	278	31
35	70	79	140	249	279	27
36	68	77	138	249	279	39
37	66	75	135	244	275	36
38	65	73	132	239	269	27
39	64	72	127	226	255	12
40	63	71	123	214	240	64
41	63	70	116	194	216	162
42	63	69	110	175	192	30

Source: Moore TR, Cayle JE. The amniotic fluid index in normal human pregnancy. Am J Obstet Gynecol. 1990;162:1168-73.

to be a better choice and the AFI method increases the rate of diagnosis of AFV abnormalities and labor inductions without improving the perinatal outcome. Though there is no constant standard, it is recommended that in cases of suspected polyhydramnios, it is preferable measure all four vertical fluid pockets and in cases of oligohydramnios to measure the single deepest vertical pocket.

OLIGOHYDRAMNIOS

Oligohydramnios means reduced liquor volume. As discussed earlier, the MVP is the best method for diagnosing oligohydramnios. In order to decide the management and predict prognosis, one needs to understand the reasons responsible for the lack of amniotic fluid in pregnancy.

The incidence is about 1-5% of pregnancies at term.[20] In pregnancies of more than 40 weeks of gestation, the incidence may be even more than 12% as the AFV declines progressively after 41 weeks of gestation.[21]

Etiology

Oligohydramnios may be due to premature rupture of membranes (PROMs) which may remain unrecognized by the mother. It can also result from some fetal abnormalities such as fetal aneuploidy, lower urinary tract obstruction, and bilateral renal agenesis. Uteroplacental insufficiency is a recognized entity which cannot be proven objectively by any investigation, but it may manifest into diminished production of amniotic fluid as in the cases of fetal growth restriction (FGR), hypertensive disorders, placental abruption, maternal thrombotic diseases, and postterm gestation. Maternal exposure to certain medications, e.g., angiotensin-converting enzyme (ACE) inhibitors,[22] nonsteroidal anti-inflammatory drugs (NSAIDs)[23] may also contribute to the condition.

Clinical Assessment and Investigations

While ultrasonography is the most common diagnostic method, detailed history and clinical examination may elicit maternal conditions like hypertension. Reduced symphysio-fundal height may be the only clinical sign, but it has a very poor sensitivity and specificity. A sterile speculum examination should be performed as soon as oligohydramnios is suspected. Any visible loss of fluid through cervical os should be documented. Targeted ultrasonography may demonstrate FGR or specific fetal anomalies. There is no consensus as to how often these ultrasonographic examinations should be performed, but it should depend on several factors such as gestation, severity of the condition, and associated fetomaternal comorbidities.

Management

In a meta-analysis performed by Chauhan et al., it was found that both antepartum and intrapartum oligohydramnios were associated with an increased risk of cesarean delivery for fetal distress and 5 minutes Apgar score < 7 but it had no impact on acidosis.[24] Furthermore, it has also been attempted to stratify cases of oligohydramnios into low-risk and high-risk pregnancies.[25] In the low-risk pregnancies with isolated oligohydramnios, there would be an increased risk of meconium aspiration syndrome, cesarean delivery for fetal distress, and admission to neonatal intensive care unit (NICU). However, the risk of stillbirth and perinatal mortality could not be evaluated in this meta-analysis. Casey et al. demonstrated the association between oligohydramnios and stillbirth, but they found it difficult to determine whether intervention would improve the outcome.[26] In the high-risk (complicated by other underlying conditions) pregnancies, there would be an increased risk of delivering smaller infants. As the oligohydramnios in such cases is probably a function of the underlying conditions, the management would depend on those specific situations.[25]

Prolonged lack of liquor from early gestation may cause multiple fetal malformations as happens in Potter sequence resulting into pulmonary hypoplasia, limb deformities, and cranial anomalies. Role of amnioinfusion in early-onset oligohydramnios has been studied extensively with inconsistent results. O'Hare et al. recently concluded that a large scale randomized controlled trial is necessary to determine the efficacy of amnioinfusion to promote lung development and assess long-term outcomes of dialysis and kidney transplant.[27]

As stated by the Fetal Medicine Foundation, UK, the standard obstetric care and delivery can be followed in fetal urinary tract abnormalities. In PROM, expectant management and vaginal delivery may be tried if cephalic presentation. For uteroplacental insufficiency, cesarean section or vaginal delivery depending on gestational age, fetal size, and degree of fetal compromise as defined by Doppler and/or cardiotocography. The prognosis of oligohydramnios depends on gestational age at diagnosis, cause, and gestational age at delivery. Preterm rupture of membranes at ≤20 weeks of gestation is associated with a poor prognosis; about 40% miscarry within 5 days of membrane rupture due to chorioamnionitis and in the remaining 60% of pregnancies, more than 50% of neonates die due to pulmonary hypoplasia. Uteroplacental insufficiency resulting in oligohydramnios at ≤24 weeks of gestation is very severe and the most likely outcome is intrauterine death.[28]

Fetuses with prolonged oligohydramnios from any cause are at increased risk for pulmonary hypoplasia. The exact pathogenesis behind this is not yet clear.

The formal diagnosis of pulmonary hypoplasia is histological and based on measurement of the postmortem lung-to-body weight ratio (LBWR). There is no reliable method with which we can assess and quantify most of these variables. Consequently, there is no current clinical indication to perform ultrasound or MRI tests in order to predict pulmonary hypoplasia.[29]

POLYHYDRAMNIOS

Excessive accumulation of amniotic fluid is called polyhydramnios. The incidence of polyhydramnios is considered to be between 0.2% and 3.9%.[30] Degree of polyhydramnios may be described as mild, moderate, and severe based on the AFI. Mild polyhydramnios has been defined as an AFI of 25–30 cm (or MVP of 8 cm or greater). Moderate polyhydramnios is meant when AFI is between 30 cm and 35 cm (MVP 12–15 cm) and severe when AFI crosses 35 cm (MVP >15 cm).[31] Every case of polyhydramnios demands a systematic approach for accurate diagnosis and management.

Etiology

Maternal diabetes leading to fetal hyperglycemia and polyuria is one of the most common causes of polyhydramnios.[30] Fetal causes would include upper gastrointestinal (GI) obstruction of any causes (commonly duodenal atresia) impairing the ability to swallow, twin-twin transfusion syndrome, high output cardiac failure as in fetal anemia, sacrococcygeal teratoma, etc. However, in about 50–60% of cases, polyhydramnios would be unexplained or idiopathic and there would be a two- to fivefold increase in perinatal morbidity and mortality.[31]

The common etiological associations of polyhydramnios in a singleton pregnancy are highlighted in Box 1 and the common fetal structural abnormalities are highlighted in Box 2.

Clinical Assessment and Investigations

Clinical findings include a tense uterus, larger fundal height for gestation, and difficulty in palpating fetal parts. However, polyhydramnios is most commonly diagnosed on ultrasound examination as incidental findings.

Maternal investigations should start with oral glucose tolerance test and hemoglobin A1c (HbA1c) for the

---

Box 1: Causes of polyhydramnios in a singleton pregnancy.

- *Maternal*:
  - Uncontrolled diabetes mellitus (pregestational and gestational)
  - Rhesus and other blood group isoimmunization leading to immune hydrops
  - Drug exposure, e.g., lithium leading to fetal diabetes insipidus
- *Fetal*:
  - Structural malformations (*see* Box 2)
  - Chromosomal and genetic abnormalities, e.g., trisomies, Beckwith-Wiedemann syndrome, fetal akinesia-dyskinesia syndrome
  - Congenital infections, e.g., toxoplasma, rubella, cytomegalovirus, parvovirus
  - Macrosomia
  - Fetal tumors, e.g., teratomas, nephromas, neuroblastomas, haemangiomas
- *Placental*: Tumors such as chorioangiomas and metastatic neuroblastomas
- Unexplained

Source: Karkhanis P, Patni S. Polyhydramnios in singleton pregnancies: perinatal outcomes and management. The Obstetrician and Gynaecologist. 2014;16:207-13.

> **Box 2:** Fetal structural abnormalities causing polyhydramnios in a singleton pregnancy.
>
> - *Central nervous system*:
>   - Anencephaly
>   - Spina bifida
>   - Encephalocele
>   - Hydrocephalus
>   - Microcephaly
>   - Dandy-Walker malformation
> - *Head and neck*: Goitre, Cystic hygroma, cleft palate
> - *Respiratory system*:
>   - Tracheal agenesis
>   - Congenital diaphragmatic hernia
>   - Congenital pulmonary airway malformation
>   - Broncho pulmonary sequestration
> - *Gastrointestinal system*:
>   - Esophageal atresia and tracheo-oesophageal fistula, duodenal and intestinal atresia
>   - Exomphalos
>   - Gastroschisis
> - *Genitourinary system*:
>   - Pelviureteric junction obstruction
>   - Barter syndrome
> - *Skeletal system*: Lethal skeletal dysplasia
> - *Cardiovascular system*: Cardiac anomalies
> - *Fetal tumors*: Sacrococcygeal teratoma
> - *Others*:
>   - Immune and nonimmune hydrops fetalis
>   - Fetal akinesia-dyskinesia syndrome
>
> *Source*: Karkhanis P, Patni S. Polyhydramnios in singleton pregnancies: perinatal outcomes and management. The Obstetrician and Gynaecologist. 2014;16:207-13.

identified diabetics. Maternal blood group, Rhesus typing, and screening for any other atypical antibodies should be performed. Testing for congenital infections, e.g., toxoplasma, parvovirus, and cytomegalovirus should also be done on maternal blood.

The mainstay of fetal investigations is ultrasonography for any structural abnormalities. The chance of finding fetal anomaly increases with increasing severity of polyhydramnios. Karyotyping or other advanced genetic testing such as chromosomal microarray should be performed depending on the type of detected anomaly.

Management

Mothers with polyhydramnios should be informed of increased risk of preterm delivery. Antenatal corticosteroids for fetal lung maturity should be administered wherever indicated. Maternal medical condition should be optimized with multidisciplinary team, like in cases of diabetes. Referral to maternal-fetal medicine is advisable in cases of suspected fetal anomaly, small for gestational age fetuses, reduced fetal movement, and persistent or worsening polyhydramnios.

Maternal complications include excessive discomfort, uterine irritability, postpartum hemorrhage, and mostly attributed to uterine overdistension. The fetal risks on the other hand include preterm PROMs, cord prolapse, placental abruption, preterm labor, and delivery. Perinatal mortality is further increased by presence of a wide range of fetal abnormalities which may not be evident on prenatal ultrasonography and appropriate postnatal workup may be necessary.

Therapeutic amniocentesis or amniodrainage has been used to treat symptomatic cases mainly to alleviate maternal respiratory discomfort. However, this procedure has its limitations in having high risk of recurrence and small chance of PROMs, chorioamnionitis, and placental abruption.

Prostaglandin synthetase inhibitors such as indomethacin and sulindac have been used for their effect on reducing fetal urinary output and by enhancing the resorption of lung fluid. However, these medications are associated with impaired renal function and premature closure of the ductus arteriosus.[32,33] Hence, they should be used only under strict supervision.

Induction of labor or cesarean section is reserved for other coexisting obstetric indications. Preparations should be in place to handle potential adverse events such as shoulder dystocia, postpartum hemorrhage, etc.

CONCLUSION

Amniotic fluid volume assessment is as an indispensable adjunct to antenatal fetal assessment; therefore, it is crucial that a standard method be determined to prevent fetal morbidity and mortality as well as other adverse pregnancy outcomes when AFV abnormalities are diagnosed. Accurate assessment and diagnosis of AFV abnormalities provides physicians with information necessary to properly manage a pregnancy longitudinally, which may improve the overall outcome of the pregnancy.

REFERENCES

1. Magann, EF, Sandlin AT, Ounpraseuth ST. Amniotic fluid and the clinical relevance of the svonographically estimated amniotic fluid volume. J Ultrasound Med. 2011;30:1573-85.
2. Wallenburg HC. The amniotic fluid I. Water and electrolyte homeostasis. J Perinat Med. 1977;5:193-205.
3. Brace RA, Wolf EJ. Normal amniotic fluid volume changes throughout pregnancy. Am J Obstet Gynecol. 1989;161:382-8.
4. Mann SE, Nijland MJ, Ross MG. Mathematic modeling of human amniotic fluid dynamics. Am J Obstet Gynecol. 1996;175:937-44.
5. Ross MG, Nijland MJ. Fetal swallowing: relation to amniotic fluid regulation. Clin Obstet Gynecol. 1997;40:352-65.
6. Espinoza J, Gonçalves LF, Romero R, et al. The prevalence and clinical significance of amniotic fluid 'sludge' in patients with preterm labor and intact membranes. Ultrasound Obstet Gynecol. 2005;25:346-52.

7. Müngen E, Tütüncü L, Muhcu M. Pregnancy outcome in women with echogenic amniotic fluid at term gestation. Int J Gynaecol Obstet. 2005;88:314-5.
8. Lind T, Kendall A, Hytten FE. The role of the fetus in the formation of amniotic fluid. J Obstet Gynaecol Br Commonw. 1972;79:289-98.
9. Abramovich DR. Fetal factors influencing the volume and composition of liquor amnii. J Obstet Gynaecol Br Commonw. 1970;77:865-77.
10. Kilpatrick SJ, Safford KL, Pomeroy T, et al. Maternal hydration increases amniotic fluid index. Obstet Gynecol. 1991;78:1098-102.
11. Pritchard JA. Fetal swallowing and amniotic fluid volume. Obstet Gynecol. 1966;28:606-10.
12. Queenan JT, Thompson W, Whitfield CR, et al. Amniotic fluid volumes in normal pregnancies. Am J Obstet Gynecol. 1972;114:34-8.
13. Magann EF, Whitworth NS, Bass JD, et al. Amniotic fluid volume of third-trimester diamniotic twin pregnancies. Obstet Gynecol. 1995;85:957-60.
14. Nabhan AF, Abdelmoula YA. Amniotic fluid index versus single deepest vertical pocket as a screening test for preventing adverse pregnancy outcome. Cochrane Database Syst Rev. 2008;(3):CD006593.
15. Manning FA, Hill LM, Platt LD. Qualitative amniotic fluid volume determination by ultrasound: antepartum detection of intrauterine growth retardation. Am J Obstet Gynecol. 1981;139:254-8.
16. Phelan JP, Smith CV, Broussard P, et al. Amniotic fluid volume assessment with the four-quadrant technique at 36-42 weeks' gestation. J Reprod Med. 1987;32:540-2.
17. Khalil A, Rodgers M, Baschat A, et al. ISUOG Practice Guidelines: role of ultrasound in twin pregnancy. Ultrasound Obstet Gynecol. 2016;47:247-63.
18. Moore TR. Superiority of the four-quadrant sum over the single-deepest pocket technique in ultrasonographic identification of abnormal amniotic fluid volumes. Am J Obstet Gynecol. 1990;163:762-7.
19. Magann E, Chauhan SP, Barrilleaux PS, et al. Amniotic fluid index and single deepest pocket: weak indicators of abnormal amniotic volumes. Obstet Gynecol. 2000;96:737-40.
20. Moore IR. Clinical assessment of amniotic fluid. Clin Obstet Gynaecol. 1997;40:303-13.
21. Sherer DM, Langer O. Oligohydramnios: use and misuse in clinical management. Ultrasound Obstet Gynecol. 2001;18:411-9.
22. Bullo ML, Tschumi S, Bucher BS, et al. Pregnancy outcome following exposure to angiotensin-converting enzyme inhibitors or angiotensin receptor antagonists: a systematic review. Hypertension. 2012;60:444-50.
23. Antonucci R, Zaffanello M, Puxeddu E, et al. Use of non-steroidal anti-inflammatory drugs in pregnancy: impact on the fetus and newborn. Curr Drug Metab. 2012;13:474-90.
24. Chauhan SP, Sanderson M, Hendrix NW, et al. Perinatal outcome and amniotic fluid index in the antepartum and intrapartum periods: a meta-analysis. Am J Obstet Gynecol. 1999;181:1473-8.
25. Rabie N, Magann E, Steelman S, et al. Oligohydramnios in complicated and uncomplicated pregnancy: a systematic review and meta-analysis. Ultrasound Obstet Gynecol. 2017;49:442-9.
26. Casey BM, McIntyre DD, Bloom SL, et al. Pregnancy outcomes after antepartum diagnosis of oligohydramnios at or beyond 34 weeks gestation. Am J Obstet Gynecol. 2003;43:129-33.
27. O'Hare EM, Jelin AC, Miller JL, et al. Amnioinfusions to treat early onset anhydramnios caused by renal anomalies: background and rationale for the renal anhydramnios fetal therapy trial. Fetal Diagn Ther. 2019;45:365-72.
28. Fetal Medicine Foundation (2019). Fetal abnormalities: amniotic fluid: oligohydramnios. [online] Available from https://fetalmedicine.org/education/fetal-abnormalities/amniotic-fluid/oligohydramnios. [Last accessed November, 2019].
29. Cavoretto P. Prediction of pulmonary hypoplasia in midtrimester preterm prelabor rupture of membranes: research or clinical practice? Ultrasound Obstet Gynecol. 2012;39:489-94.
30. Vink JY, Poggi SH, Ghidini A, et al. Amniotic fluid index and birth weight: is there a relationship in diabetes with poor glycemic control? Am J Obstet Gynecol. 2006;195:848-50.
31. Magann EF, Chauhan SP, Doherty DA, et al. A review of idiopathic hydramnios and pregnancy outcomes. Obstet Gynecol Surv. 2007;62:795-802.
32. Moise KL, Huhta JC, Sharif DS, et al. Indomethacin in the treatment of premature labor. Effects on the fetal ductus arteriosus. N Engl J Med. 1998;319:327-31.
33. Buderus S, Thomas B, Fahnenstich AH, et al. Renal failure in two preterm infants: toxic effect of prenatal maternal indomethacin treatment? Br J Obstet Gynecol. 1993;100:97-8.

16

Ultrasound in Third Trimester

Vandana Bansal, Rujul Jhaveri, Neha Singh

BACKGROUND

It is a well-established fact that antenatal ultrasound plays an important role in management of low-risk as well as high-risk pregnancies. It helps in reducing maternal and neonatal morbidity and mortality by timely diagnosis of certain fetal and maternal conditions, timely decisions and interventions, and better postnatal preparedness toward managing early neonatal problems. Third trimester starts from 28 weeks onward and assessment of fetal growth is commonly initiated at or around 28–32 weeks in pregnancies at risk.

Though, the main objective of third trimester obstetrical ultrasound examination is to provide accurate diagnostic information regarding fetal growth, amniotic fluid volume (AFV), placental localization, and Doppler flows, it may also be used as a second look for various late-onset fetal anomalies.

The rationale for such screening would be the detection of clinical condition which places the fetus or mother at high risk, which would not necessarily have been detected by other means such as clinical examination, and for which subsequent management would improve perinatal outcome.

CURRENT SCENARIO OF OBSTETRIC IMAGING IN INDIA

At present, ultrasound is used selectively in late pregnancy where there are specific clinical indications. The value of routine late pregnancy ultrasound screening in unselected populations is controversial. In Canada and the United States, a routine third trimester ultrasound scan is not offered in the low-risk pregnancy population. However, in some European countries (France, Switzerland, Belgium, and Germany), it is common practice to include routine third trimester ultrasound as part of normal prenatal care.

India has no set standards for number of ultrasounds to be done in pregnancy, their interpretation and reporting. As per the National Family Health Survey, ultrasound was performed in only 24% of pregnancies. Out of these, only 4% women in the lowest socioeconomic quintile had an ultrasound test compared with 62% among the highest wealth quintile. High-risk cases and fetal anomalies may be detected when women are delivering; thereby, there is no preparedness for outcome and complications.[1]

The Ministry of Health and Family Welfare, Government of India, has published guidelines on the use of ultrasonography during pregnancy which recommend one obstetric ultrasound should be done during pregnancy between 18 weeks and 19 weeks of pregnancy as part of routine antenatal care (ANC) package which provides opportunity to diagnose congenital anomalies, detect soft markers of aneuploidy, identify maternal pelvic pathology, confirm the number of fetuses present, the gestational age, and the location of the placenta. Additional ultrasound examinations can be done if clinically indicated. There is no mention of a third trimester ultrasound in our Indian guidelines.[1]

The World Health Organization (WHO) recommendations on ANC for a positive pregnancy experience state that one ultrasound scan before 24 weeks is recommended for pregnant women to estimate gestational age, improve detection of fetal anomalies and multiple pregnancies, reduce induction of labor for postterm pregnancy, and improve a woman's pregnancy experience. No routine

Doppler ultrasound examination in the third trimester nor any late pregnancy scan is recommended.[2]

Hence, the performance of or need for any additional third trimester scans is based on local guidelines, clinical experience, presence or absence of maternal or fetal conditions, and risk factors or related findings that are known to be associated with abnormal growth.

THIRD TRIMESTER ULTRASOUND AS A DIAGNOSTIC TOOL

After a routine midtrimester ultrasound scan, typically performed between 18 weeks and 22 weeks of gestation, an additional third trimester scan is useful for monitoring fetal well-being, amniotic fluid index (AFI), fetal presentation, placental position, cord insertion, rescreen for fetal anomalies, biometry and estimated fetal weight (EFW), and subsequent detection of fetal growth abnormalities (both growth restriction and macrosomia).

Fetal growth restriction (FGR) is an important cause of perinatal morbidity and mortality, and when detected antenatally, intensive fetal surveillance, including Doppler studies, can improve its perinatal outcome. Third trimester ultrasound assessment remains the gold standard for diagnosing FGR. Amniotic fluid abnormalities such as oligohydramnios can be both diagnosed and monitored using ultrasound. Addition of Doppler modality helps in prognostication and determining the time of delivery, especially in preterm fetuses. Also, ultrasound is used for the confirmation of breech presentation and other malpresentations, where Leopold maneuvers may not be sensitive enough. Obstetric management would change with the diagnosis of a malpresentation at term.

When fetal malformations are discovered late in pregnancy, late termination of pregnancy is permitted in few countries which justifies a policy of routine third trimester ultrasound. Also, fetal malformation diagnosed during the third trimester in a country where termination is not permitted as in India beyond 20 weeks, the location, timing, and route of delivery may be modified in order to improve the neonatal outcome.

INDICATIONS/COMPONENTS OF ULTRASOUND EXAMINATION IN THIRD TRIMESTER

A standard list of indications for which a second or third trimester ultrasound may be asked for has been enumerated by the American Institute of Ultrasound in Medicine (AIUM)-American College of Radiology (ACR)-American College of Obstetricians and Gynecologists (ACOG)-Society for Maternal-Fetal Medicine (SMFM)-Society of Radiologists in Ultrasound (SRU) guidelines on Practice Parameters for performance of standard diagnostic ultrasound examination, 2018.[3] These may be indicated at any time even in the third trimester as per the clinical situation. The starred indications may not be accurately determined in the third trimester and are more accurate in the second or the first trimesters but in developing countries like ours, this may be the first time that the patient may report for ultrasound.

Standard Second and Third Trimester Ultrasonography Examination[3]

- Screening for fetal anomalies
- Evaluation of fetal anatomy
- Estimation of gestational age
- Evaluation of suspected multiple gestation and chorionicity
- Evaluation of cervical length
- Evaluation of fetal growth
- Evaluation of a significant discrepancy between uterine size and clinical dates
- Determination of fetal presentation
- Evaluation of fetal well-being
- Suspected amniotic fluid abnormalities
- Evaluation of premature rupture of membranes and/or preterm labor
- Evaluation of vaginal bleeding
- Evaluation of abdominal or pelvic pain
- Suspected placental abruption
- Suspected fetal death
- Follow-up evaluation of a fetal anomaly
- Evaluation/follow-up of placental appearance and location, including suspected placenta previa, and abnormally adherent placenta
- Adjunct to amniocentesis or other procedure
- Adjunct to external cephalic version
- Evaluation of a pelvic mass
- Suspected uterine anomalies

IMAGING PARAMETERS FOR A STANDARD EXAMINATION IN THIRD TRIMESTER[3]

- *Fetal cardiac activity* (by video clip or M-mode), *fetal number, and presentation* should be documented. Abnormal heart rate and/or rhythm should be documented. Multiple gestations require the documentation of additional information: Chorionicity, amnionicity, comparison of fetal sizes, AFV in each gestational sac, and fetal genitalia (when visualized).
- A qualitative or semiquantitative estimate of *AFV* should be documented. Semiquantitative methods include AFI, single deepest pocket (SDP), and two-diameter pocket.

In assessing oligohydramnios, the deepest vertical pocket (<2 cm) is preferred over AFI (≤5 cm) because it results in fewer obstetric interventions without a significant difference in the perinatal outcome, and the SDP should be at least 1 cm wide. Polyhydramnios (deepest vertical pocket ≥ 8 cm or AFI ≥ 24 cm) may be associated with other pregnancy complications.

- The *placental location*, appearance, and relationship with the internal cervical os should be documented. The umbilical cord should be imaged and the number of vessels in the cord should be documented. The *placental cord insertion site* should be documented when technically possible. Color and pulsed Doppler ultrasound should be used to assess vasa previa or abnormal placental cord insertion.

- *Fetal weight estimation* can be done from measurements, i.e., biparietal diameter (BPD), head circumference (HC), abdominal circumference (AC), or average abdominal diameter, and femoral diaphysis length. Scans for growth evaluation can typically be performed at least 3 weeks apart. A shorter scan interval may result in confusion as to whether measurement changes are truly due to growth as opposed to variations in the technique itself. Currently, even the best weight prediction methods can yield errors as high as ±15%.

- Pregnancy dating should not be performed in third trimester due to reported inaccuracy by ±3 weeks.

Fetal Growth Surveillance

Symphysis-fundal height measurement is the commonly used primary screening method for small for gestational age (SGA) and intrauterine growth restriction (IUGR) worldwide. In most countries, ultrasound biometry is performed only if measurements deviate from normal or if the pregnancy is considered as high risk. However, approximately 50% of SGA infants come from low-risk pregnancies. FGR and being SGA are major causes of adverse perinatal outcome.[4]

When a growth disturbance is suspected clinically or there is a medical or obstetric condition that increases the risk of a growth disturbance, ultrasonography is the modality of choice to identify abnormal fetal growth. Ultrasound examination at 36 weeks of gestation is found to be more effective than at 32 weeks of gestation in detecting FGR and predicting related adverse perinatal and neonatal outcomes. Serial scans for interval growth are best performed at least 3 weeks after a preceding scan.[5]

Accurate estimation of gestational age is a prerequisite for determining whether fetal size is appropriate for gestational age (AGA). Dating pregnancies is best done by early ultrasound examination at 8–14 weeks [crown-rump length (CRL) <84 mm] or based on HC (if CRL > 84 mm). Dating of pregnancy once defined should not be modified as per the subsequent scans.[5]

Being a dynamic process, assessment of fetal growth requires at least two ultrasound scans separated in time. Maternal history and symptoms, amniotic fluid assessment, and Doppler velocimetry can provide additional information that may be used to identify fetuses at risk of adverse pregnancy outcome.

- Appropriate for gestational age fetus is one whose size is within the normal range for its gestational age. AGA fetuses typically have individual biometric parameters and/or EFW between the 10th percentile and 90th percentile (Fig. 1).

- Small for gestational age fetus is one whose size is below a predefined threshold for its gestational age. SGA fetuses typically have EFW or AC below the 10th percentile, although 5th centile, 3rd centile, –2 SD, and Z-score deviation have also been used as cutoffs in the literature (Fig. 2).

- Fetal growth restriction/intrauterine growth restriction fetus is one that has not achieved its growth potential. This condition can be associated with adverse perinatal and neurodevelopmental outcomes. It has been classified into *early-onset* (detected before 32 weeks of gestation) and late-onset (detected after 32 weeks of gestation) types (Figs. 3A and B).

- Large for gestational age (LGA) fetus is one whose size is above a predefined threshold for its gestational age. LGA fetuses typically have EFW or AC above the 90th percentile. Macrosomia at term usually refers to a weight above a fixed cutoff (4,000 g or 4,500 g) (Fig. 4).

Depending upon the period of onset, FGR has been classified into early-onset (detected before 32 weeks of gestation) and late-onset (detected after 32 weeks of gestation) types. Another popular traditional method of classification involves the symmetry of fetal body proportions being indicative of the underlying etiology for FGR. The concept that symmetrical FGR is due to fetal aneuploidy and progressive asymmetrical FGR is due to placental insufficiency is now challenged, with cases of fetal aneuploidy resulting in asymmetrical FGR and those of placental insufficiency resulting in symmetrical FGR. Hence, the recent International Society of Ultrasound in Obstetrics and Gynecology (ISUOG) recommendations state that the terms "symmetrical" and "asymmetrical" FGR should no longer be used, given that they do not provide additional information with regard to etiology or prognosis.[5]

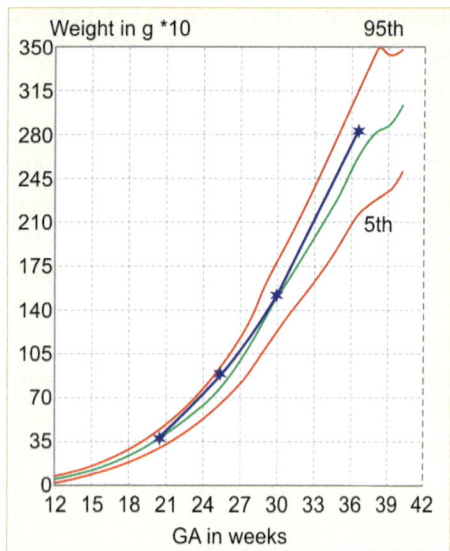
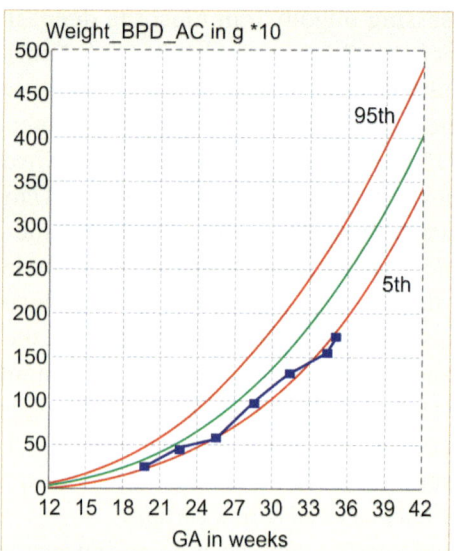

Fig. 1: Appropriate for gestational age (GA) fetus growth charts.

Fig. 2: Small for gestational age fetus growth charts (AC: abdominal circumference; BPD: biparietal diameter; GA: gestational age)

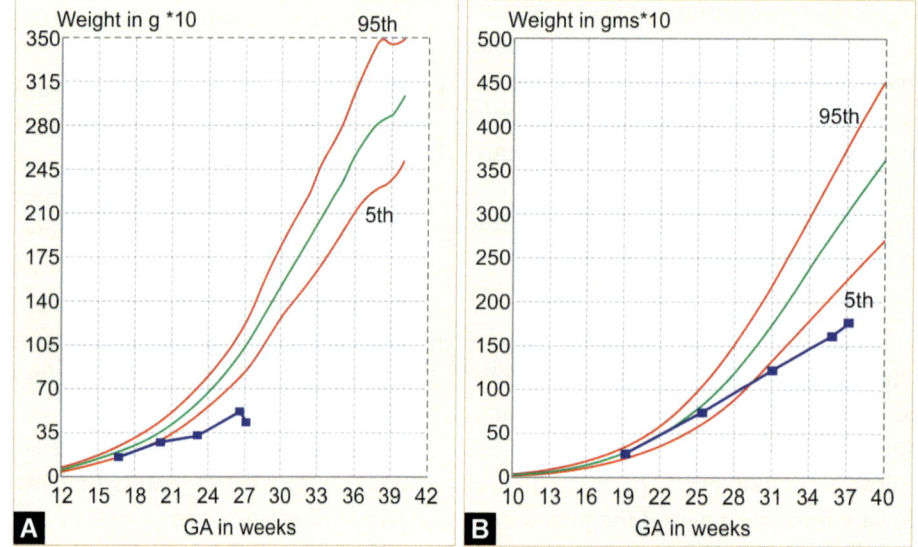

Figs. 3A and B: (A) Fetal growth restriction early-onset growth charts; and (B) Fetal growth restriction late-onset growth charts.

As per the ISUOG guidelines, EFW may be used to monitor fetal size and growth. However, the best method for SGA prediction is still unclear, with EFW having the disadvantages of large intra- and interobserver variability while using a single parameter like AC may be sensitive but not specific. They recommend that the time interval between scans should typically be at least 3 weeks to minimize false-positive rates for the detection of fetal growth disorder, but this recommendation does not preclude more frequently performed scans when clinically indicated.[5]

New fetal growth curves have been developed in an attempt to improve the detection rate of SGA, e.g., in the US, the Eunice Kennedy Shriver National Institute of Child Health and Human Development (NICHD) Fetal Growth Studies and two international, INTERGROWTH-21st and the WHO Multicentre Growth Reference Study (WHO Fetal). The INTERGROWTH-21st and WHO Fetal studies on fetal growth started with the assumption that infants and children of well-off parents represent optimal growth in size and that there would be no differences internationally in fetal growth when conditions were optimal.[6-9] Customized growth charts have also been proposed according to maternal characteristics (height, weight, parity, and ethnicity) and fetal gender.[6-9]

A cutoff point below the 10th centile for gestation for AC and/or EFW is a commonly accepted definition of FGR. However, the main drawback of using this definition is that the 10th centile cutoff value varies depending on the

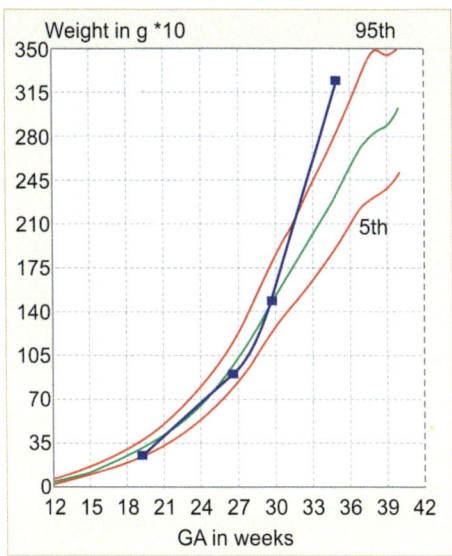

Fig. 4: Large for gestational age (GA) growth charts.

Table 1: Consensus-based definitions for early and late fetal growth restriction (FGR) in absence of congenital anomalies.[5,10]

Early FGR: GA <32 weeks, in absence of congenital anomalies	Late FGR: GA ≥32 weeks, in absence of congenital anomalies
AC/EFW <3rd centile or UA-AEDF Or 1. AC/EFW <10th centile *combined with* 2. UtA-PI >95th centile *and/or* 3. UA-PI >95th centile	AC/EFW <3rd centile Or at least two out of three of the following: 1. AC/EFW <10th centile 2. AC/EFW crossing centiles > two quartiles on growth centiles 3. CPR <5th centile or UA-PI > 95th centile

(AC: abdominal circumference; AEDF: absent end-diastolic flow; CPR: cerebroplacental ratio; EFW: estimated fetal weight; GA: gestational age; PI: pulsatility index; UA: umbilical artery; UtA: uterine artery)

Table 2: Main differences between early- and late-onset forms of FGR as per the update on diagnosis and classification of FGR proposed by Eduard Gratacos.[11]

Early-onset FGR (1–2%)	Late-onset FGR (3–5%)
Problem: Management	*Problem*: Diagnosis
Placental disease: Severe (UA Doppler abnormal, high association with pre-eclampsia)	*Placental disease*: Mild (UA Doppler normal, low association with pre-eclampsia)
Hypoxia ++: Systemic cardiovascular adaptation	*Hypoxia* ±: Central cardiovascular adaptation
Immature fetus = Higher tolerance to hypoxia = Natural history	Mature fetus = Lower tolerance to hypoxia = No (or very short) natural history
High mortality and morbidity; lower prevalence	Lower mortality (but common cause of late stillbirth); poor long-term outcome; affects large fraction of pregnancies

(FGR: fetal growth restriction; UA: umbilical artery)

chart used and there is considerable overlap between the two categories. This is because most SGA babies are not growth restricted at birth, and some babies with FGR due to placental insufficiency who are at risk of compromise or stillbirth are AGA. The lower the cutoff of AC and EFW, the higher the risk of true FGR.

An international Delphi consensus recently proposed that a cutoff of AC or EFW below the 3rd centile should be used as the sole diagnostic criterion for FGR. In case of AC or EFW below the 10th centile, the diagnosis of FGR should be considered only in association with other parameters. Observation of drop in centile or Z-score on growth charts should trigger further monitoring. A drop of more than two quartiles (or more than 50 centiles) has been recommended by consensus criteria for FGR. The ISUOG guidelines recommend the diagnostic criteria for selective FGR (sFGR) may be based on Delphi consensus criteria (Tables 1 and 2).[5,10]

A diagnosis of FGR should trigger referral to an appropriate unit for individualized management. Management will depend on the cause of FGR. In many cases, this will include assessment of fetal well-being in order to identify those fetuses requiring delivery. Antenatal testing strategies include: cardiotocography [nonstress test (NST)] by means of computerized assessment; biophysical profile (BPP) score; AFV assessment; evaluation of Doppler indices of the umbilical artery (UA), fetal middle cerebral artery (MCA), or a combination of the two (cerebroplacental or umbilicocerebral ratio); and assessment of aortic isthmus (AoI) and ductus venosus (DV) flow. Stage-based approach to management of FGR has been proposed by Gratacos (Table 3).[11]

Antepartum Fetal Surveillance

Available tests to assess fetal well-being are based upon fetal biophysical findings that include heart rate, movement, breathing, and amniotic fluid production. Tests for fetal well-being and indices can be classified as acute or chronic. Former correlate with acute changes occurring in advanced stages of fetal compromise and characterized by severe hypoxia and metabolic acidosis and usually precedes fetal death in a few days. In contrast to this, tests based on chronic changes become progressively abnormal due to gradually increasing hypoxemia and/or hypoxia. In most cases, a negative, that is, normal test result is highly reassuring, because fetal deaths within 1 week of a normal test are rare.

Biophysical Profile

Biophysical profile proposed by Manning et al. assesses five fetal biophysical variables which require 30–60 minutes

Table 3: Stage-based classification and management of FGR.

Stages	Pathophysiological correlate	Criteria (any of)	Monitoring*	GA/mode of delivery
I	Severe smallness or mild placental insufficiency	EFW < 3rd centile CPR < p5 UA-PI > p95 MCA-PI < p5 UtA-PI > p95	Weekly	37 weeks LI
II	Severe placental insufficiency	UA-AEDV Reverse AoI	Biweekly	34 weeks CS
III	Low-suspicion fetal acidosis	UA-REDV DV-PI > p95	1–2 days	30 weeks CS
IV	High-suspicion fetal acidosis	DV reverse flow cCTG <3 ms FHR decelerations	12 hours	26 weeks** CS

* Recommended intervals in the absence of severe pre-eclampsia. If FGR is accompanied by this complication, strict fetal monitoring is warranted regardless of the stage.
** Lower GA threshold recommended according to current literature figures reporting at least 50% intact survival. Threshold could be tailored according to parents' wishes or adjusted according to local statistics of intact survival.
(AEDV: absent end-diastolic velocity; AoI: aortic isthmus; CPR: cerebroplacental ratio; DV: ductus venosus; EFW: estimated fetal weight; FGR: fetal growth restriction; FHR: fetal heart rate; GA: gestational age; MCA: middle cerebral artery; PI: pulsatility index; UA: umbilical artery; UtA: uterine artery)

of examiner time. Five fetal biophysical components are: (1) Heart rate acceleration in NST, (2) Breathing, (3) Movements, (4) Tone, and (5) AFV. One study found that biophysical score of 0 was almost invariably associated with significant fetal acidemia, whereas a normal score of 8 or 10 was associated with normal pH whereas an equivocal test result (a score of 6) was a poor predictor of abnormal outcome. Observational studies have shown an association between abnormal BPP and perinatal mortality and cerebral palsy. However, as with fetal heart rate (FHR), a high false-positive rate (50%) limits the clinical usefulness of the BPP.

Amniotic Fluid Volume

Many studies have shown an association between pathological FGR and oligohydramnios. AFV is considered as a chronic parameter. AFV evaluation is based on the fact that the decreased uteroplacental perfusion may lead to diminished fetal renal blood flow, decreased urine production, thus resulting into oligohydramnios. The *AFI*, the *deepest vertical pocket*, and the *2 × 2 cm pocket* are various sonographic methods used to estimate AFV. The American College of Obstetricians and Gynecologists (ACOG) has concluded that either an AFI <5 cm or a maximum deepest vertical pocket <2 cm are acceptable criteria for diagnosis of oligohydramnios.

Modified Biophysical Profile

Modified BPP is an abbreviated BPP which combines a vibroacoustic NST (acute parameter) with AFI determination (chronic parameter). In contrast to BPP, this test requires approximately 10 minutes to perform and does not need a trained sonologist.

Fetal Doppler

With the help of Doppler velocimetry, early changes in placenta-based growth restriction are detected in peripheral vessels such as the umbilical and middle cerebral arteries. Late changes are characterized by reversal of UA flow and by abnormal flow in the DV and fetal aortic and pulmonary outflow tracts.[12]

Umbilical artery Doppler: Umbilical artery Doppler velocimetry used in conjunction with standard fetal surveillance, such as NSTs, BPPs, or both, is associated with improved outcomes in fetuses with FGR (Level A—ACOG recommendation 2016).

Measurements of UA Doppler indices should be made in a free cord loop. However, in multiple pregnancies, measurements made at fixed sites, i.e., fetal end, placental end, or intra-abdominal portion, may be more reliable. Impedance is highest at the fetal end.[12]

Umbilical artery Doppler is the only measure that provides both diagnostic and prognostic information for the management of FGR. Raised UA Doppler pulsatility index (PI), either alone or combined in the cerebroplacental ratio (CPR), has a great clinical significance for the identification of FGR. In addition to this, the progression of UA Doppler patterns to absent or reverse end-diastolic flow correlates with the risks of injury or death (Figs. 5A to D).[11]

Middle cerebral artery Doppler: Fetal MCA Doppler for peak systolic velocity (PSV) is an appropriate noninvasive means to monitor pregnancies at risk of fetal anemia when performed by trained personnel.

Middle cerebral artery Doppler also provides information about brain vasodilation, which is a surrogate

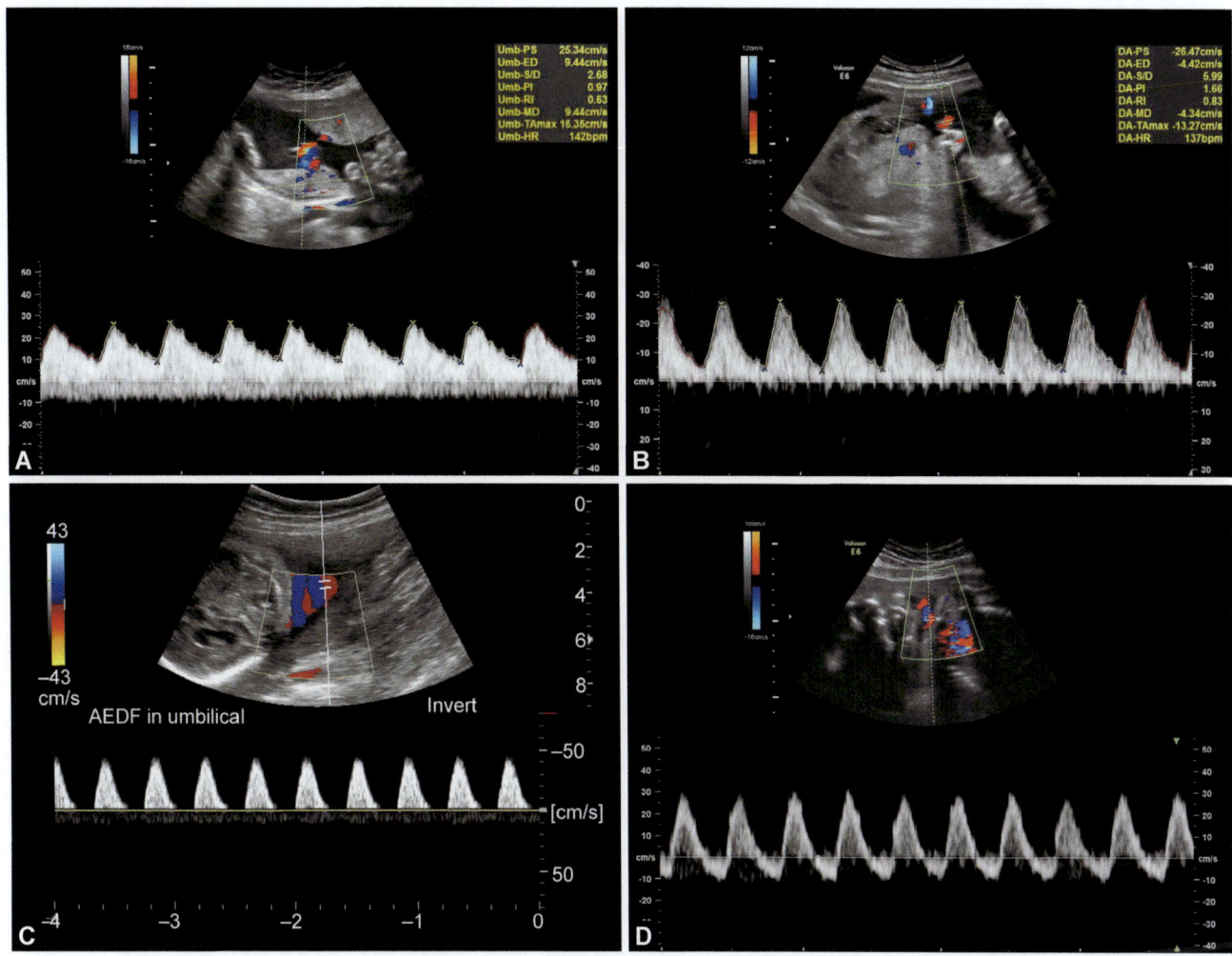

Figs. 5A to D: (A) Normal umbilical artery Doppler; (B) High resistance umbilical artery Doppler; (C) Absent diastolic flow umbilical artery Doppler; and (D) Reversed diastolic flow umbilical artery Doppler (AEDF: absent end-diastolic flow).

marker of hypoxia. There is an association between abnormal MCA-PI and adverse perinatal and neurological outcomes, but it is still unclear whether delivering before term could add any benefit. MCA is particularly valuable for the identification and prediction of adverse outcome among late-onset FGR, independently of the UA Doppler, which is often normal in these fetuses (Figs. 6A and B).[11]

While interrogating MCA for Doppler measurement, pulsed-wave Doppler gate should be placed at proximal third of the MCA, close to its origin in the internal carotid artery. Systolic velocity decreases with distance from the point of origin of MCA. The highest point of the waveform is considered as PSV (in cm/s). PI is usually calculated using autotrace measurement.[12]

Cerebroplacental ratio: Cerebroplacental ratio is the ratio between the MCA-PI and the UA-PI. It is better related to placental insufficiency. The CPR is essentially a diagnostic index and improves remarkably the sensitivity of UA and MCA alone, because increased placental impedance (UA) is often combined with reduced cerebral resistance (MCA). It is remarkable that even in the low-risk population, an abnormal CPR predicts neurobehavioral problems at 18 months of age.[11]

Ductus venosus Doppler: DV is the strongest single Doppler parameter to predict the short-term risk of fetal death in early-onset FGR. DV flow waveforms become abnormal only in advanced stages of fetal compromise. Consistently, there is a good correlation of abnormal DV waveform with late stage acidemia. Absent or reversed velocities during atrial contraction are associated with perinatal mortality independently of the gestational age at delivery, with a risk ranging from 40% to 100% in early-onset FGR. Thus, this sign is normally considered sufficient to recommend delivery at any gestational age, after completion of steroids (Figs. 7A and B).[11]

The waveform is usually triphasic, but biphasic and nonpulsating recordings, though rarer, may be seen in healthy fetuses. Doppler measurement is best achieved in

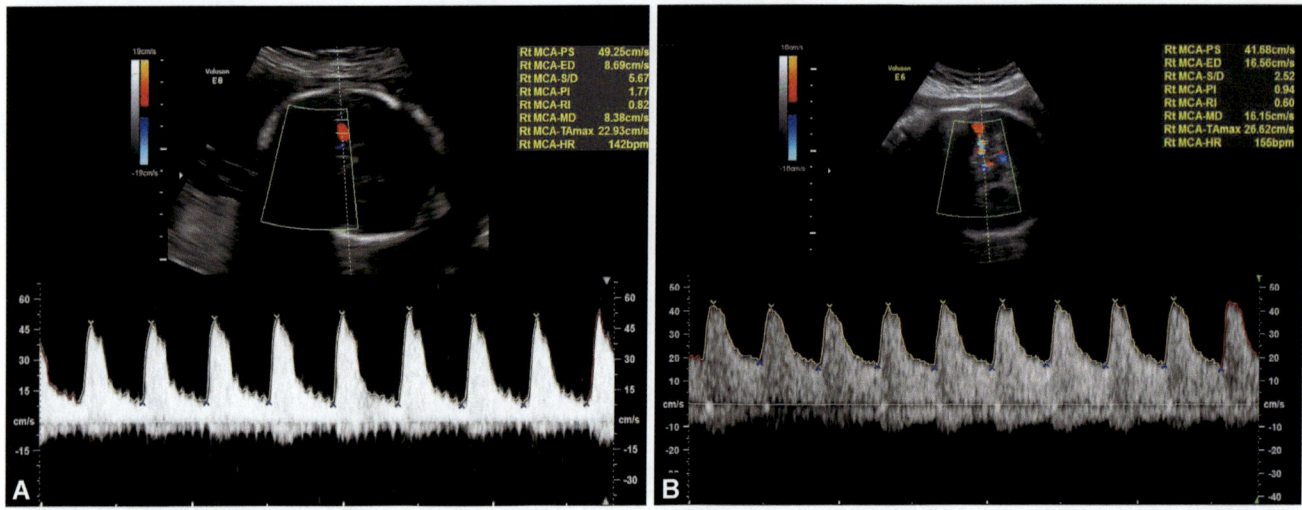

Figs. 6A and B: (A) Middle cerebral artery (MCA) normal Doppler; and (B) MCA Doppler showing brain-sparing effect.

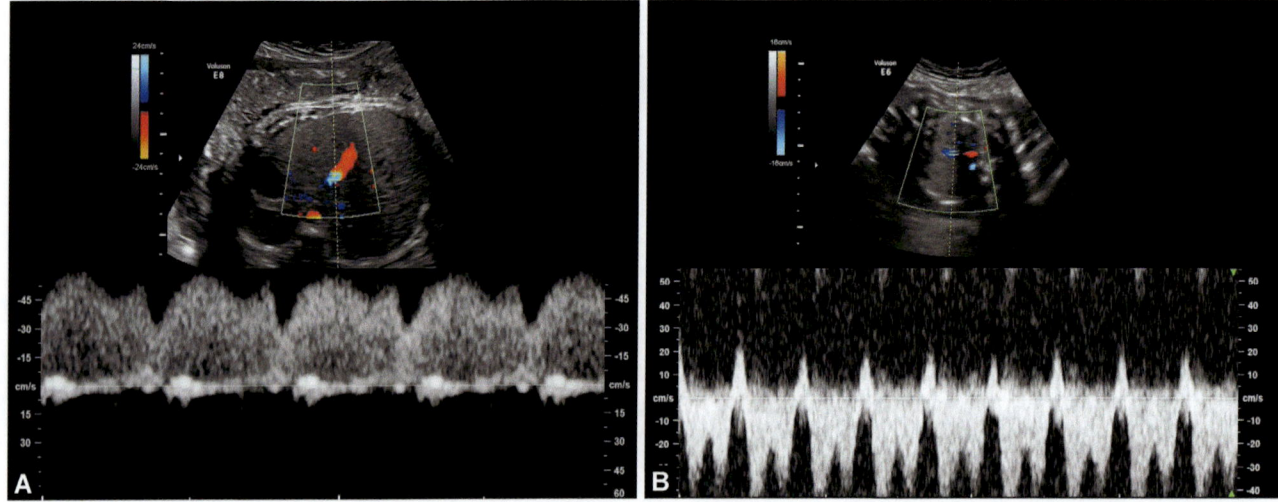

Figs. 7A and B: (A) Ductus venosus normal Doppler; and (B) Reversed a wave in ductus venosus Doppler.

the sagittal plane from the anterior lower fetal abdomen, since alignment with the isthmus can be well-controlled. Sagittal insonation through the chest is also a good option, but more demanding. The velocities are relatively high, between 55 cm/s and 90 cm/s for most of the second half of pregnancy.[12]

Aortic isthmus Doppler: The AoI Doppler is associated with increased fetal mortality and neurological morbidity in early-onset FGR. This vessel reflects the balance between the impedance of the brain and systemic vascular systems. Reverse AoI flow is a sign of advanced deterioration and a further step in the sequence starting with the UA and MCA Dopplers. AoI precedes DV abnormalities by 1 week, and consequently it is not as good to predict the short-term risk of stillbirth. In contrast, AoI Doppler seems to improve the prediction of neurological morbidity.[11]

Based upon Doppler changes, stage-based protocol for managing FGR has been proposed.[11]

Detection of Late Evolving Fetal Anomalies

An ultrasound for fetal structural anomalies in third trimester is important as some abnormalities develop or first become apparent later in pregnancy. These anomalies might be overlooked if the third trimester sonography is not done in view to detect anomalies.

Due to development of technology and state of the art sonography machines, high-resolution probes, the majority of structural anomalies are nowadays detected at 11–14 weeks of gestation or during the traditional anomaly scan at 18–20 weeks. 50% fetal anomalies are detected prior to 24 weeks, while another 50% of the malformations were detected later or remain undetected. Fetal development

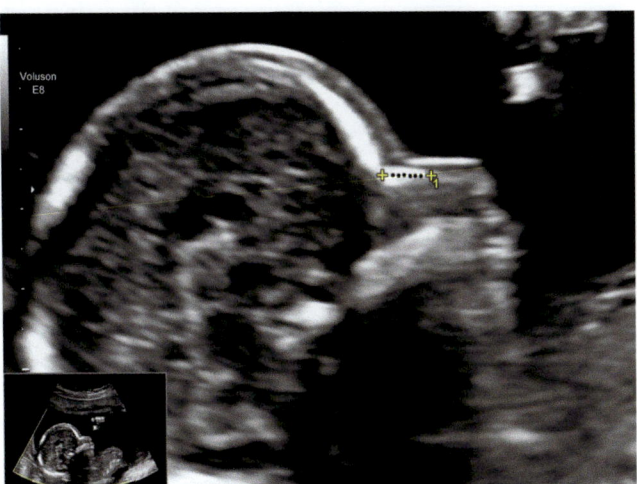
Fig. 8: Corpus callosum agenesis.

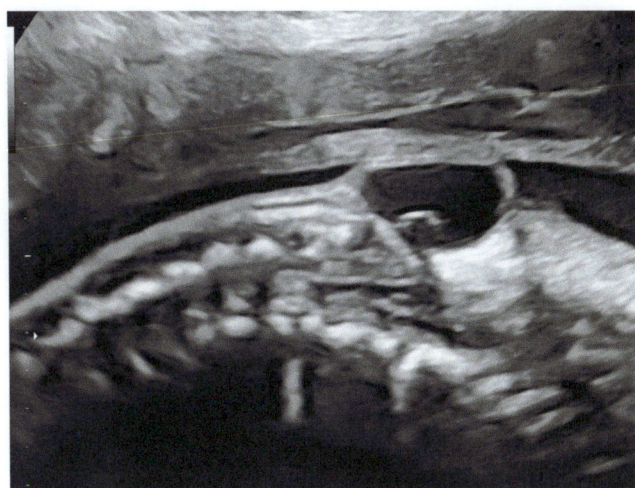
Fig. 9: Meningocele.

is a dynamic process and some fetal anomalies manifest in the third trimester. The size of various internal organs increases with gestational age that might help in detection of various anomalies in last trimester, especially those which were missed in previous examinations due to small fetal size, adverse position, or poor resolution of machines. Functions of various systems also increase as gestational age progresses. Some anomalies related to function (e.g., urogenital) are detected for the first time in the third trimester.[13]

Also, the phenotypic expression of some abnormalities become apparent only after 20 weeks, such as short limbs in the case of achondroplasia, dilated bowel in the case of bowel atresia or abnormal shape of the head in the case of craniosynostosis, or the abnormality develops only during the third trimester, such as ovarian cysts in response to maternal estrogenic stimulation or ventriculomegaly following fetal brain hemorrhage or maternal infection. Detecting these late-onset fetal anomalies have their importance in planning delivery, the location, timing, and route of delivery may be modified in order to alter perinatal care, help in parental counseling, improve neonatal outcome, and may also have medicolegal consequences.

Among the various anomalies detected in the third trimester, about 50% are comprised of central nervous system (CNS) and the urogenital system. Other organ systems that commonly manifest late anomalies are musculoskeletal and gastrointestinal (GI) systems.[13]

FETAL CENTRAL NERVOUS SYSTEM ABNORMALITIES

More than 15% of pregnancies with a fetal CNS abnormality detected in the third trimester had a previous normal second trimester scan. There are two groups of brain abnormalities that can be identified only in the third trimester; the first group consists of acquired lesions, such as stroke, hemorrhage, infection, and tumors, and the second group includes developmental anomalies, such as lissencephaly, microcephaly, and macrocephaly, which become evident during rapid brain enlargement after the end of the proliferation and migration period (2–5 months of gestation).

The most common CNS anomalies detected late is mild ventriculomegaly. It is important to note that ventriculomegaly is the endpoint of underlying structural pathology such as corpus callosum agenesis, aqueductal stenosis, Arnold–Chiari type II, or Dandy–Walker syndrome. Corpus callosum agenesis even in expert hands may be missed and may become prominent later as the growth of the fetal brain continues (Fig. 8). Open neural tube defects are usually diagnosed earlier due to technical development, intracranial signs of herniation, and addition of new markers like intracranial translucency, etc. Smaller lesions like a meningocele without cord tethering may be detected later in pregnancy or after birth due to the small size and lack of classical signs of tentorial herniation (Fig. 9).

Other CNS anomalies that specifically are diagnosed in the late trimester include vein of Galen malformation, and malformations of cortical development which include microcephaly, megalencephaly, lissencephaly/subcortical band heterotopia spectrum, cobblestone complex, heterotopia, polymicrogyria, and schizencephaly. Abnormalities of sulci-gyri may be due to single gene disorders or other genetic causes, hence the importance of detailed history cannot be overemphasized. In exceptional cases of an abnormality that is associated with severe impairment, such as severe ventriculomegaly and microcephaly, in countries in which late abortion is legal, the parents may be offered this option.

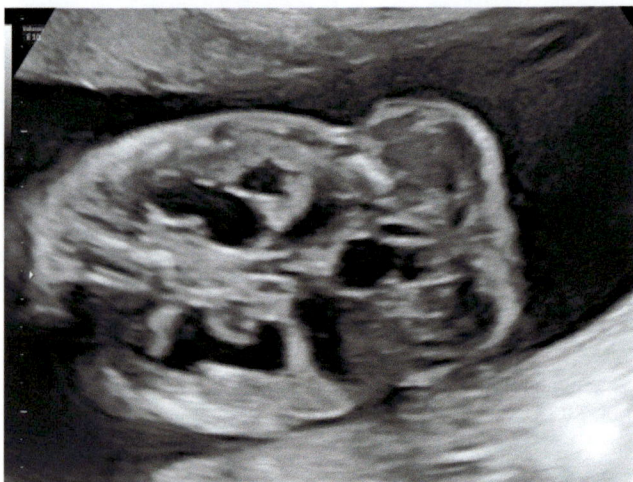

Fig. 10: Urinary tract dilatation.

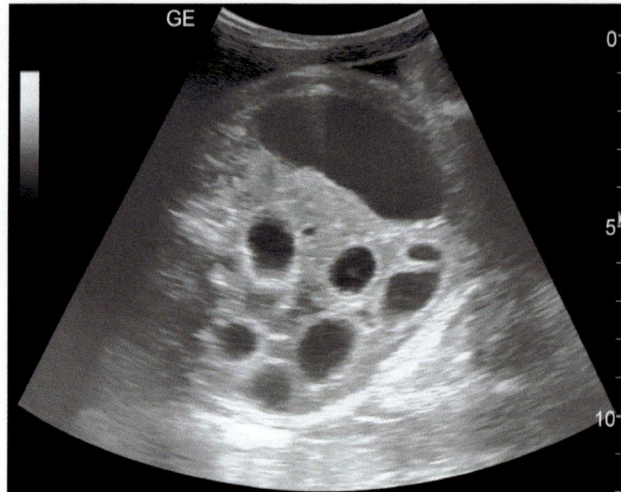

Fig. 11: Small bowel atresia.

FETAL GENITOURINARY ANOMALIES

In urogenital system, hydronephrosis is the most common genitourinary abnormality diagnosed at the third trimester scan. Such late diagnosis of hydronephrosis can be attributed to the exponential increase in fetal urine production during the third trimester of pregnancy.

Renal abnormalities include urinary tract dilatation disorders like pelviureteric junction obstruction, vesicoureteric reflux or obstruction, partial obstructive posterior urethral valves present with varying grades of hydronephrosis with/without hydroureter, and/or oligohydramnios at different gestational age depending upon the severity of obstruction and level of obstruction (Fig. 10). All urinary tract dilatation requires 3–4 weekly antenatal monitoring for worsening, oligohydramnios, cortical thickness and echogenicity, and fetal maturity, so as to decide time of delivery for balancing the risk of prematurity versus worsening renal function. This is because while section of these are functional and improve immediately in the postnatal period, about 64% may progress in the antenatal period and require postnatal care and surveillance due to risk of oliguria, urinary tract infection, and other related complications. Also, postnatal surgery is required in cases with moderate-to-severe hydronephrosis persisting in the third trimester. Hence, it is recommended to screen for renal dilatation during antenatal scans in the third trimester, even if prior scans are normal.

FETAL GASTROINTESTINAL ANOMALIES

In the GI system, intestinal obstruction is one of the most common anomalies that present in the late second and third trimesters. This obstruction may be mechanical or functional, and its prevalence depends upon the underlying condition which may be bowel atresia or stenosis, malrotation with volvulus, meconium ileus, total colonic aganglionosis, and meconium plug syndrome. Higher the obstruction earlier is the time of presentation in antenatal period by visualization of polyhydramnios and dilated bowel loops proximal to the obstruction while lower bowel obstruction in the colon or rectum may not become obvious even in the late gestation. These are usually not detected in the early trimesters since before 24 weeks of gestation, bowel loops are not recognized because there is no efficient gastric peristalsis. After 25 weeks, the echogenicity of the bowel increases to equal that of the adjacent liver. Fetal swallowing along with passive and active gastric emptying produces fluid filling of the small bowel loops and accumulation of meconium throughout the second and third trimesters. To distinguish between the proximal and distal segments, the "double bubble" sign and presence of polyhydramnios indicate a proximal segment obstruction. The "double bubble" sign which includes a dilated fluid-filled stomach adjacent to a dilated proximal intestinal segment indicates a contiguous obstruction, such as duodenal atresia. However, in colonic obstructions, there is no bowel dilatation generally, because fluid is resorbed in the upstream of small bowel and colonic loops.

Prenatal diagnosis of bowel obstruction and referral to tertiary center with early neonatal surgical correction reduce morbidity due to aspiration pneumonia or further abdominal distension with respiratory embarrassment if undiagnosed (Fig. 11).

CONGENITAL LUNG MALFORMATIONS

Congenital pulmonary airway malformation (CPAM) and bronchopulmonary sequestration (BPS) are fetal

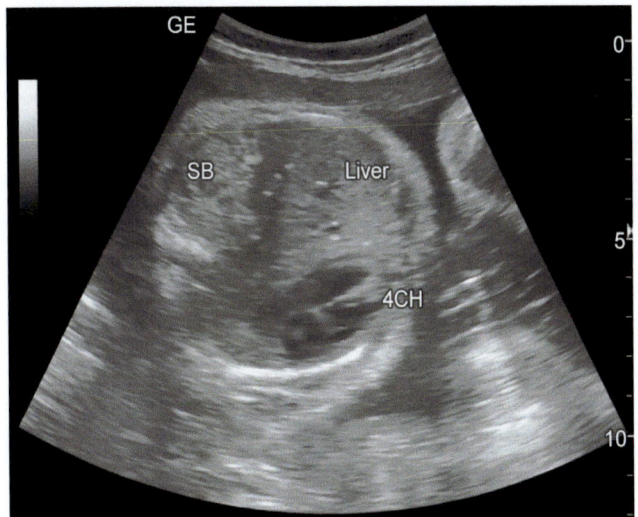

Fig. 12: Congenital diaphragmatic hernia.

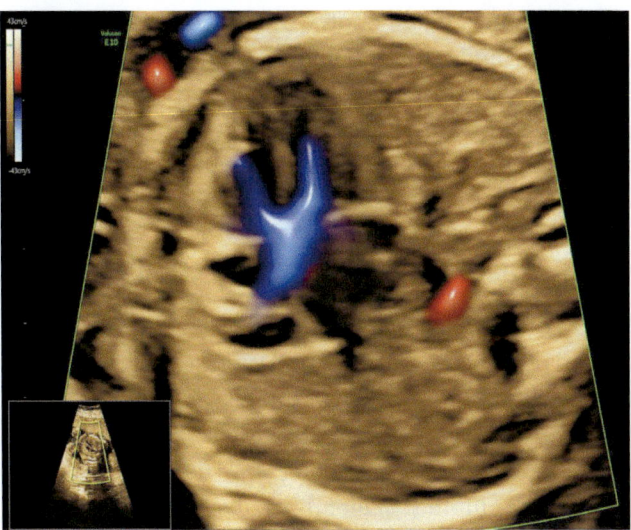

Fig. 13: Fallot's tetralogy.

lung masses that are nearly 100% fatal when associated with hydrops. The natural history of this lung lesion may be progression/regression or remains stable antenatally and hence requires monitoring in the third trimester for worsening or development of hydrops. Congenital pulmonary airway malformation volume ratio (CVR) helps determine the risk of development of hydrops and is an important parameter which is to be considered when counseling such patients. CVR is the volume of the CPAM mass normalized for gestational age. A CVR of ≤1.6 at presentation suggests that the risk of hydrops developing is low in the absence of a dominant large cyst. A CVR >1.6 or a CPAM with a dominant large cyst increases risk of developing hydrops.

Congenital diaphragmatic hernia is a malformation with important implications due to high mortality. If diagnosed before 26 weeks of gestation with associated liver herniation and a low lung-to-head circumference ratio (LHR < 1), they have a relatively poor prognosis with conventional therapy after birth. LHR is the ratio of opposite normal lung area to the head circumference at that gestation (Fig. 12). The mainstay of management includes meticulous initial evaluation of LHR and extent of liver herniation, chromosomal analysis, antenatal monitoring of the fetus for signs of worsening, cardiac dysfunction and development of hydrops under expert fetomaternal unit care, delivery near term at a tertiary care center with neonatal intensive care unit (NICU) setup, standard protocols for management of neonate at birth including initial intubation, stabilization, and treatment of pulmonary hypertension, and then surgical management. Fetuses with diaphragmatic hernia are best delivered in centers with facilities for pediatric surgery.

CARDIAC ANOMALIES

Perinatal morbidity and mortality improved significantly when cardiac malformations are diagnosed prenatally, because adequate perinatal management could be instituted in tertiary care units. Relatively, nonlethal with good postsurgical results include isolated ventricular septal defects, isolated transposition of great vessels, Fallot's tetralogy with good size pulmonary artery, total anomalous pulmonary venous connections, and milder varieties of coarctation of aorta may become obvious at later gestation (Fig. 13). This may be explained by some influencing factors like lack of the operator expertise, higher-resolution ultrasound equipment, suboptimal fetal presentation, and growing body mass indices of the mothers as well as the higher frequency of abdominal scars due to the worldwide increasing rates of cesarean sections. Such unfavorable conditions may alter the quality of the ultrasound evaluation, especially the conditions for fetal echocardiography. It is also well known that antenatal development of the heart can lead to changes of the ventricular inflow and outflow and stenosis or hypoplasia can progress and might not be detectable at earlier stages in development. Also, rare conditions like cardiac soft tissue tumors such as rhabdomyoma are almost always detected in the late trimester.

These cases need detailed evaluation and counseling for further prognostication by a team of obstetrician, perinatologist, neonatologist, geneticist, and a pediatric cardiologist. Further antenatal monitoring is necessary by an expert fetal medicine/fetal cardiac specialized center for worsening of cardiac function, signs of heart failure or development of hydrops, and deciding the timing/

mode of delivery at a center with good NICU for initial assessment and stabilization. In some cases of progressive heart abnormality, such as coarctation of the aorta and pulmonary or aortic stenosis, it may be advisable for delivery to be scheduled in a center with pediatric cardiac expertise.

FETAL MUSCULOSKELETAL ABNORMALITIES

Diseases of the musculoskeletal system like achondroplasia, though rare, manifest in the third trimester after 26 weeks. Only the most severe forms can be seen before the third trimester due to signs like clover-leaf skull, small chest circumference, or multiple long bone fractures. Although these are nonlethal skeletal dysplasia without mental impairment, it is nevertheless of great importance to prepare the parents and to inform them prenatally.

As per recent study on 52,400 study population on the value of routine ultrasound at 35–37 weeks of gestation in the diagnosis of fetal abnormalities, the incidence of fetal abnormality was 1.9% including 67.7% were diagnosed during the first and/or second trimester, 24.8% were detected for the first time at 35–37 weeks, and 7.4% were detected for the first time postnatally.[13]

Prenatal diagnosis, even if diagnosed late in gestation, may have a significant impact on the perinatal management of the fetus with a surgically correctable congenital anomaly. A routine ultrasound during the third trimester is, therefore, justified for study of fetal morphology for detection of anomalies, especially anomalies of GI tract, urinary tract, and CNS. When these anomalies are diagnosed prenatally, optimal perinatal and postnatal care can be planned. The delivery can be advised in a multispeciality hospital with a NICU. This allows the affected families with valuable insight into the need for delivery in an appropriate setting, by the safest mode of delivery, at the gestational age appropriate to minimize effects of the anomaly. It helps for planning of immediate postnatal surgery or close follow-up by team of specialists.

Role of Third Trimester Ultrasound in Obese Pregnant Women

Obesity, particularly when presents with a pannus, may hamper fundal height measurements by limiting the ability to palpate the pubic symphysis and uterine fundus as well as by potentially falsely increasing the measurements due to inclusion of the pannus. This may lead to overestimation of LGA. As a consequence, few studies recommend serial ultrasound for assessment of growth and liquor in otherwise low-risk obese women to begin at or after 32 weeks. Prenatal identification of liquor and growth abnormalities enables managing obstetrician to timed interventions in order to reduce incidence of stillbirth.[14]

INTRAPARTUM ULTRASONOGRAPHY

The use of ultrasound has been proposed to aid in the management of labor. Traditionally, the assessment and management of a woman in labor is based upon clinical findings. However, clinical examination of head station and position is inaccurate and subjective, especially when caput succedaneum impairs palpation of the sutures and fontanels.

Several studies have demonstrated that ultrasound examination is more accurate and reproducible than clinical examination in the diagnosis of fetal head position and station and in the prediction of arrest of labor. Ultrasound in labor can be performed using a transabdominal approach, mainly to determine head and spine position, or a transperineal approach, for assessment of head station and position at low stations.[15]

REFERENCES

1. Ministry of Health and Family Welfare, Government of India (2011). Guidelines on Use of Ultrasonography during Pregnancy. [online] Available from http://www.nrhmhp.gov.in/sites/default/files/files/Approved-%20Guidelines%20on%20use%20of%20Ultrasonography.pdf [Last accessed December, 2019].
2. World Health Organization (WHO) (2016). WHO recommendations on antenatal care for a positive pregnancy experience. [online] Available from https://apps.who.int/iris/bitstream/handle/10665/250796/9789241549912-eng.pdf;jsessionid=13B3B8CCBEEEF0BF76E4F5D463B4CBE4?sequence=1 [Last accessed December, 2019].
3. AIUM-ACR-ACOG-SMFM-SRU Practice Parameter for the Performance of Standard Diagnostic Obstetric Ultrasound Examinations. J Ultrasound Med. 2018;37:E13-24.
4. Committee on Practice Bulletins—Obstetrics and the American Institute of Ultrasound in Medicine. Practice Bulletin No. 175: Ultrasound in Pregnancy. Obstet Gynecol. 2016;128:e241-56.
5. Salomon LJ, Alfirevic Z, Da Silva Costa F, et al. ISUOG Practice Guidelines: ultrasound assessment of fetal biometry and growth. Ultrasound Obstet Gynecol. 2019;53:715-23.
6. Buck Louis GM, Grewal J, Albert PS, et al. Racial/ethnic standards for fetal growth: the NICHD Fetal Growth Studies. Am J Obstet Gynecol. 2015;213:449.e1-449.e41.

7. Stirnemann J, Villar J, Salomon LJ, et al. International estimated fetal weight standards of the INTERGROWTH-21st Project. Ultrasound Obstet Gynecol. 2017;49:478-86.
8. Kiserud T, Piaggio G, Carroli G, et al. The World Health Organization Fetal Growth Charts: A Multinational Longitudinal Study of Ultrasound Biometric Measurements and Estimated Fetal Weight. PLoS Med. 2017;14:e1002220.
9. Gardosi J, Francis A, Turner S, et al. Customized growth charts: rationale, validation and clinical benefits. Am J Obstet Gynecol. 2018;218:S609-18.
10. Gordijn SJ, Beune IM, Thilaganathan B, et al. Consensus definition of fetal growth restriction: a Delphi procedure. Ultrasound Obstet Gynecol. 2016;48:333-9.
11. Figueras F, Gratacós E. Update on the diagnosis and classification of fetal growth restriction and proposal of a stage-based management protocol. Fetal Diagn Ther. 2014;36:86-98.
12. Bhide A, Acharya G, Bilardo CM, et al. ISUOG practice guidelines: use of Doppler ultrasonography in obstetrics. Ultrasound Obstet Gynecol. 2013;41:233-9.
13. Ficara A, Syngelaki A, Hammami A, et al. Value of routine ultrasound examination at 35–37 weeks' gestation in diagnosis of fetal abnormalities. Ultrasound Obstet Gynecol. 2019. [Epub ahead of print].
14. Harper LM, Jauk VC, Owen J, et al. The utility of ultrasound surveillance of fluid and growth in obese women. Am J Obstet Gynecol. 2014;211:524.e1-8.
15. Ghi T, Eggebø T, Lees C, et al. ISUOG Practice Guidelines: intrapartum ultrasound. Ultrasound Obstet Gynecol. 2018;52:128-39.

17

Fetal Intervention

Vandana Bansal

INTRODUCTION

Prenatal diagnosis of fetal disorders and structural malformations is becoming increasingly important. Approximately 3% of all pregnancies result in the delivery of an infant with a genetic disorder or birth defect. Such anomalies are also the biggest cause of infant mortality.

Down syndrome is the most common cause of intellectual disability and accounts for about 15–30% of cases. In India, the birth prevalence is reported to vary from one in 1,230 to one in 1,361.[1]

Fetal medicine (also known as perinatology) is a subspecialty which deals with the diagnosis of fetal illnesses and abnormalities, assessment of fetal growth and well-being, and maintenance of in-utero fetal health and treatment. Advances in the last 3 decades in imaging sciences (e.g., high-resolution ultrasound, MRI), molecular genetics, and in-utero surgical techniques have made it possible to accurately diagnose many conditions prenatally, so as to offer curative or ameliorative treatments in the antenatal period itself which were previously considered treatable only in neonatal period.

Prenatal screening, prenatal diagnosis, and fetal therapy are the main areas of interest in the field of perinatal medicine.

- *Prenatal screening*: Serum beta-human chorionic gonadotropin and pregnancy-associated plasma protein A in combination with ultrasonography (USG) for nuchal translucency in the first trimester, targeted imaging for fetal anomalies and quadruple screen in the second trimester, and fetal growth, Doppler, and biophysical profile in the third trimester.
- *Prenatal diagnosis*: Chorionic villous sampling, amniocentesis, cordocentesis, placental biopsy, and fetal skin/urine/liver biopsy.
- *Fetal therapy*: Medical therapy (hypothyroidism, congenital arrhythmias), surgical treatment (ultrasound-guided procedures, e.g., vesicoamniotic shunt placement, fetoscopic procedures, e.g., laser ablation in twin-to-twin transfusion syndrome (TTTS), and open fetal surgery, e.g., meningomyelocele, congenital diaphragmatic hernia, and sacrococcygeal teratoma).

Over the past several decades, we have developed an understanding of the genetic basis of an increasing number of diseases. Safe and effective fetal diagnostic techniques are being developed, and earlier detection of various fetal disorders is expanding therapeutic options. With prenatal diagnosis of fetal abnormalities, the parents, obstetric team, geneticist, and other subspecialists can discuss options ranging from abortion to intrauterine medical and surgical treatments. In concert with the neonatologists, the optimal time, mode, and place of delivery can be determined. Parents can be prepared for short- and long-term postnatal expectations. If appropriate, genetic counseling can assist with further reproductive planning and recurrence risk.

GENETIC COUNSELING

Genetic counseling is an integral part of genetic testing and screening programs, including prenatal testing. Clinical genetics is concerned with the diagnosis and management of the medical, social, and psychological aspects of hereditary disorder. Common indications include parents with previous child affected with a potential or known genetic condition or adults with an abnormality or family history of a condition such as cancer or neurodegenerative disorders.

Genetic evaluation consists of validation of the diagnosis of index case, detailed family history and pedigree analysis, recurrence risk estimation, helping proband/family in decision making, and taking appropriate action such as genetic testing and follow-up. Patients who undergo genetic testing are also informed about prenatal screening and diagnostic testing options available during pregnancy.[2]

Detecting or defining risk for disease in an asymptomatic low-risk population is the goal of screening. Screening is intended to identify populations who have an increased risk for a specific disorder for whom diagnostic testing may be warranted. Screening is currently available and should be offered in pregnancy for a number of genetic (single gene or Mendelian) disorders, chromosomal aneuploidy, and structural birth defects in the fetus regardless of maternal age or family history.[3]

It is very important to explain the optional nature of all prenatal testing and to emphasize this fact that a low-risk screening test result does not guarantee a healthy child and a high-risk screening test result does not mean the fetus has the disorder. Distinction should be made clear between a diagnostic and a screening test. A screening test identifies an increased likelihood of a fetal abnormality in an apparently normal pregnancy whereas a diagnostic test confirms or refutes the existence of an actual anomaly in a fetus believed to be at increased risk.

Pregnancies which are screen positive for a disorder need to undergo invasive testing for confirmation of the disorder in question. It is currently recommended that both screening and diagnostic testing options should be offered to all pregnant women regardless of their age or perceived risk.[4]

Prenatal genetic diagnostic testing is intended to determine, with as much certainty as possible, whether a specific genetic disorder or condition is present in the fetus. In contrast, prenatal genetic screening is designed to assess whether a patient is at increased risk of having a fetus affected by a genetic disorder.[4]

INVASIVE PRENATAL DIAGNOSIS

Five percent of all pregnant women are offered a choice of invasive prenatal testing. Originally, prenatal genetic testing focused primarily on Down syndrome (trisomy 21), but now it is able to detect a broad range of genetic disorders.[4]

All diagnostic interventions are directed toward some form of fetal tissue sampling for genetic, biochemical, hematological, and histological processing. The type of diagnostic test offered is likely to vary depending upon the timing of any initial screening test that is performed, gestational age, nature of the problem, and the information needed.

Prerequisites

Women should be counseled by trained professionals prior to any prenatal diagnostic tests. The indication, details of the procedure, expected risks, and benefits should be explained clearly. The results generated from the study of the amniotic fluid/chorionic villus sampling (CVS)/fetal blood sampling (FBS) sample [cytogenetic study, fluorescence in situ hybridization (FISH), polymerase chain reaction (PCR), microarray, etc.], and the limitations of the results and the processes for any long-term sample storage should be communicated clearly to the women. If alternative invasive sampling is offered, the relative advantages and disadvantages must be explained clearly in terms that the woman will understand. A formal written consent for the invasive procedure must be taken (including Form F and G which is a requirement in India).

An ultrasound examination must be done prior to any invasive testing to determine gestational age, viability, identify any fetal abnormalities, position of the placenta, and assess the route and position of target. The center performing the invasive tests must be recognized by the local authorities [Pre-Conception and Pre-Natal Diagnostic Techniques (PCPNDT) registered center in India].

Prophylaxis with anti-D immunoglobulin must be offered within 72 hours following each procedure in mothers who are Rhesus negative. Antibiotics/tocolysis are not essential.

INDICATIONS FOR AMNIOCENTESIS OR CHORIONIC VILLUS SAMPLING[5]

Currently valid indications for invasive prenatal testing include increased risk for fetal chromosomal abnormality, increased risk for hereditary genetic or metabolic disease, and increased risk for some perinatal infections. Various invasive techniques for prenatal diagnosis are amniocentesis, CVS, and FBS.

- *Increased risk of fetal aneuploidy*:
  - High-risk aneuploidy screening test results from first trimester combined screening/noninvasive prenatal screening (NIPS)/second trimester triple or quadruple test
  - Structural anomalies or soft markers associated with aneuploidy
  - Previous fetus or child affected by aneuploidy
  - Parental aneuploidy or mosaicism for aneuploidy or parental carrier of chromosomal balanced translocation or inversion.

    Advanced maternal age >35 years alone should not be considered an indication.[5] Conception by assisted reproductive technique in itself is again not considered a valid indication for invasive prenatal diagnosis.

- *Increased risk for a known genetic or biochemical disease of the fetus*:
  - History of family hereditary disease with a known mutation or biochemical change
  - Male fetus and carrier status of pregnant woman for a disease with X-chromosomal inheritance, e.g., hemophilias
  - Couples carrier for an autosomal recessive disorder, e.g., thalessemias, inborn errors of metabolism.
- *Maternal transmissible infectious disease to confirm or exclude fetal infection*:
  - History of maternal primary infection or seroconversion involving toxoplasma, cytomegalovirus (CMV), or rubella
  - Fetus showing markers of infection on ultrasound.
- *Maternal request* under certain circumstances, e.g., acute parental anxiety after extensive counseling. It is generally not considered a valid indication or as a standalone criterion.

AMNIOCENTESIS

Amniocentesis is the most common invasive prenatal diagnostic procedure performed worldwide. Amniocentesis refers to transabdominal aspiration of amniotic fluid (around 15–30 mL) from the uterine cavity using 20–22 G spinal needle under continuous ultrasound guidance avoiding the placental cord insertion site and the placenta if technically feasible. It involves aspirating 20 mL of amniotic fluid for obtaining fetal skin cells for culture for fetal karyotyping and other genetic studies (Fig. 1). It is recommended to perform amniocentesis at or beyond 15+0 completed weeks of gestation as large randomized controlled trials have reported higher rate of total fetal losses, fetal talipes, and postprocedure amniotic fluid leakage in cases of early amniocentesis done prior to 14 weeks.

Complications include risk of fetal loss varying from 0.1% to 1%, postprocedure membrane rupture in 1–2%, chorioamnionitis (<0.1%), needle injury to the fetus, and maternal sepsis in very rare circumstances.[5] The risk of amniotic fluid leakage following amniocentesis remains higher up to 24 weeks. However, in women with iatrogenic leak following amniocentesis, spontaneous sealing of the membranes is commonly seen.

Lower fetal loss rates have been documented with better operator experience of more than 100 procedures per annum. If more than two punctures have been attempted, it is suggested that the procedure can be postponed by 24 hours. Use of 20 G or 22 G needle is associated with similar loss rates. Large caliber needle is associated with faster fluid retrieval. Maximum outer needle gauge size of 0.9 mm (20 gauge) should be used to perform amniocentesis.[6]

The presence of fetal structural anomalies itself places the pregnancy at higher background risk of miscarriage and the risk increases further following amniocentesis. A bloody or brown discolored tap reflects intra-amniotic bleeding and is associated with a higher postprocedure fetal loss.

Several risk factors have been suggested to increase the risk of fetal loss following amniocentesis, although their association has not been proven consistently. Plausible risk factors include uterine fibroids, Müllerian malformations, chorioamniotic separation, retrochorionic hematoma, previous or current maternal bleeding, maternal body mass index >40 kg/m², multiparity (>3 births), manifest vaginal infection, and history of three or more miscarriages.

The frequency of maternal cell contamination reported in experienced hands is about 0.35%. Maternal cell contamination increases when the amniotic fluid is blood stained (Fig. 2). This may be reduced with transmembrane

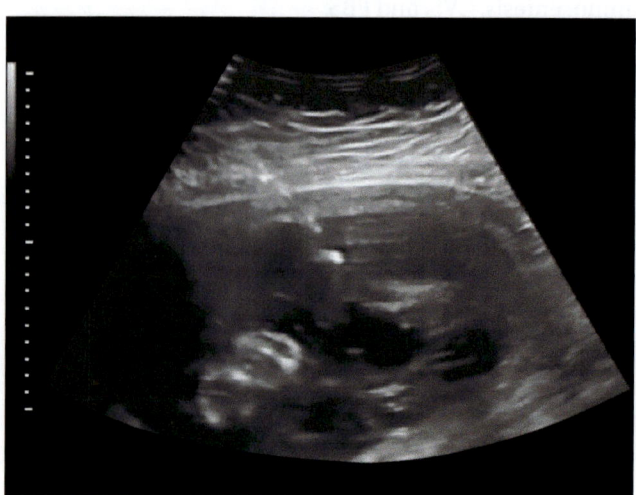

Fig. 1: Amniocentesis.

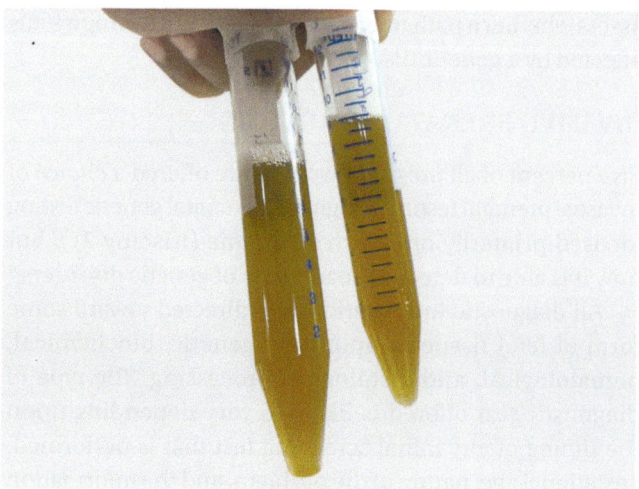

Fig. 2: Old blood-stained amniotic fluid.

needle passage rather than transplacental approach, more operator experience, and less number of attempts. In addition, contamination can be minimized by discarding the first 2 mL of amniotic fluid.

Amniotic fluid obtained is centrifuged and cultured and complete karyotype report is available in 12–21 days. Failure of amniocytes to culture is reported in 0.1% of procedures and is more with advanced gestational age at amniocentesis and a blood-stained tap.

Laboratory Aspects

Various tests that can be done from the amniotic fluid may include regular karyotype or a chromosomal microarray or single gene menu including Sanger sequencing, next generation sequencing (NGS), multiplex ligation-dependent probe amplification (MLPA), whole exome or a clinical exome, and depending on the requirement PCR-based tests for fetal infections.

Rapid results are available by using other techniques such as FISH or quantitative fluorescence PCR (QF-PCR). However, results generated by these newer methods should be interpreted with an understanding of their limitations, which include diagnosis of only a limited number of chromosomal abnormalities and the inability to diagnose mosaicism.

Fluorescence in situ hybridization should be considered a screening test due to false-positive and false-negative results having been reported with FISH. Any clinical decision should not be based solely on FISH, but after confirmatory diagnostic results or consistent clinical information, e.g., abnormal ultrasound findings or a positive screening result.[4]

Conventionally, chromosomal FISH for the common five aneuploidies and karyotype analysis is performed.

Another technology-driven revolution in chromosomal analysis is chromosomal microarray analysis (CMA) that is a molecular cytogenetic technique to visualize chromosomes at a very high resolution. In prenatal samples, cytogenetic microarray is considered an option even in fetuses with normal USG evaluation. This will help in primary prevention of numerous well-delineated sporadic microdeletion/duplication syndromes. Individually, these are rare but account for a significant proportion of intellectual disability. CMA detects such copy number variations in 1% of prenatal samples with any indication and 3–4% of fetuses with malformations. One limitation of CMA is that it detects some copy number variations of unknown significance in about 1% of cases making counseling and prognostication difficult.

As per the American College of Obstetricians and Gynecologists (ACOG) guidelines, "CMA" should be made available to any patient choosing to undergo invasive diagnostic testing. In the case of an ultrasound finding of fetal structural abnormality, CMA is recommended as a primary test, unless the abnormality is "strongly suggestive" of a particular aneuploidy, in which case karyotype may be offered before CMA.[4]

Like all prenatal testing and screening methods, CMA also needs good supportive counseling facilities. CMA has made its place in all invasive prenatal diagnosis and is here to stay and replace traditional karyotyping.

CHORIONIC VILLUS SAMPLING

Chorionic villus sampling is the withdrawal of trophoblastic cells from the placenta performed between 11 weeks and 14 weeks of gestation by transabdominal or transcervical route according to operator's experience, preference, or placental location using 18–20 G needle under continuous ultrasound guidance (Fig. 3). Once the needle has reached the target within the placenta, samples are aspirated manually by back and forth movements while maintaining the vacuum. The amount of villi obtained in the sample is checked visually and a minimum amount of 5–10 mg villi must be obtained (Fig. 4). Chorionic tissue has ample amount of deoxyribonucleic acid (DNA) material and is especially useful for DNA-based tests. In addition, cytogenetic study from chorionic tissue culture takes less turnaround time.

It is recommended not to perform CVS before 10 completed weeks of gestation, due to higher risk of fetal loss and complications such as limb reduction defects/oromandibular hypoplasia reported in literature. The limbs and mandible are more susceptible to vascular disruption before 10 weeks.

Complications include fetal loss (0.2–2%), vaginal bleeding (10%), amniotic fluid leakage (<0.5%), and

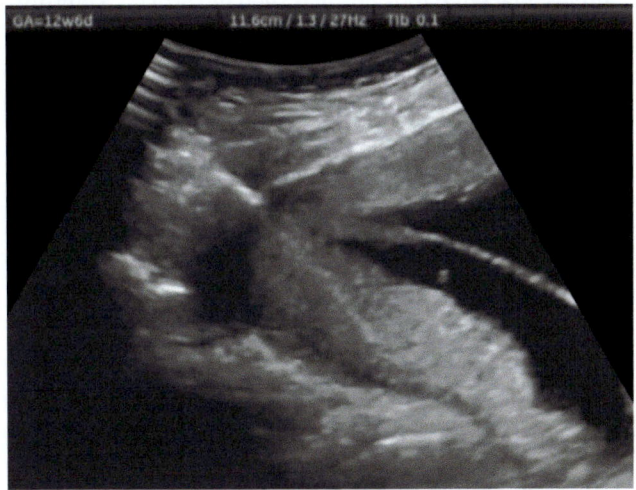

Fig. 3: Chorionic villus sampling.

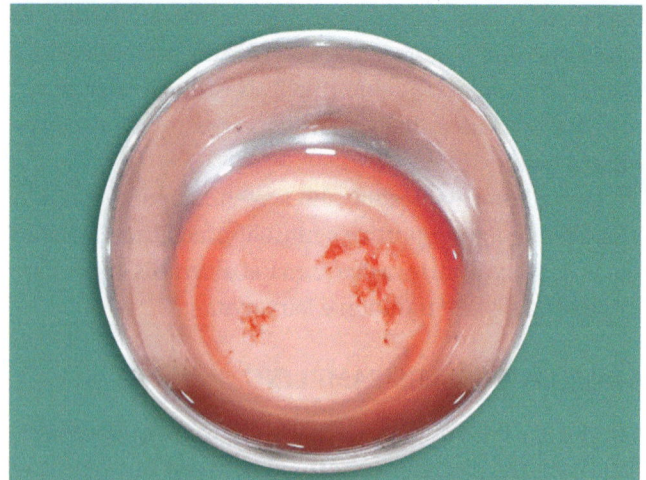

Fig. 4: Visual assessment of chorionic villi aspirated.

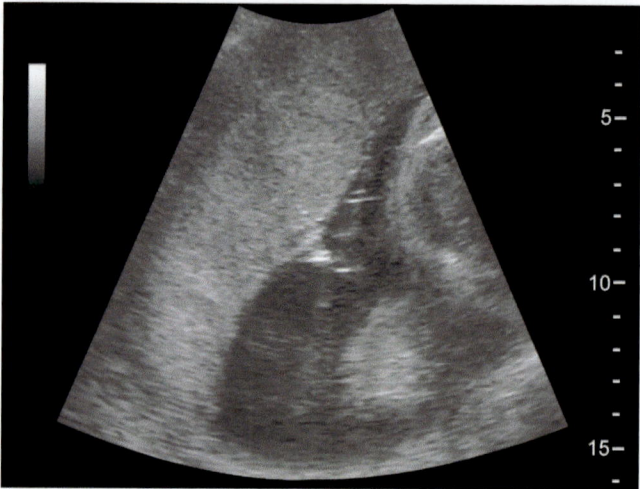

Fig. 5: Fetal cord blood sampling.

chorioamnionitis (1–2 in 3,000).[5] Fetal loss rates increase with number of needle insertion and gestational age less than 10 weeks. Fetal loss rates are slightly higher with transcervical route as compared to transabdominal route. Presence of fetal structural malformation or an increased nuchal translucency or a low pregnancy-associated plasma protein-A (PAPP-A) in the maternal serum screen is associated with a background increased risk of miscarriage even before a CVS. Risk of miscarriage decreases obviously with better operator experience. Experts as per the International Society of Ultrasound in Obstetrics and Gynecology (ISUOG) guidelines on invasive procedures suggest that an operator's competence should be reviewed when loss rates exceed 8/100 and sampling failure exceeds 5/100 consecutive CVS.[4] Association of CVS with development of pre-eclampsia and fetal growth restriction later in pregnancy, possibly due to placental damage, has not been confirmed in meta-analysis.

Failure of trophoblast culture may be seen in 0.5% of samples. Placental mosaicism is seen in 1% of CVS cultures. Hence, in few such cases, a repeat invasive procedure of amniocentesis or cordocentesis may be required to differentiate true fetal mosaicism from confined placental mosaicism.

Benefit of CVS over amniocentesis is an early diagnosis, so that decisions about pregnancy can be taken earlier.

FETAL BLOOD SAMPLING

Cordocentesis refers to ultrasound-guided puncture of umbilical cord (umbilical vein), for either diagnostic (FBS) or therapeutic (intrauterine transfusion or drug instillation) purposes performed beyond 18+0 completed weeks of gestation (due to increased fetal loss rate if performed earlier) using 20–22 G needle under continuous ultrasound guidance. Fetal blood can be sampled transabdominally under USG guidance either from the placental cord insertion site, fetal intrahepatic portal vein, or a free loop of cord (Fig. 5). Needle should reach the umbilical vein and avoid the umbilical artery. Fetal origin of the blood should be confirmed by mean corpuscular volume or by Kleihauer–Betke test.

The risk of fetal loss is between 1% and 2%.[5] Complications include amniotic fluid leak, chorioamnionitis, cord hematoma, transient bradycardia, bleeding from the needle site, fetomaternal hemorrhage, and rarely fetal demise. Increased risk of fetal loss may be associated with fetal anomalies, hydrops, fetal growth restriction, and gestational age of less than 24 weeks at sampling.

Specific Indications for Fetal Blood Sampling[5]

- Fetal blood sampling is specially indicated in fetus at higher risk for hematological disorders such as hemophilia and hemoglobinopathy.
- Identify genetic disorders where amniocentesis or CVS are inconclusive or unsuccessful such as placental mosaicism.
- Suspected fetal anemia—Rh sensitized, parvovirus, chronic fetomaternal hemorrhage, and hydrops (quantification of fetal anemia or platelet/lymphocyte count)
- Alloimmune thrombocytopenia
- Along with intrauterine transfusion in Rh isoimmunized
- Along with therapeutic procedures—arrhythmias, fetal thyroid disease
- No amniotic fluid is available for sampling (anhydramnios).

Full karyotype, blood typing, platelet antigen status, genetic testing, infection, and plasma or serum studies for metabolites or hormones were among the common indications for FBS in the past and currently this practice has been replaced by easier and safer invasive techniques such as CVS and amniocentesis and newer rapid techniques of analysis such as FISH and QF-PCR.

Advantage of FBS is its ability to obtain full cytogenetics study faster within 3–5 days at a lower cost, especially in pregnancy near 20 weeks where decisions have to be made early. Length of chromosomes in fetal blood is longer as compared to amniocytes and chorionic tissue. Hence, better identification of smaller structural abnormalities in the chromosomes can be made. Direct cord blood sampling eliminates the problem of pseudomosaicism encountered in CVS or amniotic fluid sample. In cases where hematological disorders are suspected, direct hematological and biochemical analysis is possible. Risk of culture failure is less, especially in late gestation.

Prenatal Testing in Multiple Pregnancies

It is recommended that, in the case of multiple pregnancies, a CVS or amniocentesis is performed by a specialist who has the expertise to subsequently perform a selective termination of pregnancy if required. A high level of expertise in ultrasound scanning is essential for operators undertaking amniocentesis or CVS in multiple pregnancies, because chorionicity must be determined, fetuses have to be "mapped" with great care as per their positions, placental localization, and cord insertions. Labeling is greatly assisted by the presence of obvious fetal abnormality (such as hydrocephalus or heart defect) or discordant fetal gender. This is essential to ensure that separate samples are taken for each fetus and clearly labeled as such. However, to minimize the risk of chromosomal abnormality being assigned to the wrong twin, invasive procedures in multiple pregnancy should only be performed by a specialist who is able to proceed to selective termination of pregnancy. Most clinicians will use two separate puncture sites when performing amniocentesis or CVS in multiple pregnancies.[5]

FETAL THERAPY AND ITS PRINCIPLES

Fetal therapy is defined as any fetal intervention, whether medical or surgical, that attempts to treat a disorder in utero with an aim to improve perinatal outcome.

In the past, once a disorder was diagnosed prenatally, options available were either termination of pregnancy or continuation till term and have the appropriate pediatric specialist and neonatal care team ready to manage the neonate with the birth defect. However, many such abnormalities are progressive in utero and by the time the neonate is delivered, the disorder is either uncorrectable or correctable with residual disease which may compromise quality of life or the fetus may deteriorate to death in utero.

With technological advancement in ultrasound, we have not only been able to diagnose disorders in utero but also understand fetal development process and the natural history of disease detected prenatally. Fetal therapeutic interventions were aimed at correcting in utero progression of disorder, so as to reduce damage to the fetus and subsequently improve long-term outcome.

Diseases which are amenable to in utero intervention may be structural abnormality, cardiac defects or rhythm disorder, fetal metabolic, hematological, and hormonal disorders, or abnormalities of placental vessels.

Most fetal therapies whether medical or surgical are interim procedures intended to allow the fetus to remain in utero until it is mature enough to survive delivery, neonatal period, and postnatal surgical procedure.

Fetal therapy may be categorized into:
- Fetal medical therapy
- Fetal surgery

Routes of fetal interventions may be:
- Noninvasive transplacental route
- Ultrasound-guided interventions
- Fetoscopic surgery
- Open fetal surgery

Fetal Medical Therapy

Transplacental Route

Route where maternal administration crosses placenta and treats the fetus. It is a noninvasive intervention.
- *Steroids for lung maturity* in fetuses at risk for preterm delivery are the best known pharmacological intervention for preventing hyaline membrane disease and reduce the incidence of intraventricular hemorrhage.[7]
- *Transplacental transport of folic acid supplementation* has a protective effect on neural tube defect.
- *Maternal administration of intravenous immunoglobulin (IVIg)* to mothers who is alloimmunized against fetal platelets antigen inherited from father to the fetus.
- *Maternal administration of magnesium sulfate (Magsulf)* in pre-eclampsia and extreme preterm for neuroprotection and reducing risk of cerebral palsy.[8]
- *Congenital adrenal hyperplasia*: Differentiation of external genitalia starts at 7–8 weeks, hence all mothers of fetuses at risk of congenital adrenal hyperplasia (parents carrier, previous affected fetus) are initiated on 0.25 mg dexamethasone orally as early as 7–9 weeks which transfers to the developing fetus transplacentally. Steroids are continued through pregnancy only in female fetuses found to be affected at CVS.

- *Maternal human immunodeficiency virus (HIV)*: Maternal administration of zidovudine started at 14 weeks of gestation and continued throughout pregnancy, intrapartum period, and to the neonate reduces rate of vertical transmission.
- *Thyroid disorders*:
  - *Hyperthyroidism* in the fetus may occur due to transplacental transfer of thyroid-stimulating antibodies from a mother with Graves' disease to the fetus. This may be diagnosed on ultrasound by the presence of fetal tachycardia, fetal growth restriction, and hydrops and confirmed on cordocentesis for thyroid-stimulating hormone (TSH) values. The hyperthyroid fetus is then treated by maternal administration of higher doses of propylthiouracil or methimazole. If the mother becomes hypothyroid, supplementation with thyroxine may be needed.
  - *Hypothyroid fetus*: Fetus in utero becomes hypothyroid in mothers who are thyrotoxic on antithyroid drugs, mothers who have received radioactive radioiodine in pregnancy, and euthyroid mother with fetal dysgenesis/agenesis of thyroid gland. Increased levels of TSH in the amniotic fluid or fetal cord blood are diagnostic. Intra-amniotic instillation of L-thyroxine (500 μg) every 2 weeks or 200 μg weekly may help in regression of goiter, polyhydramnios, and normalization of hormonal levels.
- *Fetal arrhythmias*:
  - *Supraventricular tachycardia*: Most fetal arrhythmias are intermittent and benign in nature. Persistent supraventricular tachycardia may evolve into fetal hydrops and hence must be treated in utero or delivered if pregnancy is close to term.

    Transplacental treatment of fetus is done by administering digoxin to the mother under supervision of an adult cardiologist. Mother should be admitted and investigated with electrocardiogram (ECG), renal function, and electrolyte prior to the loading dose as the impact of the drug on the mother should be monitored. Digoxin is widely accepted as the first-line antiarrhythmic drug for fetal therapy. Recently, sotalol, flecainide, and amiodarone are being used as second-line treatment when either digoxin is ineffective or when correction is attempted after hydrops develops.
  - *Complete heart block* in the fetus is seen in association with maternal autoimmune disease (systemic lupus erythematosus, Sjögren syndrome) with maternal serum positive for anti-Ro and/or anti-La antibodies. These antibodies cause fetal myocarditis and damage the conduction fibers leading to dissociation of atrial and ventricular rhythm. Prior to any prenatal intervention in a complete heart block, structural cardiac anomalies associated in about 50% of cases such as atrioventricular canal defect, ventricular septal defects, and transposition of great vessels must be ruled out. Maternal administration of steroids (dexamethasone 4 mg) or beta 2-stimulants transplacentally to the fetus have been reported as effective with variable results.[9]

Ultrasound-guided Medical Intervention

Intrauterine transfusion: Hemolytic disease of the fetus and newborn is due to maternal alloantibodies directed against paternal antigen on fetal cells resulting in hemolysis of fetal red blood cell (RBC) causing anemia. Intrauterine transfusion of blood to these anemic fetuses is one of the best fetal therapies available with extremely good results.

Rh-negative isoimmunized mother with previously affected fetus or those with Rh antibodies titers above critical levels are monitored noninvasively by Doppler of middle cerebral artery peak systolic velocity (MCA PSV) to identify moderate-to-severe anemia prior to development of hydrops. MCA PSV correlates well with the degree of fetal anemia. A cutoff value of MCA PSV of 1.5 multiples of median (MoM) for the period of gestation or evidence of hydrops on ultrasound indicates severe anemia (hematocrit < 30%) requiring intrauterine transfusion.

If untreated, the anemic fetus would develop hepatosplenomegaly, cardiomegaly, placentomegaly, polyhydramnios, and end-stage hydropic fetus which may die in utero or postnatally of cardiac failure or develop kernicterus with its sequelae.

Under ultrasound guidance, intrauterine transfusion is done for double-packed (hematocrit of 75–80%) fresh O-negative blood, leukodepleted, CMV, cross-matched with mothers blood into the intravascular (cord insertion site or hepatic portal vein), or intraperitoneal compartment. Volume of blood to be transfused is calculated depending on the initial fetal hematocrit, donor hematocrit, and fetoplacental blood volume. In experienced hands, intrauterine transfusion is considered relatively safe with survival rates of about 90% for red cell alloimmunization.[10]

Intrauterine transfusion may also be used in anemic fetuses secondary to parvovirus infection, large fetomaternal hemorrhage, twin anemia polycythemia syndrome, intrauterine fetal demise of single fetus in monochorionic twins, and placental and fetal tumors such as chorioangioma and sacrococcygeal teratoma.

Multifetal pregnancy reduction and selective fetal reduction: With increasing use of assisted reproduction and advanced maternal age, there is a boom of higher-order multiple gestations in the past 2 decades.

The risk of preterm delivery (<37 weeks) for singleton is about 10% and it increases to 50% for twins and 80% for triplets. Average gestational age at delivery decreases from 35 weeks for twins to 32 weeks for triplets and 29 weeks for quadruplets. Risk of spontaneous loss of entire pregnancy is 25% for quadruplets, 15% for triplets, and 8% for twins. Rate of fetal growth restriction reported is 14–25% for twins and increases to 50–60% for triplets and quadruplets. Higher preterm and growth restriction in higher-order multiple births are major contributors to neonatal major handicap, cerebral palsy, learning disability, and death before 1 year of age.[11]

Multifetal pregnancy reduction (MFPR) is defined as first or early second trimester procedure for reduction of one or more normal fetuses, so as to increase the likelihood of survival and reduce morbidity of remaining fetuses. In addition, it reduces maternal morbidity.

The inherent risk of pregnancy loss in MFPR is directly proportional to the higher starting number of fetuses, number of fetuses reduced, and finishing fetal numbers. The risk reduces with the experience and expertise of the operator. The average risk of pregnancy loss due to the procedure at <26 weeks is about 4–5%.[12]

Preprocedure assessment and counseling: A detailed ultrasound is performed before MFPR to confirm gestational age, determine number of fetuses, labeling them, assessing growth of each fetus, chorionicity determination, early evaluation for structural defects, and screening for aneuploidy by nuchal translucency.

Determining chorionicity is most important before fetal reduction as MFPR with intracardiac potassium chloride (KCl) can only be done in dichorionic fetuses. Presence of the twin peak sign in the initial evaluation would confirm dichorionicity.

Detailed nondirective counseling is extremely necessary prior to the procedure and the benefits, risks, and alternatives should be explained. An informed consent is to be documented.

Choosing the fetus to be reduced: Fetal reduction is done on the fetus that, on initial evaluation, is relatively smaller in size (early fetal growth restricted) or structurally abnormal or fetus with increased nuchal translucency. However, if all fetuses are similar in above assessment, then the fetus that is easily approachable, fundal, and away from the cervix is targeted for reduction.

Technique: Although the procedure can be done from 8 weeks to 20 weeks, the ideal timing for the procedure is between 11 weeks and 13 weeks. The advantages of pregnancy reduction after 11 weeks (crown-rump length > 45 mm) include:
- Most spontaneous fetal loss would have already occurred
- Procedure is technically easier
- Identification of many structural anomalies and aneuploidy screening can be done
- Risk of procedure loss rate is least

Route: Multifetal pregnancy reduction can be done transabdominal or transvaginal depending on the expertise of the operator. However, pregnancy loss rates are higher in transvaginal route than transabdominal (13.3% vs. 3.5%).[13] Hence, transvaginal route is rarely used unless there is severe maternal obesity or approach to the fetus to be reduced requires it.

Procedure: Under ultrasound guidance and under aseptic precautions, a 20–22 G spinal needle is inserted into the heart or thorax of the fetus and 0.2–0.5 mL KCl is injected (Fig. 6). Needle is not withdrawn till asystole is achieved.

Risks:
- Amniotic fluid leak
- Chorioamnionitis
- Damage of the fetus without death
- Death of rest of the fetuses if chorionicity determination was inappropriate
- Threatened miscarriage and bleeding
- Loss of entire pregnancy

Postprocedure: In view of risk for chorioamnionitis, a broad-spectrum antibiotic is given prior to the procedure

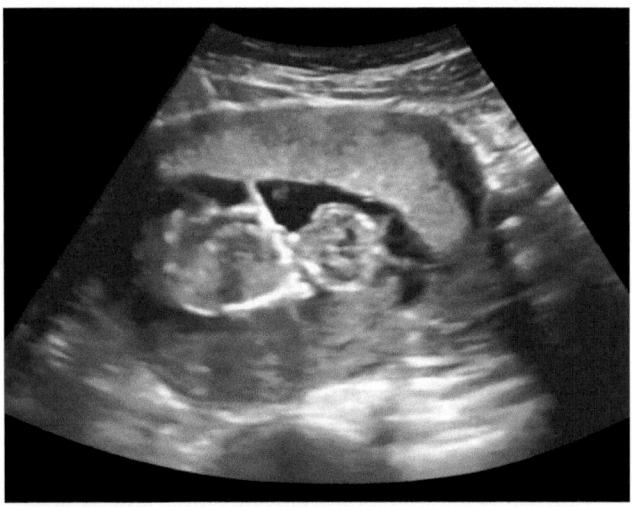

Fig. 6: Fetal reduction using potassium chloride (KCl).

and continued for 5 days. Giving progesterone/tocolysis are individual decisions. Patient is advised on restricted activity for few days and to report if fever/bleeding/leaking/pain in abdomen.

Reduction in monochorionic fetuses: In monochorionic twins, intracardiac KCl will crossover to the other fetus through vascular communications and cause fetal demise of the co-twin also. In these cases, if indicated, selective cord occlusion or radiofrequency ablation or ultrasound-guided/fetoscopic laser is the treatment of choice, but carries a higher risk of pregnancy loss.

Selective feticide: This is a term used distinctly for reduction done in a twin fetus for discordant fetal anomaly. Selective feticide is indicated in fetuses whose anomaly is nonlethal, but with morbidity or if the defect has a potential for affecting the other fetus and course of pregnancy.

Fetal Surgery

Distinct advantages of fetal surgery are:
- Intervene before progressive damage
- Surgical healing is better with no scars
- Fetus has the ideal postoperative environment in the mother's womb

Three approaches are used for fetal surgical intervention:
1. Open fetal surgery
2. Fetoscopic surgery
3. Percutaneous ultrasound-guided surgery using shunts

Principles of Fetal Surgery

Prenatal intervention is justified only if:
- Accurate diagnosis is made
- Disease is severe enough to warrant risk of intervention
- The malformation interferes with organ development
- If alleviated will allow normal development
- Fetus cannot be safely delivered at that point of time.

Prerequisites for Fetal Surgery

- *Nondirective counseling*: Although the final goal of fetal intervention is to improve the health of the fetus, any fetal intervention in utero has implications on the mother's health. Hence, the women and the family should be informed in detail about the risks and benefits. The informed consent should involve thorough discussion of the options available including fetal intervention, postnatal therapy, palliative nature of the therapy, residual disease and its long-term implications, and also options of pregnancy termination.
- Coexisting anomalies and chromosomal abnormalities are ruled out.
- Prenatal diagnostic procedure is done to determine the functional status of the organ system, which needs treatment.
- *Tertiary level obstetric, anesthetic, and neonatal* care available

Conditions Amenable to Surgery with Proven Results

- Pleuroamniotic shunt in primary hydrothorax
- Twin-to-twin transfusion syndrome
- Twin reversed arterial perfusion sequence
- Ovarian cyst aspiration

Conditions Amenable to Surgery with Mixed Results

- Vesicoamniotic shunt for obstructive uropathy
- Thoracoamniotic shunt for congenital pulmonary airway malformation [CPAM, initially called congenital cystic adenomatoid malformation (CCAM)]
- Fetal tracheal occlusion for congenital diaphragmatic hernia
- Surgery for meningomyelocele
- Surgery for sacrococcygeal teratoma

Conditions Amenable to Surgery with Disappointing Results

- Ventriculomegaly—aqueductal stenosis
- Structural cardiac defects—balloon valvuloplasty/septoplasty

Open Fetal Surgery

Open fetal surgery was first attempted in 1960. It involves an initial hysterotomy under general anesthesia where the fetus is extracted partially without disconnecting from the placenta and undergoes fetal surgery intrapartum for the disorder. Fetus is then returned back to the amniotic cavity and the uterus with membranes is resutured. Mother has to be under high doses of intravenous tocolysis for the procedure as well as subsequently to tide over the extremely high risk of preterm labor. Subsequently, the mother will need a second surgery [lower segment cesarean section (LSCS)] for delivery of the baby.

Conditions correctable with open fetal surgery are:
- Meningomyelocele
- Repair of congenital diaphragmatic hernia
- Ligation of sacrococcygeal teratoma

Fetal Surgery for Meningomyelocele

Meningomyelocele can cause hydrocephalus as well as motor impairment and loss of bowel and bladder control. These have been postulated to aggravate due to exposure of spinal cord to the trauma of amniotic fluid in utero. Covering of meningomyelocele (initially in sheep and later in human fetus) has been shown to reduce the need for ventriculoperitoneal shunts, slow the progress of ventriculomegaly, resolution of hindbrain hernia, and improved motor outcome in short-term follow-up of 30 months.[14]

Surgery for Sacrococcygeal Teratoma

Sacrococcygeal teratoma causes large arteriovenous shunting of blood leading to high output cardiac failure, hydrops, and death. Traditionally, the tumor was resected by open technique followed by fetoscopic route. Attempts have been made toward percutaneous minimal invasive coagulation of tumor vessels.

Risks involved with open surgery include:
- High chances of preterm labor
- Premature rupture of membrane
- Bleeding per vaginum
- Chorioamnionitis
- Pulmonary edema and complications of anesthesia
- Need for LSCS for present as well as all subsequent pregnancies

Fetoscopic Fetal Surgery

Open fetal surgery gave way to fetoscopic surgeries as they were relatively less invasive than open fetal surgery. Fetoscopic surgery is done under epidural/local anesthesia. It requires specialized fetoscopic instruments, atraumatic ports, and working fluid media (saline/Ringer). There is no mandatory need for LSCS later as compared to open surgery.

Indications

- *Fetoscopic tracheal occlusion for treatment of congenital diaphragmatic hernia (Fetendo technique)*: The aim is to temporarily plug the trachea using clips or balloon, so as to cause obstruction to lung secretion and subsequently cause expansion of lungs pushing the herniated abdominal viscera back into the abdomen.
  An ex utero intrapartum treatment (EXIT) to remove the clips and intubate the trachea is performed at term during LSCS while the partially delivered fetus is still receiving placental supply.
- Fetoscopic balloon valvuloplasty of critical aortic stenosis in the fetus has been attempted to prevent progression to hypoplastic left heart syndrome with mixed results.
- About 10–15% of all monozygous twins have TTTS where there are unbalanced vascular anastomosis between both the fetuses. Without treatment, perinatal mortality reaches 63–80%. Fetoscopic surgery has reemerged as the treatment of choice for TTTS where selective laser photocoagulation of communicating vessels is done.[15]
- Fetoscopic cord occlusion/ligation of acardiac twin is also a successful surgical modality. Twin reversed arterial perfusion sequence is seen in 1% of monozygous twins and is associated with cardiac failure in the pump twin with perinatal mortality as high as 55%. Recently, intrafetal interstitial laser in the acardiac fetus under ultrasound guidance using laser fibers inserted via 18-gauze needle has become the treatment of choice as it is simple, safer, and more effective.
- Fetoscopic fulguration of posterior urethral valves.

Limitations of Fetoscopic Surgery

- Invasive
- Limited depth and field of vision
- Intra-amniotic bleed may obscure vision
- Risk of preterm labor and premature rupture of membranes slightly more than USG-guided procedures, but less than open fetal surgery
- Maternal and fetal injury with the trocar
- Potential teratogenic effect of light and heat

Percutaneous Ultrasound-guided Fetal Shunts

Ultrasound-guided interventional procedures are done under local anesthesia.

Complications

Complications are low as compared to above procedures and include:
- Preterm, premature rupture of membranes
- Fetal injury
- Shunt block or displacement
- Chorioamnionitis

Indications

- *Primary pleural effusion (chylothorax)*: Extrinsic compression on the developing lungs may lead to pulmonary hypoplasia and hydrops. Pleuroamniotic shunt is a double pigtail catheter which is placed under ultrasound guidance with one end of the shunt in the pleural cavity and other end in the amniotic cavity. About 60% survival rates have been achieved in carefully selected cases of primary pleural effusion.[16] Another approach in fetal chylothorax is performing pleurodesis by administering OK-432 in the pleural cavity.
- *Obstructive uropathy*: Severe bilateral obstruction to outflow of urine may cause backpressure changes

leading to nonfunctional dysplastic kidneys in utero and pulmonary hypoplasia due to oligohydramnios (Potter's syndrome). Vesicoamniotic shunts aim to release backpressure effect in the urinary tract, restore urinary outflow, and improve liquor and pulmonary development.

Intervention justified only if the obstruction is severe, bilateral, causing progressive oligohydramnios, and deteriorating renal function on serial ultrasound remote from term. Some amount of residual renal function must be preserved before intervention. Fetal karyotype must be done and any other disorders ruled out.

Renal function is assessed by fetal vesicocentesis where initially urine in the distended fetal bladder is completely aspirated. Subsequent urine sample is analyzed for sodium, chloride, and β2 microglobulin. Nonfunctional kidneys are salt wasters and β2 microglobulin of >2 mg/L is the best predictor of poor renal function.

Ultrasound-guided vesicoamniotic shunt is done under local anesthesia using double pigtail shunt where one end is in the fetal bladder and other end in the amniotic fluid. The PLUTO trial compared conservative treatment with vesicoamniotic shunts in singleton fetuses less than 28 weeks. Survival seemed to be better in the intervention group at 28 days of life. However, the authors concluded that there was substantial short- and long-term morbidity in both groups due to poor renal residual function.[17]

Relieving obstruction temporarily may prolong gestational age at delivery, improve pulmonary maturity, but renal damage already done and its sequel may remain. The child may subsequently develop chronic renal failure requiring dialysis.

Other options are open or fetoscopic fulguration of posterior urethral valves.

- *Ventriculoamniotic shunts* have been evaluated for decompression in obstructive hydrocephalus, but have poor results and have been abandoned.
- *Congenital pulmonary airway obstruction (CPAM/CCAM)*: The natural history of this lung lesion may be progression/regression or remains stable antenatally. Large cysts involving a large part of the lung may cause lung compression, mediastinal shift, hydrops, and fetal mortality. These progressive, macrocystic, and large lung cysts may be drained via a cystoamniotic shunt under ultrasound guidance and thus help in regression and improve lung growth.

CONCLUSION

With the advent of high-resolution ultrasound, better training and expertise, and improved understanding of fetal development, the 11-13+6 weeks scan provides much more information and has become a window for detection of aneuploidy, anomalies, cardiac defects, genetic and nongenetic syndromes, and pregnancy complications. However, to maintain high level of quality in these screening methods, adherence to strict standardized technique and extensive training and auditing cannot be overstated.

The objective of prenatal genetic testing is to detect health problems that could affect the woman, fetus, or newborn and provides the patient and her obstetrician with enough information to allow a fully informed decision about pregnancy management. Prenatal genetic testing cannot identify all abnormalities or problems in a fetus, and any testing should be focused on the individual patient's risks, reproductive goals, and preferences. It is important that patients understand the benefits and limitations of all prenatal screening and diagnostic testing, including the conditions for which tests are available and the conditions that will not be detected by testing. It is also important that patients realize that there is a broad range of clinical presentations, or phenotypes, for many genetic disorders, and that results of genetic testing cannot predict all outcomes. Prenatal genetic testing has many benefits, including reassuring patients when results are normal, identifying disorders for which prenatal treatment may provide benefit, optimizing neonatal outcomes by ensuring the appropriate location for delivery and the necessary personnel to care for affected infants, and allowing the opportunity for pregnancy termination.

Prenatal medical therapy has good postintervention results with minimal risk to the mother. Intrauterine transfusion in Rh-isoimmunized anemic fetus has a survival rate as high as 70–80%. Fetal reduction procedures are extremely important for risk reduction in patients with higher-order pregnancies.

However, fetal surgeries have a potential risk to mother and fetus and need an extensive presurgical counseling of parents and family. It necessitates careful case selection, well-coordinated team, and extensive expertise in the field and hence is limited to few specialized centers in India and worldwide.

Fetoscopy has reevolved with its use in treating complications of monochorionic twins. Fetoscopic laser ablation of unbalanced communicating vessels in TTTS is today the most common fetal surgical procedure carried out.

REFERENCES

1. Phadke SR, Puri RD, Ranganath P. Prenatal screening for genetic disorders: suggested guidelines for the Indian scenario. Indian J Med Res. 2017;146:689-99.
2. Norton ME, Scoutt LM, Feldstein VA. Genetics and prenatal genetic testing. In: Norton ME (Ed). Callen's Ultrasonography in Obstetrics and Gynecology, 6th edition. Philadelphia: Elsevier; 2016. pp. 24-52.
3. Creasy RK, Resnik R, Iams JD, et al. Prenatal diagnosis of congenital disorders. In: Resnik R, Creasy R, Iams J, Lockwood C, Moore T, Greene M (Eds). Creasy and Resnik's Maternal-Fetal Medicine: Principles and Practice, 7th edition. Philadelphia: Elsevier; 2013. pp. 417-64.
4. American College of Obstetricians and Gynecologists' Committee on Practice Bulletins—Obstetrics, Committee on Genetics, Society for Maternal–Fetal Medicine. Practice Bulletin No. 162: Prenatal Diagnostic Testing for Genetic Disorders. Obstet Gynecol. 2016;127:e108-22.
5. Ghi T, Sotiriadis A, Calda P, et al. ISUOG Practice Guidelines: invasive procedures for prenatal diagnosis. Ultrasound Obstet Gynecol. 2016;48:256-68.
6. Royal College of Obstetricians and Gynaecologists (RCOG) (2010). Amniocentesis and Chorionic Villus Sampling: Green-top Guideline No.8. [online] Available from https://www.rcog.org.uk/globalassets/documents/guidelines/gtg_8.pdf. [Last accessed November, 2019].
7. National Institutes of Health (NIH) (1994). The Effect of Corticosteroids for Fetal Maturation on Perinatal outcomes. [online] Available from https://consensus.nih.gov/1994/1994antenatalsteroidperinatal095html.htm. [Last accessed November, 2019].
8. The Antenatal Magnesium Sulphate for Neuroprotection Guideline Development Panel (2010). Antenatal Magnesium Sulphate Prior to Preterm Birth for Neuroprotection of the Fetus, Infant and Child: National Clinical Practice Guidelines. [online] Available from https://cdn.auckland.ac.nz/assets/liggins/docs/Antenatal%20magnesium%20sulphate%20prior%20to%20preterm%20birth%20for%20neuroprotection%20of%20the%20fetus,%20infant%20&%20child,%20National%20clinical%20practice%20guidelines.pdf. [Last accessed November, 2019].
9. Breur JM, Visser GH, Kruize AA, et al. Treatment of fetal heart block with maternal steroid therapy: case report and review of the literature. Ultrasound Obstet Gynecol. 2004;24:467-72.
10. Oepkes D, Adama van Scheltema P. Intrauterine fetal transfusions in the management of fetal anemia and fetal thrombocytopenia. Semin Fetal Neonatal Med. 2007;12:432-8.
11. American College of Obstetricians and Gynecologists Committee on Practice Bulletins-Obstetrics, Society for Maternal-Fetal Medicine, ACOG Joint Editorial Committee. ACOG Practice Bulletin #56: Multiple gestation: complicated twin, triplet, and high-order multifetal pregnancy. Obstet Gynecol. 2004;104:869-93.
12. Evans ML, Berkowitz RL, Wapner RJ, et al. Improvement in outcome of multifetal pregnancy reduction with increased experience. Am J Obstet Gynecol. 2001;184:97-103.
13. Timor-Tritsch IE, Bashiri A, Monteagudo A, et al. Two hundred and ninety consecutive cases of multifetal pregnancy reduction: comparison of transabdominal versus the transvaginal approach. Am J Obstet Gynecol. 2004;194:2085-9.
14. Adzick NS, Thom EA, Spong CY, et al. A randomized trial of prenatal versus postnatal repair of myelomeningocele. N Engl J Med. 2011;364:993-1004.
15. Ville Y. Treatment of twin-to-twin-transfusion syndrome. The end of a long-standing misunderstanding. Ultrasound Obstet Gynecol. 2003;22:64.
16. Smith RP, Illanes S, Denbow ML, et al. Outcome of fetal pleural effusions treated by thoracoamniotic shunting. Ultrasound Obstet Gynecol. 2005;26:63-6.
17. Morris RK, Malin GL, Quinlan-Jones E, et al. Percutaneous vesicoamniotic shunting versus conservative management for fetal lower urinary tract obstruction (PLUTO): a randomised trial. Lancet. 2013;382:1496-506.

18

Gastrointestinal Tract Anomalies

Parul Choudhary Vali, Jayprakash Shah

INTRODUCTION

Fetal abdomen is a Pandora box with various organs and systems. But here we will be discussing the normal appearance and anomalies of gastrointestinal (GI) tract only. Fetal GI tract's appearance varies in ultrasound throughout the pregnancy; also, some organs may appear differently during the same ultrasound examination due to normal physiological acts of swallowing, gastric emptying, and intestinal peristalsis. Another point to be kept in mind is that antenatal detection of GI anomalies is a difficult task because of frequent absence of any ultrasound detectable signs before the third trimester. For better understanding of GI anomalies, the chapter is divided as given in Table 1.

ESOPHAGEAL ATRESIA

Normal Appearance

Normal esophagus can be visualized on sagittal view as well as axial view.

Sagittal View of Thorax

Esophagus is visible as a tubular structure behind the trachea composed of four parallel echogenic lines corresponding to the apposition of anterior and posterior walls of esophagus (Fig. 1). When fetus swallows amniotic fluid, it appears as an anechoic structure because of filling of esophagus.

Axial View of Thorax

In this view, esophagus is not visualized until immediately after fetal swallowing. In this situation, it is visualized as small anechoic structure behind the heart on four-chamber view, for short time, and disappears when swallowing stops. It may be mistaken for an abnormal vessel. Here, color or power Doppler can be used to exclude its vascular origin.

Table 1: Gastrointestinal (GI) tract malformations.

Obstruction of GI tract:	Intra-abdominal cyst of GI origin:	Hepatobiliary system anomalies:	Echogenic bowel
• Esophageal atresia • Duodenal atresia • Jejunoileal atresia • Meconium ileus • Meconium peritonitis • Anal atresia	• Enteric duplication cyst • Mesenteric cyst • Meconium pseudocyst • Hepatic cyst • Splenic cyst • Choledochal cyst	• Agenesis of ductus venosus • Persistent right umbilical vein	

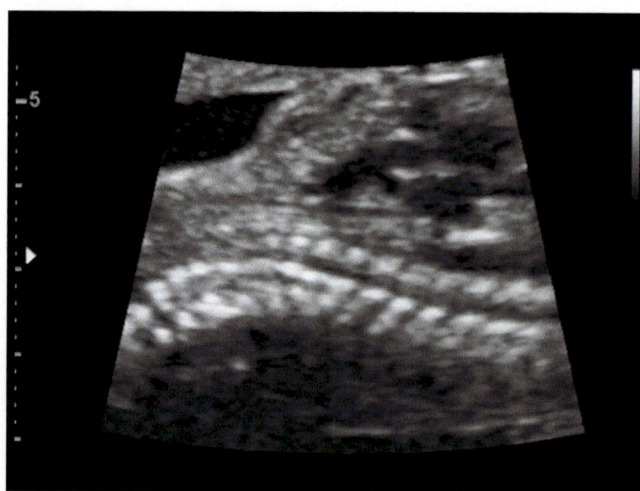

Fig. 1: Sagittal view of upper thorax showing normal esophagus as four parallel echogenic lines behind the trachea.

Gastrointestinal Tract Anomalies

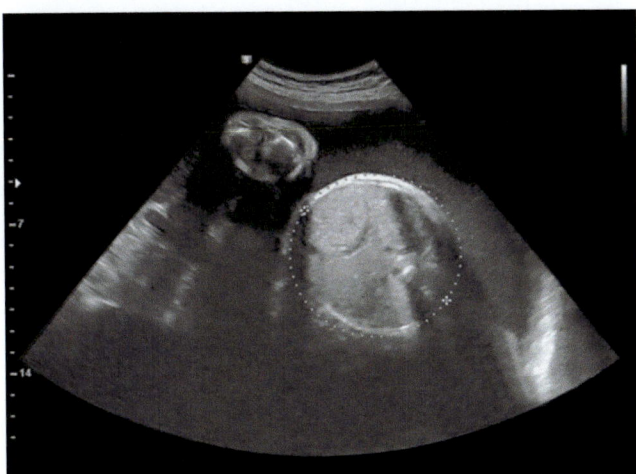

Fig. 2: Axial view of abdomen showing absence of stomach with increased amniotic fluid as an indirect sign, suggestive of esophageal atresia.

Table 2: Associated system anomalies with esophageal atresia.

System affected	Percentage of anomalies (%)
Cardiovascular	29
Anorectum	14
Genitourinary	14
Gastrointestinal (excluding anorectum)	13
Vertebral and skeletal	21
Respiratory	13
Genetic	4
Others	11

Incidence

The incidence is 1/2,500–1/4,000 live births.[1]

Ultrasound Appearance

It can be in form of indirect signs, where you suspect high probability of esophageal atresia, but indirect signs do not confirm it. Direct signs represent the atresia with or without fistula as direct visualization and are practically confirmative of esophageal atresia.

Indirect Signs

Absence of Stomach

It is suspected when stomach bubble is continuously smaller than normal or may be not visible with polyamnios in second or early third trimester (Fig. 2). The problem with this sign is that first proper quantification criteria for stomach size are not available and second stomach may not be completely absent because of its frequent association with tracheoesophageal (TE) fistula. Also, even when TE fistula is not associated, gastric secretion may produce a small amount of fluid in stomach. Overall sensitivity of ultrasonography is 42% and positive predictive value of this sign is 56%.[2] Unexplained early symmetric intrauterine growth restriction (IUGR) is common with TE fistula.

- Absence of stomach does not confirm esophageal atresia.
- Presence of stomach does not rule out esophageal atresia.
- Usually, diagnosis is made after 20 weeks of pregnancy.

Direct Signs

Dilatation of blind-ending esophagus (esophageal pouch) in fetal neck and mediastinum on sagittal view of thorax are seen with "type C" TE fistula (gross classification). Absence of this sign does not rule out esophageal atresia.

A break in the continuity of the four echogenic lines on sagittal view of thorax and upper mediastinum is very difficult to visualize.

Differential Diagnosis

Nonvisualization of Stomach

- *Stomach just emptied in duodenum*: Physiological emptying cycle is 50–60 minutes. Rescan may be performed after an hour.
- Situs inversus
- Diaphragmatic hernia
- Anterior abdominal wall defect
- Heterotaxy syndrome

Small Stomach—Any Condition Leading to Poor Swallowing of Amniotic Fluid by Fetus

- Severe oligoamnios
- Facial and neck abnormalities—cleft lip, severe micrognathia, large goiter, and teratoma
- Neuroarthrogryposis—decreased swallowing leads to small stomach.

Associations (Table 2)

Over 50% of infants with esophageal atresia have additional one or the other anomalies.[3]

Other associations are as follows:
- CHARGE syndrome (Coloboma, Heart disease, Atresia choanae, Retarded growth and development, Genital hypoplasia, and Ear anomalies or deafness)
- Potter syndrome (renal agenesis, pulmonary hypoplasia, and typical dysmorphic facies)
- Schisis syndrome (omphalocele, cleft lip and/or palate, genital hypoplasia).

Genetic defects include trisomy 21, trisomy 18 and 13q deletion.

Prenatal Management and Counseling

When esophageal atresia is suspected:
- Thorough anatomical scan is to be performed to rule out any associated anomalies of any system.
- Fetal karyotyping is advised as it is associated with trisomy 21 and 18.
- Delivery should be planned in a tertiary care center as early corrective surgery and neonatal intensive care unit (NICU) admission may be required.
- Parents should be counseled regarding the outcome of the baby. The survival rate of the esophageal atresia-TE fistula repair in a term baby with no associated anomalies is about 95%.[4]

Postnatal Treatment

- Once fetus is stabilized and fit for operation.
- If it is not fit for major surgery, gastrostomy can be done and feeding can be given to neonate till fit for surgery.

DUODENAL ATRESIA

Incidence

The incidence is 1/5,000–1/10,000 live births.[5]

Ultrasound Diagnosis

Classical double bubble with connection between two bubbles associated with early polyhydramnios is seen in late second and early third trimesters. One bubble is on the left side and other bubble is in the center or right side in transverse section of abdomen at abdominal circumference (AC) level (Fig. 3), and there shall be connection visible between two bubbles.

At the time of anomaly scan, when double bubble is not fully formed and polyamnios is not present, doubt may arise when we see persistent dilated stomach and slight dilatation of the duodenum.

Differential Diagnosis

All the cystic structures in the middle or right upper abdomen such as enteric duplication cyst (EDC), choledochal cyst, and hepatic cyst are differential diagnosis. The differentiating feature is the communication between the two cysts in case of duodenal atresia (Box 1).

Associations

Multiple associated anomalies with duodenal atresia6 are given in Table 3.

Prenatal Management and Counseling

- Thorough anatomical scan is to be performed to rule out any associated anomalies.
- Fetal karyotyping is mandatory as there is a high risk of trisomy 21.
- Fetal echocardiography should be performed because of high association with cardiac anomalies.
- In selected cases, amniodrainage may be performed for severe polyamnios.

Box 1: Differential diagnosis of duodenal atresia.
- Prominent stomach with prominent incisura angularis
- Annular pancreas
- Proximal jejunal atresia
- Ladd's band gastric duplication
- Duodenal stenosis

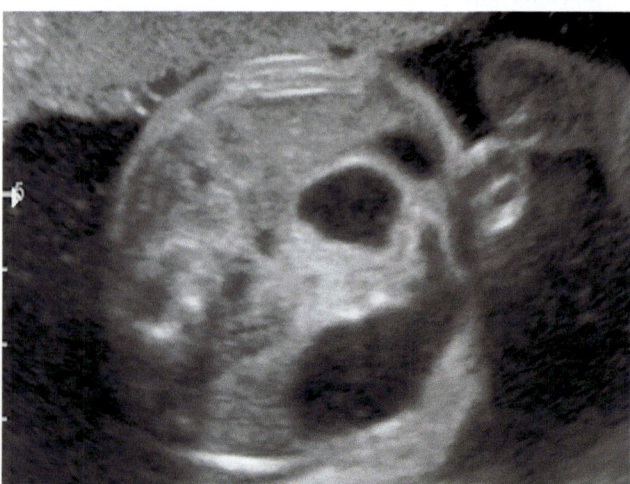

Fig. 3: Axial scan of abdomen showing the two anechoic cystic structures, the "double bubble", where one bubble is on the left and the other one is in the center, slightly toward right.

Table 3: Anomalies associated with duodenal atresia.

Associated anomalies	Percentage (%)
Down syndrome	46
Cardiac anomalies	31
Malrotation	10
Bowel atresia	7
Vertebral anomalies	5
Tracheoesophageal fistula	5
Renal anomalies	5
VACTERL	5
Anorectal	3

(VACTERL: vertebral defects, anal atresia, cardiac defects, tracheoesophageal fistula, renal anomalies, and limb abnormalities)

- Delivery should be planned in a tertiary care center where NICU and pediatric surgery is available.
- Parents should be counseled about the good prognosis in isolated cases with 90% survival rate after surgery in isolated cases.[7]

Postnatal Treatment

Surgical procedures for duodenal atresia include duodenoduodenostomy or duodenojejunostomy. Additional surgical procedures may be required in associated intestinal, pancreatic, and/or biliary malformations.

SMALL BOWEL ATRESIA

Normal Appearance

Small bowel appears during the second trimester as small hypoechoic areas with echogenic wall and shows peristalsis in the form of continuously changing appearance. While using high-frequency transducer, individual loops of bowel can often be discerned and can be visible precisely but will be more echogenic. During the third trimester, fluid can be seen within bowel lumen, but the transverse diameter of small intestine should be up to 7 mm and continuous visible length of bowel is never more than 15 mm.

Incidence

The incidence is 1/2,500–1/5,000 live births.[8]

Ultrasound Appearance

Small bowel obstruction by ultrasound is usually seen after 25 weeks. It is suspected when you come across dilatation of small bowel with visible peristalsis and transverse diameter is measuring more than 7 mm. These dilated loops are located in the center of abdomen just behind cord entry, anterior to the spine and kidneys and superior to the bladder. Increased bilateral peristalsis is visible in the dilated segment. In fact, in suspected bowel obstruction, you are not seeing the atretic or obstructed segment but it is indirectly picked up by dilated segments. In case of jejunal atresia, dilated bowel loops are usually not more than four in number and polyamnios is seen earlier (Fig. 4). Dilated bowel loops are almost of same size. In ileal obstruction, one can see dilated loops of different sizes with more than four dilated loops and relatively late polyamnios (Fig. 5). In the later stage of long-standing small bowel obstruction, perforation of bowel with ascites, meconium pseudocyst, and later calcified areas in peritoneal cavity can appear and these are important landmarks to understand outcome in cases of small bowel obstruction.

Differential Diagnosis

Differential diagnosis among volvulus, meconium ileus, and Hirschsprung's disease is extremely challenging. In volvulus, rapid onset of dilatation of the bowel in 3–4 days can roughly give us an idea. In meconium ileus, presence of intra-abdominal calcifications following intestinal perforation leading to meconium peritonitis may give us a clue.

Associations

Around 25% of cases of bowel atresia may be associated with other intestinal anomalies such as malrotation, intussusception, intestinal duplication, and volvulus.

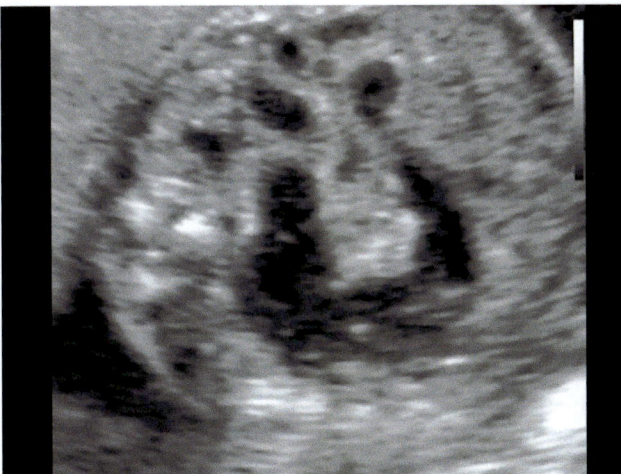

Fig. 4: Axial view of abdomen showing multiple dilated loops of almost same size, 3–5 in number suggestive of jejunal atresia. It may mimic as if it is duodenal atresia.

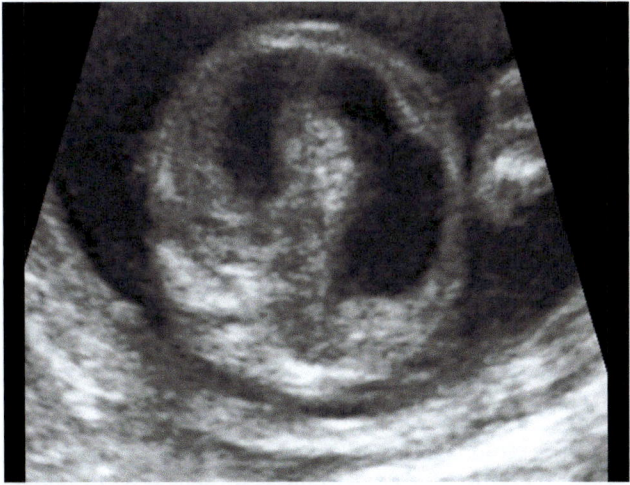

Fig. 5: Axial view of abdomen showing dilated loops of bowel with wide connection and on real-time with peristalsis suggestive of jejunoileal atresia.

Chromosomal association is low. But there is 10% risk of cystic fibrosis which increases to 90% if meconium peritonitis is associated.

Prenatal Management and Counseling

- Karyotyping is not routinely indicated as association with chromosomal abnormalities is low.
- Delivery should be planned in tertiary care center as earliest surgery needs to be carried out in most of the cases.
- Amniodrainage may be performed in certain selected cases of polyamnios endangering preterm delivery.
- The final outcome is generally good except for relatively rare cases of multiple atresia and apple-peel atresia as the total length of the bowel is reduced in these two, leading to malabsorption (short bowel syndrome). Also, if volvulus, perforation, and meconium peritonitis are associated, it increases the postoperative mortality.

Poor prognostic signs include:
- Intra-abdominal calcification—suggestive of meconium ileus complicated by perforation and meconium peritonitis
- Polyhydramnios—due to delayed anastomosis and longer hospital stay
- Multiple atresia and apple-peel atresia—leads to short bowel syndrome
- Congenital volvulus

Postnatal Treatment

The surgical treatment includes removal of atretic segment and end-to-end intestinal anastomosis. In more complex cases, initial ileostomy followed by anastomosis is performed as a two-stage operation.

MECONIUM ILEUS

Meconium ileus is characterized by ileal mechanical obstruction caused by thickened meconium. This obstruction often leads to ileal perforation and meconium peritonitis.

Incidence

It is unknown in fetus.

Ultrasound Appearance

On ultrasound, it is visualized as one or more dilated loops of intestine that characteristically show hyperechoic content (Fig. 6), and hyperechoic bowel walls are usually evident after 24 weeks of gestation. Walls may appear normal

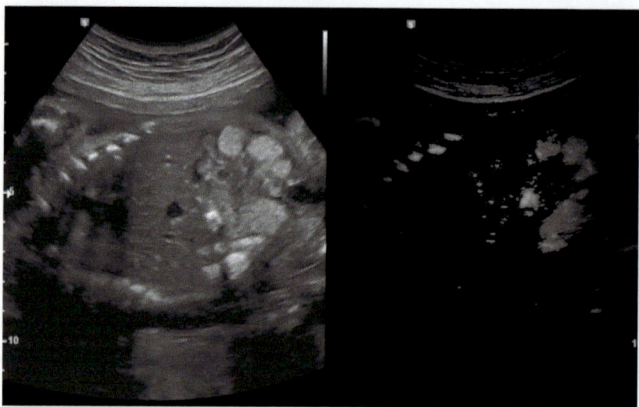

Fig. 6: Dilated loops of bowel with hyperechoic content seen on the right side; we can see the hyperechoic content of bowel after reducing the gain too. This ultrasound image is suggestive of meconium ileus.

also. Diffuse intra-abdominal calcifications may be seen if meconium peritonitis occurs due to perforation. The first evidence of meconium ileus is echogenic bowel seen in mid-trimester in a significant number of cases.

Differential Diagnosis

Main differential diagnosis is small bowel atresia but the differentiation between the ileal or jejunal may be impossible prenatally. Presence of meconium peritonitis and echogenic meconium in ileal loops may point toward meconium ileus.

Associations

Cystic fibrosis is almost ubiquitous. Though meconium ileus has low chromosomal association, the first sign of meconium ileus—"echogenic bowel"—carries a 9% risk of chromosomal anomalies.

Prenatal Management and Counseling

- If echogenic bowel is seen in mid-trimester, karyotyping and fetal DNA (deoxyribonucleic acid) for cystic fibrosis should be performed.
- Delivery should be planned in a tertiary care center.
- Meconium ileus itself is a poor prognostic sign, especially when associated with meconium peritonitis because of its extremely high association with cystic fibrosis. Its association with meconium peritonitis increases the complexity of operation. The survival and long-term outcome depend on the clinical severity of the underlying cystic fibrosis.

Postnatal Treatment

After delivery, contrast-enhanced computed tomography (CECT) scan should be performed to ascertain intestinal perforation. If bowel atresia is associated along with meconium ileus, bowel resection with end-to-end anastomosis should be performed. If no bowel atresia is associated, then a simple saline, water-soluble contrast enema or N-acetyl cysteine may induce meconium passage.

MECONIUM PERITONITIS

Meconium peritonitis is the end result of prenatal bowel perforation following bowel atresia, meconium ileus, gastroschisis, intussusception, volvulus, and intrauterine fetal infections, especially cytomegalovirus (CMV).

Incidence

It is a rare abnormality.

Ultrasound Appearance

It can present as simple or complex peritonitis.
- Simple peritonitis—only peritoneal calcification is seen.
- Complex peritonitis—peritoneal calcification is associated with meconium pseudocyst, ascites, polyamnios, and/or bowel dilatation.

Differential Diagnosis

- *Hepatic calcification*: It can be vascular, parenchymal, or peritoneal. In meconium peritonitis, we see only peritoneal calcification.
- *Enterolithiasis*: In enterolithiasis, calcification is present in bowel lumen, whereas in meconium peritonitis calcification is present in the wall of bowel.

Associations

Association with extra GI malformations and chromosomal malformations is low.

Cystic fibrosis in complex peritonitis ranges between 15% and 45% in neonatal series. Cystic fibrosis is uncommon in simple peritonitis.

Prenatal Management and Counseling

- First step of prenatal management is to rule out fetal infection and check fetal DNA for cystic fibrosis. If it comes out to be negative, the etiology is bowel atresia, volvulus, or intussusception.
- Delivery should be planned in a tertiary care center

Prognostic Factors

- Simple peritonitis—good outcome
- Complex peritonitis—guarded outcome because of high association with cystic fibrosis

Postnatal Treatment

Surgical intervention is usually required in complex peritonitis. In simple peritonitis, surgical intervention is not necessary.

ANAL ATRESIA AND ANORECTAL MALFORMATIONS

Ultrasound Diagnosis

Most of the anorectal malformations, especially imperforate anus, remain undiagnosed prenatally. Overdistension of rectum or sigmoid colon with the maximal diameter of rectum more than the adjacent full urinary bladder gives us a clue to the diagnosis. In some cases, hyperechoic meconium is also visualized. Intraluminal calcifications in case of long-standing meconium and alkaline urine from associated urorectal malformation, if present, are also seen.

Amniotic fluid is normal except in the cases of associated urorectal malformation where amniotic fluid is reduced. If polyamnios is seen, it is due to associated anomalies of other organs.

In cases with persistent cloaca, a septated or bilateral pelvic cystic mass is visualized representing hydrocolpos or hydrometrocolpos and bladder obstruction (megacystis).

Associations

Urogenital malformations have high association with anorectal atresia because of common embryological association. Other common associated anomalies are vertebral anomalies, GI anomalies, and cardiac anomalies.

There is a high risk of chromosomal anomalies, especially trisomy 18 and 13.

High-risk syndromes are as follows:
- *VACTERL association*: Vertebral anomalies, anal atresia, cardiac defects, tracheoesophageal fistula, renal agenesis, and limb anomalies
- *Sirenomelia*: Anorectal malformation, renal agenesis, fusion of inferior limbs, severe vertebral anomalies, and genital anomalies
- *Caudal regression syndrome*: Anorectal malformations, renal agenesis, sacral agenesis, lumbar vertebral anomalies, femoral hypoplasia, and talipes
- *OEIS syndrome*: Omphalocele, exstrophy of bladder, imperforate anus, and spinal anomalies.

Prenatal Management and Counseling

- Detailed anatomical scan is performed to rule out associated anomalies, especially urogenital malformations, vertebral, and GI malformations.

Gastrointestinal Tract Anomalies

- Fetal echocardiography should also be performed because of high association with cardiac anomalies.
- Karyotyping is also recommended because of high association with trisomy 18 and 13.
- Delivery should be planned in a tertiary care center where proper diagnostic workup and surgical treatment of bowel obstruction can be performed because the baby will require immediate postnatal evaluation and treatment.
- In isolated cases of anorectal malformation, prognosis is good.

Poor prognostic factors include:
- Sirenomelia, OEIS complex, and caudal regression (lethal because of renal agenesis)
- VACTERL association and other syndromic association
- Vertebral, GI, and other associated anomalies

Postnatal Management

All the fetuses should carefully be evaluated for urogenital anomalies. Single perineal orifice indicates persistent cloaca.

Plain X-ray of spine is done to rule out any associated vertebral anomalies and to assess the sacrum, which has a direct bearing on the prognosis in imperforate anus.

Surgical Repair of Anorectal Malformations

In low imperforate anus: Y-V anoplasty or a limited posterior sagittal anorectoplasty can be performed.

In intermediate and high levels of imperforate anus: A diverting colostomy is to be performed initially and then anorectal reconstruction is to be carried at 4–8 weeks of age.

AGENESIS OF DUCTUS VENOSUS

Normal Anatomy

Fetal ductus venosus is a slender trumpet-like shunt, connecting the intra-abdominal umbilical vein to inferior vena cava (IVC) at its inlet to the heart. The hepatic vein joins the IVC and the ductus venosus in the subdiaphragmatic vestibulum, an inverted funnel-shaped vascular space just below the diaphragm. The vestibulum continues through the diaphragm and joins the right atrium.

Ultrasound Appearance

Ductus venosus agenesis is shown in Figure 7.

Types of Ductus Venosus Agenesis[9]

- *Extrahepatic*: Here umbilical venous drainage bypasses the liver [the umbilical vein directly connects to the iliac

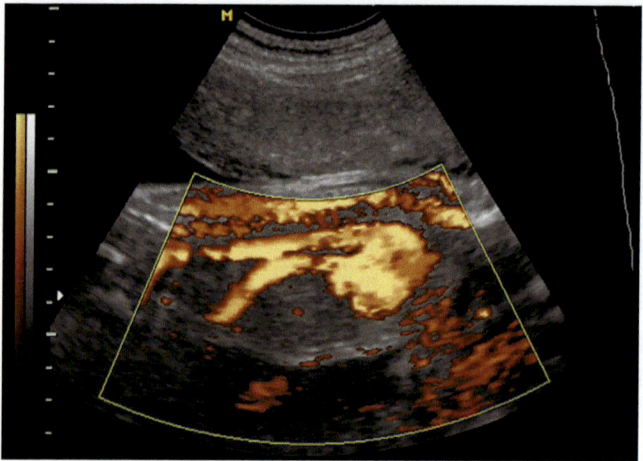

Fig. 7: The umbilical vein is directly connecting to the inferior vena cava instead of joining a subdiaphragmatic vestibulum. It is an extrahepatic type of ductus venosus agenesis. It is the second most common variety.

vein, the IVC (Fig. 7), the renal vein, the right atrium or, rarely, the left atrium or the coronary sinus].
- *Intrahepatic*: In intrahepatic type, umbilical venous drainage does not bypass the liver (the umbilical vein connects to the portal sinus in its usual way without giving rise to the ductus venosus).

Umbilical vein directly connecting to the right atrium is the most common variety followed by the one draining to the IVC. Intrahepatic variety is not very common.

Associations

- It is significantly associated with other anomalies, especially cardiac malformations, fetal hydrops, and agenesis of portal venous system. These associations are more common with extrahepatic type.[9]
- Chromosomal association is high (trisomy 21 and 18 and Turner syndrome).
- Nonchromosomal syndrome association is also high.

Prenatal Management and Counseling

- Fetal karyotyping is recommended because of high association with chromosomal abnormalities.
- Thorough anatomical scan and fetal echocardiography are to be performed to rule out associated anomalies. Portal venous system should be evaluated.
- Isolated absent ductus venosus (ADV) has good outcome.

Postnatal Treatment

In isolated cases, no treatment is required usually.

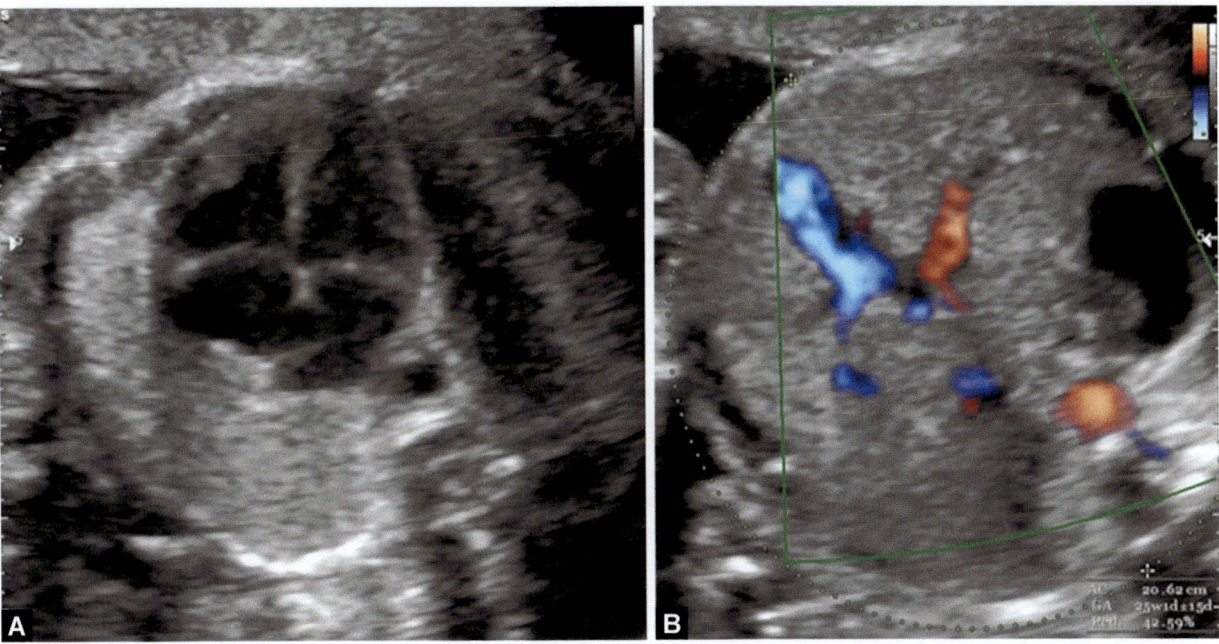

Figs. 8A and B: The situs is confirmed and the stomach is on left and heart is pointing toward left. But the umbilical vein instead of turning toward the right side is turning toward the stomach on the left side suggestive of persistent right umbilical vein.

PERSISTENT RIGHT UMBILICAL VEIN

Incidence

The incidence is from 1:526 to 1:1228.[10]

Ultrasound Appearance

The main feature is umbilical vein turning to left and toward the stomach. Gallbladder will be on the left of the umbilical vein (Figs. 8A and B). In some cases, it may not drain into portal vein and drains directly into IVC or fetal heart (extrahepatic).

Associations

In nearly 25% of cases, it is associated with other anomalies. GI malformations, heart anomalies, and urinary tract anomalies are seen associated with it. Chromosomal abnormalities are also seen associated.

Prenatal Management and Counseling

- Thorough anatomical scan needs to be performed.
- In isolated cases with connection to portal system, prognosis is very good and considered as a normal variant.

Postnatal Treatment

In isolated cases, no treatment is required.

ENTERIC DUPLICATION CYST

Enteric duplication cysts are rare, congenital anomalies found anywhere along the GI tract from the mouth to the rectum; they are most commonly found in the ileum.

Incidence

The incidence is 1:4,500 live births.[11]

Ultrasound Appearance

The typical ultrasound features of an EDC are:
- An inner hyperechoic epithelial lining containing the mucosa of the alimentary tract and the outer hypoechoic layer of smooth muscle closely attached to the GI tract by sharing a common wall. This is known as muscular rim sign or gut signature. However, the double-wall sign in other cystic lesions (mesenteric cyst and Meckel's diverticulum) may be seen.[11]
- Cyst wall also shows the peristalsis. It appears as a transient change of the shape and contour of the cyst because of a concentric contraction of the cyst wall when the transducer stays still on the cyst for a while.

Postnatal Treatment

Treatment of asymptomatic EDCs remains controversial. The clinical behavior of EDCs is unpredictable. EDCs tend to increase in size gradually and can cause symptoms and

Gastrointestinal Tract Anomalies

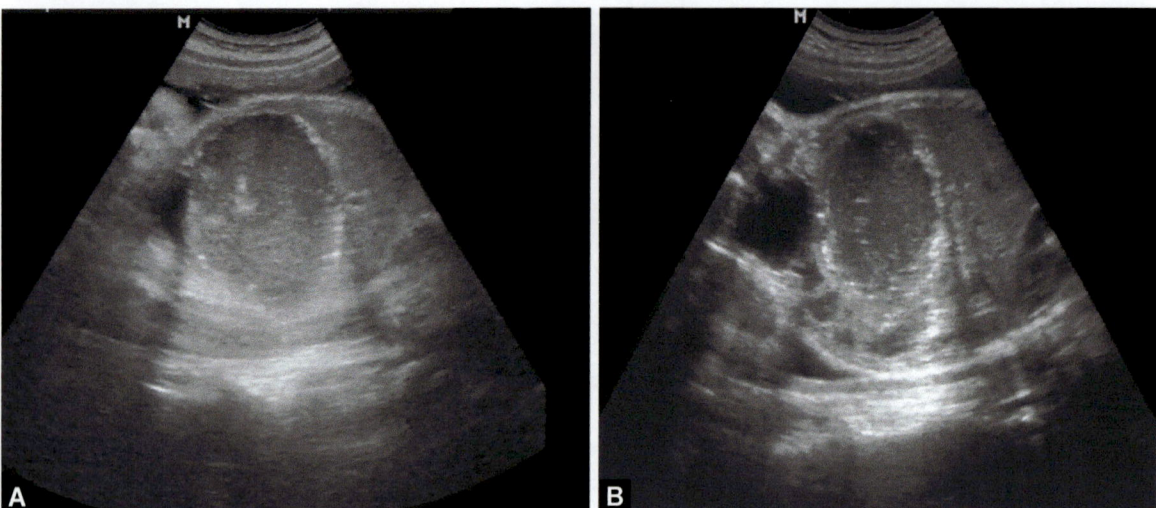

Figs. 9A and B: A cyst in the lower abdomen with irregular borders and increased echogenicity of wall suggestive of meconium pseudocyst.

complications that might be fatal, such as obstruction and massive bleeding. Also, early excision is associated with less morbidity and a shorter length of stay compared to excision in symptomatic patients.

Cyst excision alone could be considered, but if there is a communication, sometimes a resection of the adjacent bowel is necessary. It is important to ensure that the cyst is entirely resected because recurrence or malignant changes may occur.

MESENTERIC CYST

These are the cysts arising in the mesentery of the small bowel.

Ultrasound Appearance

These are seen as unilocular or multilocular hypoechogenic cysts with very thin walls. Peristalsis is not seen.

MECONIUM PSEUDOCYST

It results due to formation of fibrous wall around the leaked meconium, from perforation of bowel, during the prenatal period.

Ultrasound Appearance

- The pseudocyst has irregular echogenic borders with calcifications on its wall (Figs. 9A and B).
- Bowel dilatation is present.
- Polyamnios and ascites may also be seen.

Postnatal Treatment

Emergent surgery may need to be performed.

HEPATIC CYST

Hepatic cysts are very rare.

Ultrasound Appearance

Right upper quadrant cystic mass anterior to gallbladder, demonstrating no peristalsis or blood flow.[12]

SPLENIC CYST

It is very rare.

Ultrasound Appearance

It is commonly observed in the upper left quadrant of the fetal abdomen above the stomach, visualized from mid-trimester onward.

CHOLEDOCHAL CYST

It is the cystic dilatation of the bile duct. It is very rare.

Ultrasound Appearance

It appears as a simple anechoic cystic mass in upper right quadrant of abdomen near gallbladder, usually seen in the third trimester.

ECHOGENIC BOWEL

Hyperechogenicity has been defined by most authors as bowel of similar or greater echogenicity than the surrounding bone.

Ultrasound Diagnosis

This grading system of echogenic bowel (Table 4) is given by Slotnick et al.[13]

Table 4: Grading of echogenic bowel.[13]	
Grade 0	Normal
Grade 1	Increased echogenicity, but less echogenic than bone
Grade 2	Echogenicity equal to bone
Grade 3	Echogenicity greater than bone

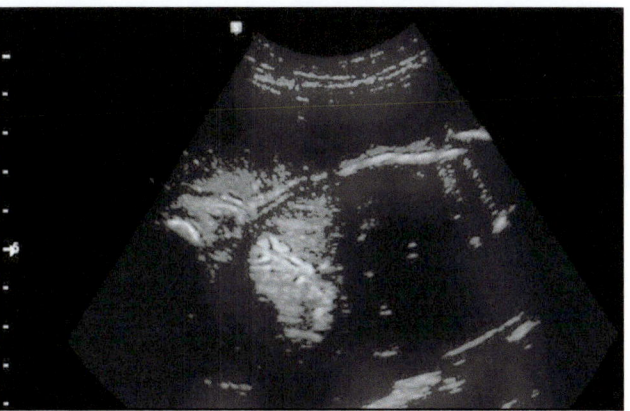

Fig. 10: Increased echogenicity of the bowel wall even after reducing the gain, the echogenicity is grade 2, i.e., echogenicity is equal to the bone suggestive of echogenic bowel.

Whenever echogenic bowel is suspected (Fig. 10), the gain setting should be lowered,[13] the frequency of probe should be reduced, and harmonics should be off, to enable the comparison with bone and to ensure that bowel hyperechogenicity is real. This should help to minimize a false-positive diagnosis of hyperechogenicity.

Associations

The causes of echogenic bowel are as follows:
- *Fetal aneuploidy* in 9%,[14] especially trisomy 21 and less frequently trisomy 18 or 13, Turner syndrome and triploidy. It is thought to be due to decreased bowel motility with increased water absorption from the meconium.
- *Oligohydramnios*: Echogenic bowel is also thought to be due to decreased amniotic fluid content of meconium.
- Hirschsprung's disease (increased frequency in fetuses with Down syndrome) could produce hyperechogenic bowel due to hypoperistalsis.
- *Bowel atresia*: Echogenic bowel is thought to be due to decreased amniotic fluid content of the meconium.
- *Intrauterine growth restriction*: The association of echogenic bowel with IUGR may be caused in part by ischemia from redistribution of blood flow.
- *Intra-amniotic hemorrhage*: Echogenic bowel is probably due to swallowed blood products resulting in a hypercellular meconium.
- *Cystic fibrosis*: Echogenic bowel has been reported to be found on ultrasound in 50–78% of fetuses affected with cystic fibrosis.[15,16] The association of echogenic bowel with fetuses affected with cystic fibrosis is thought to be caused by changes in the consistency of meconium in the small intestine as a result of abnormalities in pancreatic enzymes.
- *Other less common associations*: CMV, toxoplasmosis, and parvovirus. The association of congenital infections with echogenic bowel has been reported to be from 0% to 10%. The most commonly detected infectious agent is CMV.

Prenatal Management and Counseling

- Thorough history should be taken regarding any bleeding episode and any history of infections.
- Hyperechoic bowel should prompt a complete and careful fetal anatomical survey and look for features of intra-amniotic bleed such as particulate matter floating in amniotic fluid, chorioamniotic separation, and echogenic material in fetal stomach.
- It is reasonable to consider karyotyping even if no other ultrasound findings are detected.[14]
- Direct fetal DNA testing for cystic fibrosis should always be considered when prenatal karyotyping is performed to exclude aneuploidy. Conversely, if parents are willing to avoid invasive procedure, parental carrier status may be initially determined and amniocentesis is only offered to couples in which both are carriers of an identifiable mutation.[14]
- Maternal serological testing for infections should be considered.
- Serial sonographic assessment of fetal growth.
- Counseling and treatment will depend upon the etiology of echogenic bowel.

Postnatal Treatment

Treatment depends upon the etiology of the echogenic bowel.

REFERENCES

1. Sfeir R, Michaud L, Salleron J, et al. Epidemiology of esophageal atresia. Dis Esophagus. 2013;26(4):354-5.
2. Stringer MD, McKenna KM, Goldstein RB, et al. Prenatal diagnosis of esophageal atresia. J Pediatr Surg. 1995;30: 1258-63.
3. Chittmittrapap S, Spitz L, Kiely EM, et al. Oesophageal atresia and associated anomalies. Arch Dis Child. 1989;64:364-8.
4. Houben CH, Curry JI. Current status of prenatal diagnosis, operative management and outcome of esophageal atresia/trachea-esophageal fistula. Prenat Diagn. 2008;28:667-5.

5. Gossman W, Eovaldi BJ, Cohen HL. Duodenal Atresia and Stenosis. StatPearls Publishing LLC; 2003.
6. Choudhry MS, Rahman N, Boyd P, et al. Duodenal atresia: associated anomalies, prenatal diagnosis and outcome. Pediatr Surg Int. 2009;25(8):727-30.
7. Escobar MA, Ladd AP, Grosveld JL, et al. Duodenal atresia and stenosis: long-term follow-up over 30 years. J Pediatr Surg. 2004;39:867-71.
8. Palidini D, Volpe P. Ultrasound of Congenital Fetal Anomalies: Differential Diagnosis and Prognostic Indicators. Florida: CRC Press; 2014. p. 277.
9. Berg C, Kamil D, Geipel A, et al. Absence of ductus venosus-importance of umbilical venous drainage site. Ultrasound Obstet Gynecol. 2006;28:275-81.
10. Weichert J, Hartge D, Germer U, et al. Persistent right umbilical vein: a prenatal condition worth mentioning? Ultrasound Obstet Gynecol. 2011;37:543-8.
11. Nebot CS, Salvado RL, Palacios EC, et al. Enteric duplication cysts in children: varied presentations, varied imaging findings. Insights Imaging. 2018;9(6):1097-106.
12. Kumru P, Arisoy R, Erdogdu E, et al. The prenatal diagnosis and perinatal outcome of fetal intra-abdominal cysts. Zeynep Kamil Tip Bülteni. 2015;46(2):69-75.
13. Slotnick RN, Abuhamad AZ. Prognostic implications of fetal echogenic bowel. Lancet. 1996;347(8994):85-7.
14. Sepulveda W, Sebire NJ. Fetal echogenic bowel: a complex scenario. Ultrasound Obstet Gynecol. 2000;16:510-14.
15. Hill LM. Ultrasound of fetal gastrointestinal tract. In: Callen PW (Ed). Ultrasonography in Obstetrics and Gynecology. Philadelphia: WB Saunders; 2000. pp. 457-87.
16. Boue A, Muller F, Nezelof C, et al. Prenatal diagnosis in 200 pregnancies with a 1-in-4 risk of cystic fibrosis. Hum Genet. 1986;74(3):288-97.

19

Imaging in Labor

Girija Wagh, Rohan Wagh, Mahima Arya

INTRODUCTION

Intrapartum imaging has added value to increase the safety of the mother and the baby and can be a useful tool to ensure better outcomes. Till the recent past, only handheld Dopplers were the progress as far as imaging is concerned and much of the labor would be conducted based on antepartum imaging in form of ultrasound. In today's era, bedside ultrasound, especially in acute settings with added color Doppler assessments, has become important, especially in placental abnormalities and compromised fetuses. Additionally, some workers have also used dynamic sonography to assess progress of labor. MRI can also be used in some special situations such as placenta accreta or other variants of morbidly adherent placenta (MAP).

In this write up, we will deal with the various aspects of intrapartum imaging with a case scenario at the end.

Aspects of imaging as mentioned below:
- Imaging in acute setting such as MAP or placental abruption
- To assess the fetal well-being
- To assess the progress of labor
- Additional assessment, if any

IMAGING IN MORBIDLY ADHERENT PLACENTA AND PLACENTAL ABRUPTION

Ultrasonography is not sensitive for detection of placental abruption, but is high specific as positive findings are associated with increased maternal morbidity and worse perinatal outcome.

Ultrasonography criteria for diagnosis of placental abruption include:
- Preplacental collection under chorionic plate
- "Jello"-like movement of chorionic plate with fetal activity
- Retroplacental collection
- Marginal hematoma
- Subchorionic hematoma
- Increased placental thickness of more than 5 cm

Placental abruption can occur intrapartum in patients of severe pre-eclampsia, commonly pregnancies with fetal growth restriction, premature rupture of membranes (PROM), prolonged PROM, in twin pregnancies, and sometimes with no obvious antecedent cause. During labor, presence of uterine contractions may obliterate the classic triad of pain, uterine tenderness, and vaginal bleeding which help in diagnosing abruption. High index of suspicion, clinical vigilance, decelerations, and sinusoidal pattern of tracing on electronic fetal monitoring (EFM) may help suspect abruption. Sonography and color Doppler can help to confirm the diagnosis, assess the fetal condition thus help in delivery decision-making. However, ultrasound may miss the diagnosis in about 40–50% of patients.

The trial of labor can be considered in pregnancies with placenta previa when placental lower edge is 2 cm away from the internal os. This must, however, be taken with caution in a posterior low-lying placenta. Premature deliveries and possibility of postpartum hemorrhage should be borne in mind. Additionally, it has to be remembered that MAP can be associated with a low-lying placenta. Ultrasonography is a valuable tool in assessing the placental position, the distance from the internal os of the bleeding edge of the placenta, placental bed separation to some extent, and MAP. Ultrasonography also helps in planning the incision in eventuality of cesarean delivery.

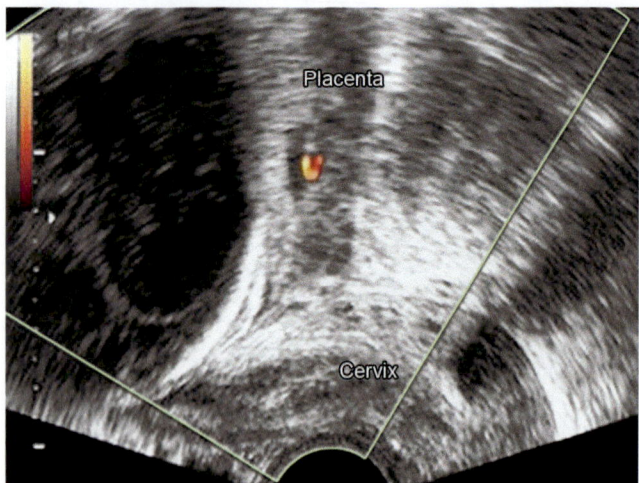

Fig. 1: Transvaginal ultrasound of placenta previa minor posterior showing the lower margin of the placenta reaching the margin of the cervix with no encroaching on the internal os, no lacunae, or hypervascularity.

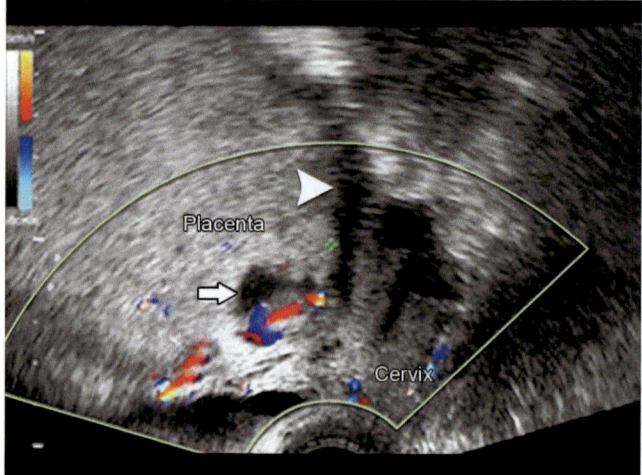

Fig. 2: Transvaginal Doppler ultrasound of placenta previa minor showing the lower margin of the placenta reaching the margin of the cervix with no encroaching on the internal os, and there is placental lacunae (arrow) with preserved clear retroplacental zone (arrowhead).

On transvaginal sonography (TVS), the low-lying placenta is diagnosed as under:
- Complete placenta previa, when internal cervical os is covered by placental tissue.
- Central placenta previa, when internal os is not visualized by TVS (Figs. 1 and 2).
- Low-lying placenta, when the lower edge is within 3 cm from the internal cervical os

Presence of placental lacunae and lack of clear zone in the placental bed raises the suspicion of MAP. There are certain ultrasonographic criteria which help in assessing severe intrapartum hemorrhage.[1,2]
- Placental lacunae of equal to larger than 1 × 1 cm to the placental parenchyma
- Lack of clear zone between the myometrium and placenta
- Placenta located on a previous cesarean scar
- Os covered by placenta, more than 2 cm
- Retroplacental hypervascularity on color Doppler (Figs. 3 and 4)

ASSESSMENT OF FETAL WELL-BEING

Intrapartum monitoring has always been done based on clinical assessment and aided by electronic monitoring, partographs, and rarely use of ultrasonography to assess associated morbidities. Today ultrasound, especially the three-dimensional (3D), is used to assess dystocia. The ergonomics of the intrapelvic passage of the fetus is assessed by use of ultrasonography by assessing various dimensions and quantifying the progress. This is fascinating new facet of intrapartum imaging still in its inception and not completely accessible for obvious reasons.

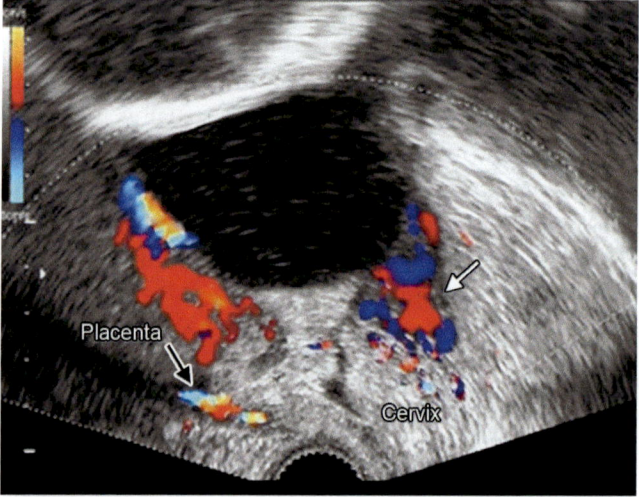

Fig. 3: Transvaginal Doppler ultrasound of placenta previa with focal accreta showing the placenta covering the internal os of the cervix, with placental lacuna, loss of subplacental sonolucent line, retroplacental hypervascularity (black arrow), and increased cervical vasculature (white arrow).

Indications of Ultrasound

- Slow progress and arrest of labor in the second stage
- To confirm the fetal head and position before instrumental vaginal delivery
- Assessment of fetal head and malpresentation

Doppler ultrasound examination during labor is usually undertaken in high-risk mothers and compromised babies to help understand the pathophysiology of the fetoplacental unit and fetal adaptive mechanisms. It helps in identifying acute fetal asphyxia and consequent effects on fetal dynamics. Intrapartum Doppler is technically difficult due to:
- Lack of easy accessibility
- The dynamic nature of intrapartum situation.

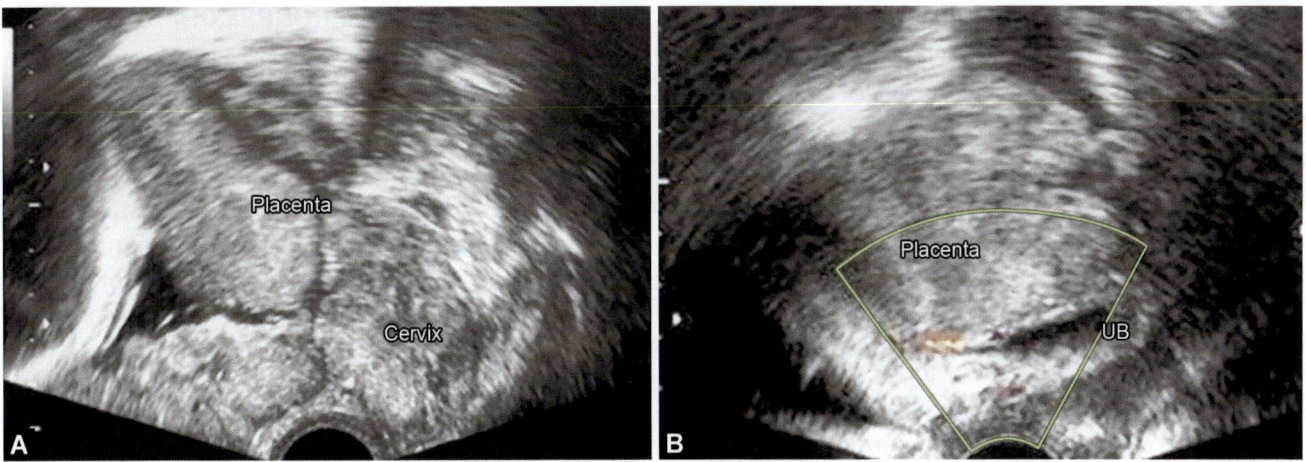

Figs. 4A and B: (A) Transvaginal ultrasound of placenta previa grayscale; and (B) Doppler shows the placenta covering the internal os of the cervix with loss of subplacental sonolucent line and mild retroplacental hypervascularity.

The following are the reasons which may confound intrapartum color Doppler assessment:
- Changing maternal circulating parameters due to contractions and change in the position of the transducer and the fetus.
- Excessive maternal respiratory movements during contractions preventing continuous recording of Doppler signal.
- Reduced amniotic fluid volume, especially after rupture of membranes preventing assessment of fetal vessels.
- Deeply engaged fetal head prevents assessment of fetal cerebral vessels.

The sites which are explored by intrapartum ultrasonographic Doppler are uterine arteries, umbilical vessels, and fetal circulation.

During the uterine contraction, there is a mean reduction of 40–60% in blood flow velocity in response of maximum reduction of intrauterine pressure of approximately 60 mm Hg. It is observed that the systolic peak decreases by only 20% while the diastolic peak is low or absent. Thus, there is significant reduction in the perfusion pressure in the uterine artery blood flow at the maximum peak of the uterine contraction. During the diastole, the intrauterine pressure exceeds maternal diastolic pressure and the uterine artery perfusion blood pressure disappears. A progressive reduction is observed when correlated with increase in intrauterine pressure from 10 mm Hg to 60 mm Hg. Thus, it has been found that when intrauterine pressure reaches 80 mm Hg, there is no diastolic flow while systolic blood flow continues even at intrauterine pressure of 130 mm Hg. The uterine diastolic flow reflects blood flow in the arcuate and the spiral arterioles.

In special conditions such as premature delivery and pre-eclampsia, these assessments would be relevant. It has been observed in premature delivery, even in the absence of painful uterine contractions, there can be suppression or reversal of the diastolic flow. This finding, therefore, supports the use of tocolysis. Systolic blood pressure of 130 mm Hg is enough as minimum blood flow in the intervillous space. In pre-eclampsia, due to incomplete trophoblastic invasion of uterine spiral arterioles, there is chronic deficiency in uteroplacental vascularization. The unchanged flow velocimetry of hypertension maintains the blood flow in intervillous space during uterine contractions and this must be remembered when using antihypertensive medications. In presence of prelabor with abnormal uterine Dopplers, the fetal prognosis is reserved. Umbilical artery is the last vessel before placental obstacle as placenta is the only organ at the other end of the umbilical artery. Before the rupture of membranes, the umbilical artery perfusion remains the same as it was in prelabor. This may continue further because if the fetal head covers the cervical orifice, it maintains the intrauterine pressure. It is proposed that fetal heart rate (FHR) of 140–160 bpm is a sign that umbilical Dopplers are normal and has been found that the umbilical artery resistance index (RI) values during labor are remarkably stable. Despite the active phenomenon such as delivery, umbilical circulation maintains its independence. There are no significant changes observed in the umbilical RI in the context of all four stages of uterine contraction. This can be deciphered by EFM as well, as there is a progressive umbilical diastolic flow diminution during intrapartum deceleration and fetal bradycardia. The diastolic flow completely disappears when the FHR is 80 bpm. It has been found that there is a prolonged significant diastole in response to fetal bradycardia of 100 bpm depicting a compensatory mechanism. The intrapartum variations in the umbilical artery diastolic flow in a situation of changed FHR are more of cardiogenic in origin than due to increased placental resistance. So, it is observed that despite increase in uterine contraction pressure from 10 mm Hg to 60 mm Hg, the umbilical artery flows remain stable. The systolic peak of the umbilical artery represents the cardiac ejection volume and the residual diastolic flow represents the placental resistance.

Thus, it has been found that intrapartum Doppler ultrasound is valuable when there is occurrence of FHR decelerations which are indicative of decreased oxygen supply and associated with reversed diastolic flow. This helps in assessing risk of fetal acidosis. This observation also impresses that spontaneous or oxytocin-induced labor should be avoided in cases of intrapartum null diastolic flow in uterine arteries because uterine contractions may cause a dangerous decrease in the oxygen perfusion in the intervillous spaces and decelerations will be present which are indicative of reduced umbilical blood flow. Fetuses with late decelerations are known to have hypoxemia and Doppler velocimetry reveals high standard deviation (SD) index both during and in between uterine contractions. About 90% of the times, umbilical vein pulsations are seen in fetuses with late decelerations which are indicative of momentary overloading of the right heart.

There is a progressive increase in aortic blood flow until 36 weeks of gestation with a slight reduction starting from 39 weeks. There are no changes in the aortic Doppler vein when the FHR is normal; however, decrease in the aortic flow has been seen in the presence of fetal decelerations. Redistribution of fetal heart blood flow favoring the cerebral blood vessels does not alter the aortic spectrum of perfusion. Major vasoconstriction of the aorta is associated with increased risk of hemorrhagic enterocolitis in the fetus. Increased vascular resistance in the aorta leads to dilatation of the arteriolar duct leading to pulmonary hypertension, right heart decompensation, and decreased cardiac blood flow.

Very few studies have evaluated intrapartum cerebral perfusion. If FHR remains normal during the uterine contraction, the perfusion in the middle cerebral artery (MCA) remains unchanged. Fetal head pressure can cause absent or reversed diastolic flow, especially during the second stage of labor and iatrogenically due to the ultrasound probe pressure, especially in presence of oligohydramnios. Repeated decelerations are known to trigger compensatory cerebrodilatation till these adaptive phenomena are overcome. Once the reserve is overcome, the reduction in FHR results in decrease of vascular cerebral blood flow. Intrapartum color Doppler evaluation can help in delivery decisions and assessment of compromised fetuses, especially in high-risk situations.

ASSESSMENT OF THE PROGRESS OF LABOR

Ultrasound in active labor is not widely used at the present time and much of labor progress is assessed by clinical assessment. It has been proposed that ultrasound allows objective measurement and precise documentation which can aid the clinical assessment. Many studies have revealed that the transvaginal digital assessment has been shown to have a mean category error of 30% for resident doctors and 34% for obstetricians when assessed on labor simulators. Additionally, majority of errors were observed in assessment of midpelvic station. Dynamic and accurate documentation of various parameters of labor can be achieved by:

- Assessing the head station (relationship between the presenting part with the ischial spine).
- By measuring the midline angle (MLA) which would help to identify the rotation of the presenting part.
- By assessing the head direction, especially when planning an operative vaginal delivery.

There are two approaches in which ultrasound in labor can be performed:
1. Transabdominal approach to determine head and spine
2. Transperineal approach for assessment of head station and position at low stations.

Also, quantitative sonographic parameters have been proposed to assess head parameters. The important parameters that are assessed as follows:

- Position of fetal occiput (Figs. 5 and 6)
- Fetal head descent
- Fetal head attitude
- Station

A series of sonographic parameters have been proposed to describe the fetal head position and these have been documented to have inter- and intraobserver variation.[3] This is done by transabdominal imaging in axial and sagittal planes by placing the ultrasound probe on the maternal abdomen. After determining the position of fetal spine, the probe is moved toward the maternal suprapubic region to visualize the fetal head. The landmarks which identify fetal occiput position are depicted in Table 1.

At low fetal head stations, transperineal ultrasound approach may be combined to determine precise position. Apart from the classical positions and diameters which are clinically measured in sonographic approach, additional quantitative measurements have been proposed such as the angle of progression (AOP) or descent, the progression distance (PD), the head–symphysis distance (HSD), and the MLA. These are best identified by 3D reconstruction of the sonographic data and 3D ultrasound is needed to assess them with precision. Parameters such as MLA,

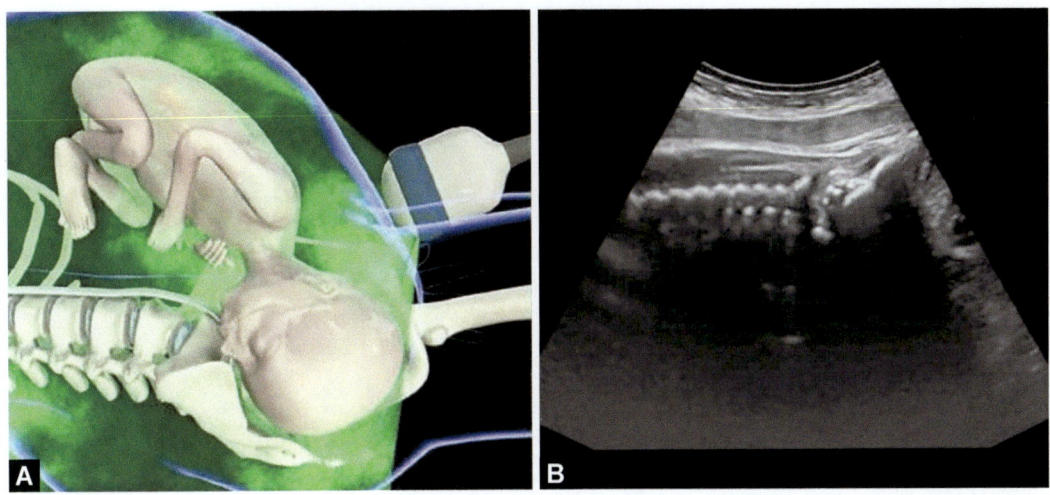

Figs. 5A and B: Transabdominal ultrasound imaging (sagittal plane) in fetus with occiput anterior position.

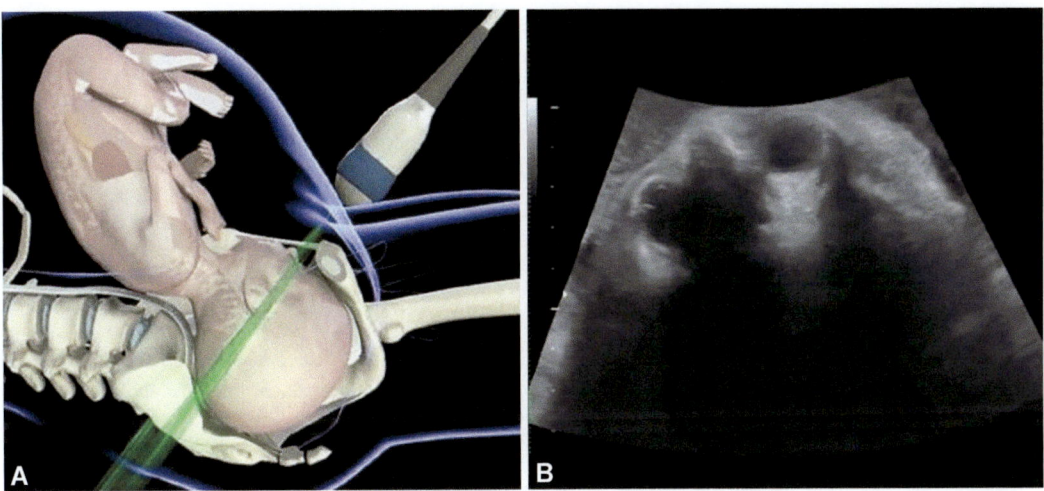

Figs. 6A and B: Transabdominal ultrasound imaging (transverse plane) in fetus with occiput posterior position.

head–perineum distance (HPD), the AOP, the HSD, and PD help in assessing the fetal distance.
- *Midline angle*: MLA is the angle between the anteroposterior axis of the maternal axis and the line (echogenic) interposed between the two cerebral hemispheres. This angle helps in determining the station as well as the rotation.
- *Head-perineum distance*: HPD is the shortest distance of outer bony limit of the fetal skull to the perineum and represents the birth canal yet to be traversed by fetus (Figs. 7A to C). It is measured by placing the probe between the labia majora in the posterior fourchette angled till the skull contour is clear.
- *Angle of progression*: AOP is the accurate and reproducible measurement for assessment of fetal head descent (Figs. 8A to C). It is the angle between the long axis of the pubic bone and the tangential line from the lowest edge of the pubis extended to the deepest bony part of the fetal skull. It is found that at station 0 (when the occiput at the ischial spines), it corresponds to AOP of 116°.
- *Head-symphysis distance*: HSD is recently proposed to aid fetal head station and progression (Figs. 9A and B). It is the distance between the lower edge of maternal symphysis pubis and fetal skull along

Table 1: Ultrasound landmarks to identify fetal occiput position.

Positions	Landmarks
Anterior	Cervical spine
Posterior	Two fetal orbits
Transverse	Midline cerebral echo

Note: The choroid plexus is used to determine fetal head position as it diverges toward the occiput.

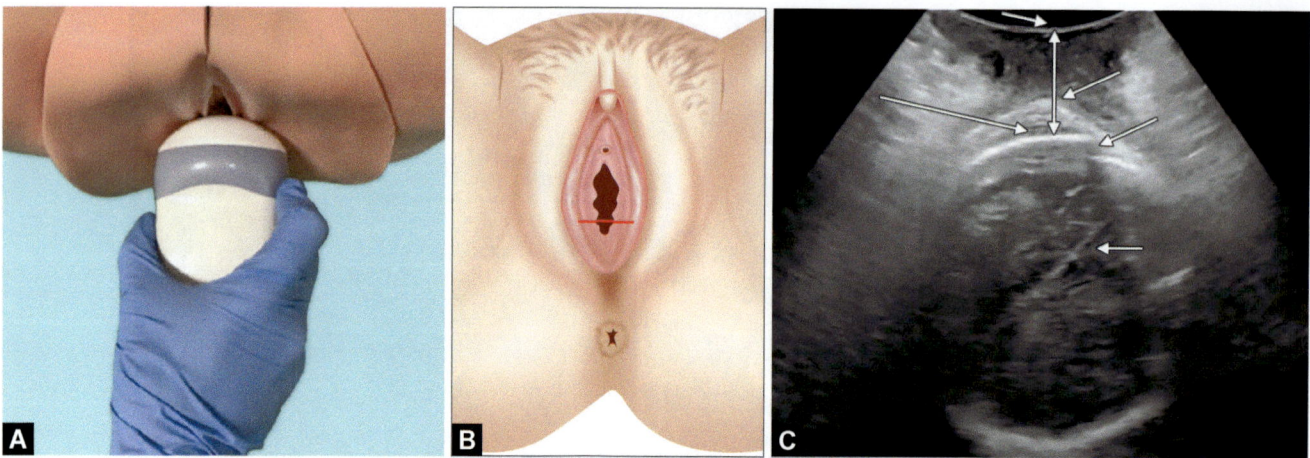

Figs. 7A to C: Measurement of head–perineum distance (HPD), showing placement of transducer and how distance is measured (red line and white arrows).
Courtesy: S Benediktsdóttir, I Frøysa, and JK Iversen.

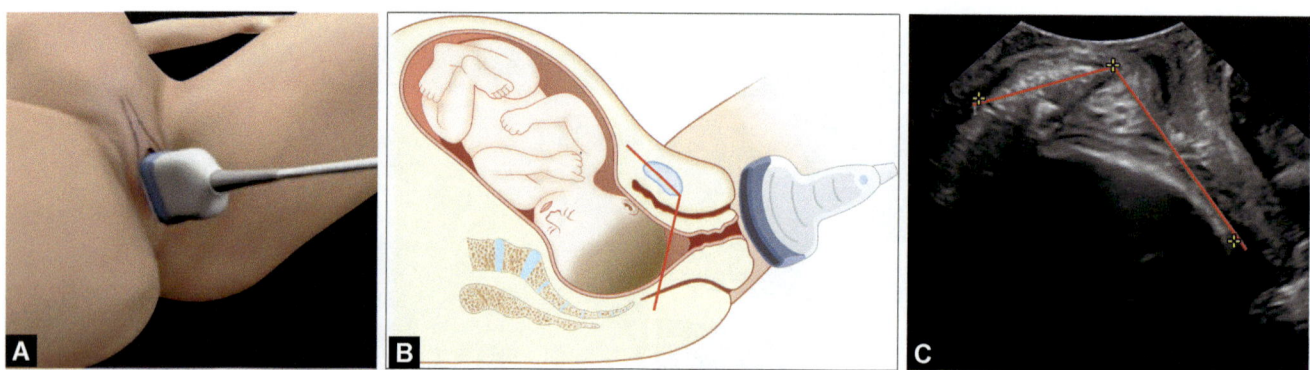

Figs. 8A to C: Measurement of angle of progression, showing placement of transducer and how angle is measured.
Courtesy: A Youssef, EA Torkildsen, and TM Eggebø.

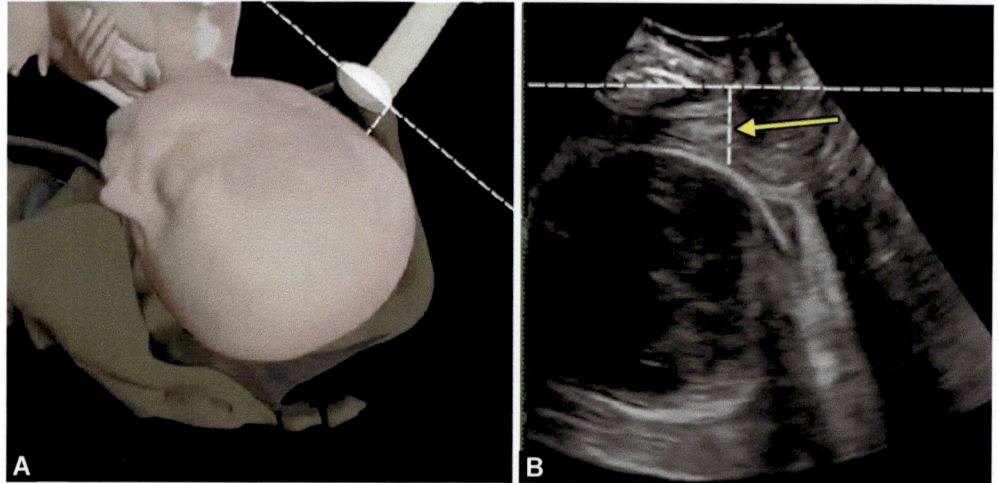

Figs. 9A and B: Measurement of head–symphysis distance (HSD) showing placement of transducer and how distance is measured (yellow arrow).
Source: Reproduced from Youssef A, Maroni E, Ragusa A, et al. Fetal head-symphysis distance: a simple and reliable ultrasound index of fetal head station in labor. Ultrasound Obstet Gynecol. 2013;41(4):419-24.

the infrapubic line. It is the indirect marker of fetal head descent and can be measured only at the lower stations.

- *Progression distance*: It is an objective parameter of fetal head engagement assessed before the onset of labor (Figs. 10A and B). It is defined as the minimum distance from

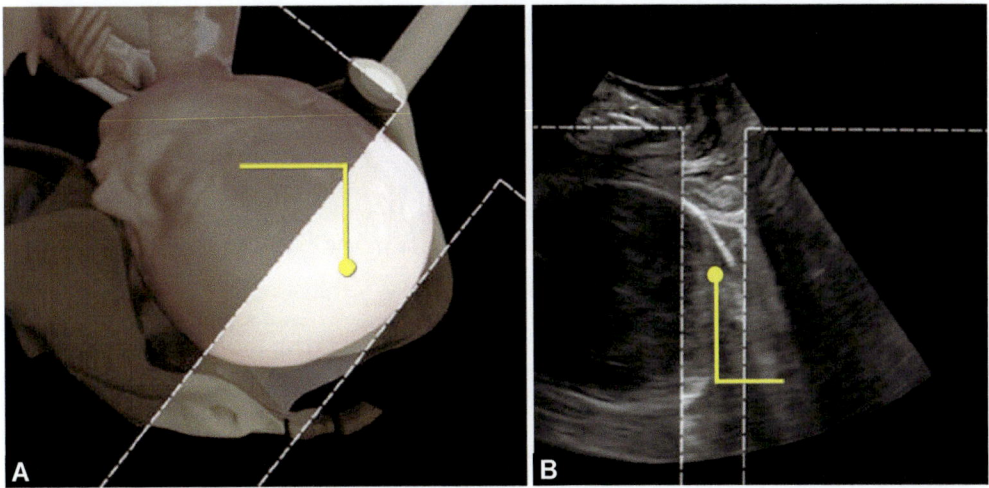

Figs. 10A and B: Measurement of progression distance. The yellow lines depict the progression distance.
Source: Reproduced from Youssef A, Maroni E, Ragusa A, et al. Fetal head-symphysis distance: a simple and reliable ultrasound index of fetal head station in labor. Ultrasound Obstet Gynecol. 2013;41(4):419-24.

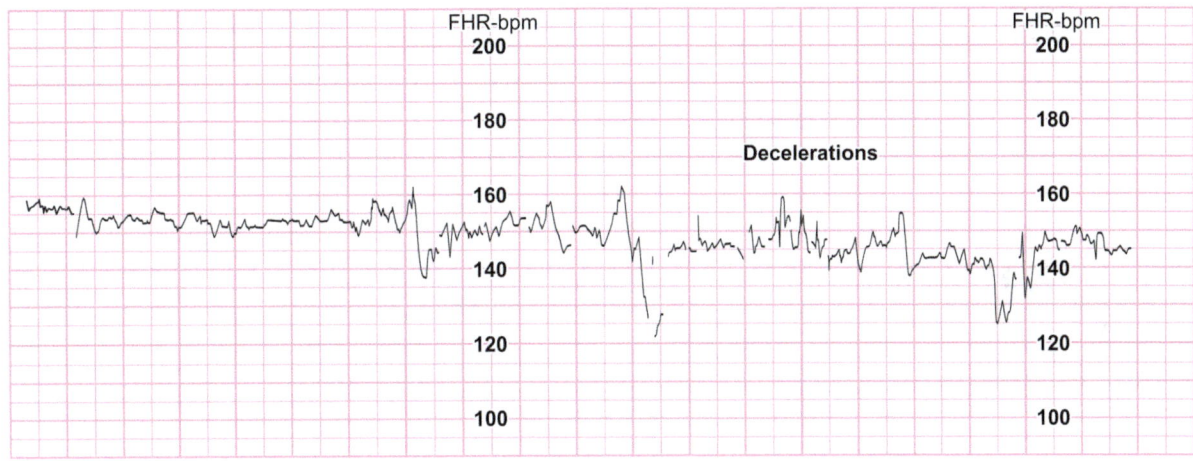

Fig. 11: Admission test was performed on electronic fetal monitoring (EFM).

the infrapubic line and the presenting part. The presenting part here is defined as the most distal part of the fetal skull.

At present times, there is no consensus regarding the indications, timings, and the parameters to be obtained when using intrapartum ultrasound.

CASE SCENARIO

Mrs S, 21-year-old, 38 weeks primigravida, married since 1 year came to hospital for routine antenatal care (ANC) visit. She gave history of decreased fetal movements from 2 to 3 days. Admission test was performed on EFM as depicted in Figure 11.

Patient was advised left lateral position, intranasal oxygen, and hydration. Repeat nonstress test (NST) as described in Figure 12.

Thus, patient was admitted for NST monitoring. Ultrasonography was performed suggestive of single live intrauterine pregnancy of 37 weeks 4 days ± 2 weeks. Amniotic fluid index (AFI) reduced to 5–6 cm. Placenta—fundoposterior and estimated fetal weight of 2,977 g. Biophysical profile score was 6/10 with fetal breathing of 2/2, gross body movements of 0/2, fetal tone of 2/2, AFI of 0/2, and uterine artery Doppler within normal limits having score of 2/2. Patient was monitored 2 hourly. Fetal heart sound (FHS) and NST were repeated after 6 hours. In view of decelerations as depicted underneath, patient was taken up for cesarean section (Fig. 13).

Cesarean section was done uneventfully. Baby boy of 2.9 kg was delivered with Apgar score of 8 and 9. Thin meconium-stained liquor was noted intraoperatively. Thus, a combination of EFM and ultrasound imaging aided in offering the appropriate approach in this case. Induction

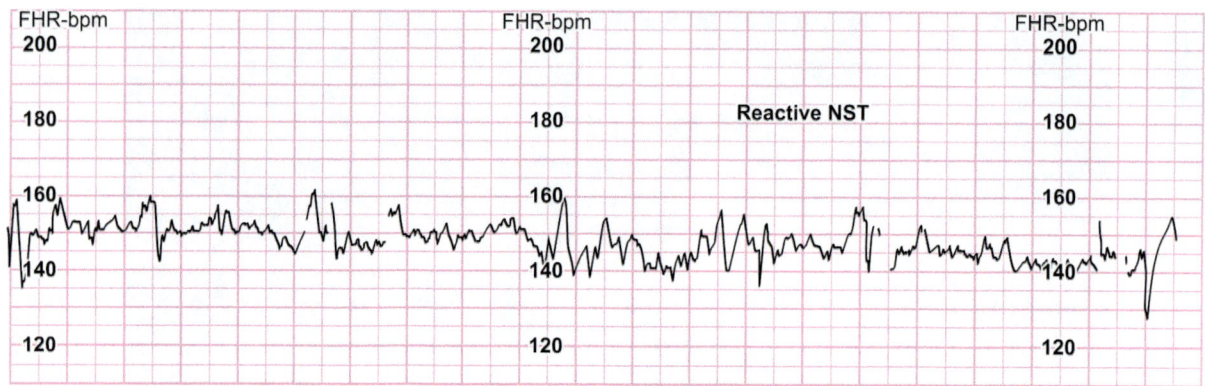

Fig. 12: Reactive nonstress test (NST).

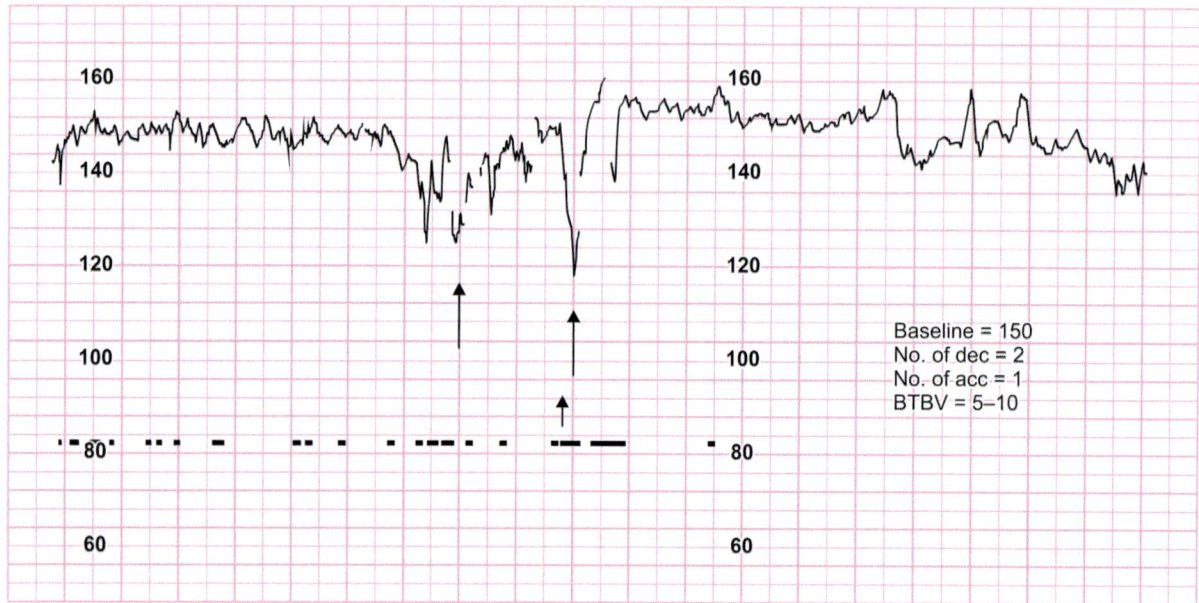

Fig. 13: NST showing decelerations.

of labor may have resulted in birth of an asphyxiated baby.

Imaging during third stage of labor may be essential in retained placenta. With the rising incidence of MAP, retained placenta always may not be an entrapped placenta. Manual removal of placenta is always better undertaken under imaging guidance. This will definitely help in assessing a previously missed MAP or identifying other causes of retained placenta.

CONCLUSION

Imaging during labor adds values to clinical judgment to help delivery and is the new evolution in intrapartum imaging.

REFERENCES

1. Hasegawa J, Matsuoka R, Ichizuka K, et al. Predisposing factors for massive hemorrhage during cesarean section in patients with placenta previa. Ultrasound Obstet Gynecol. 2009;34(1):80-4.
2. Ebrahim MA, Zaiton F, Elkamash TH. Clinical and ultrasound assessment in patients with placenta previa to predict the severity of intrapartum hemorrhage. Egyptian J Radiol Nuclear Med. 2013;44(3):657-63.
3. Youssef A, Maroni E, Ragusa A, et al. Fetal head-symphysis distance: a simple and reliable ultrasound index of fetal head station in labor. Ultrasound Obstet Gynecol. 2013;41(4):419-24.

Role of MRI in Pregnancy

Neeta Singh, Mandakini Pradhan

INTRODUCTION

An obstetrician in today's world has multiple options of imaging the mother and the fetus. Though ultrasonography (USG) is the most commonly used imaging modality, since last two decades magnetic resonance imaging (MRI) has emerged as an alternative modality to evaluate mother and fetus in specific circumstances. USG has the limitation of interobserver variability and poor visibility in cases of maternal obesity and oligohydramnios. Gravid uterus may obstruct visibility of maternal intra-abdominal structures and hence MRI may be useful in certain set of clinical conditions when required for maternal indications, even though USG may be a better modality in nonpregnant condition.

INDICATIONS OF MRI

Indications of MRI during pregnancy may be nonobstetric, gynecological, and obstetric which are as follows:
- *Nonobstetric causes*:
  - *Acute abdominal pain*: Most common nonobstetric cause of acute abdomen during pregnancy is appendicitis. During pregnancy, appendix is pushed superiorly and visualization of this structure may be difficult due to gravid uterus leading to delay in diagnosis by USG and increased morbidity and mortality of mother and fetus. Some authors suggest MRI to be the test of choice for this condition during pregnancy due to its high sensitivity and specificity.
    Various bowel conditions such as inflammation, obstruction, and diverticulitis can be diagnosed easily with MRI. Hepatobiliary conditions such as cholelithiasis, pancreatitis, pancreatic pseudocyst, and splenic vein thrombosis can be diagnosed with higher sensitivity. If urolithiasis is clinically suspected but USG fails to demonstrate a uretic stone due to gravid uterus, MRI may be resorted.
  - *Thrombosis*: Thrombosis in hepatic, mesenteric, gonadal, and pelvic veins can be diagnosed during pregnancy using MRI.
  - *Intracranial lesions*: In cases of evaluation of pre-existing intracranial lesions or in clinical setting of stroke, new-onset severe headache and clinical suspicion of tumors MRI may be preferred over ionizing radiations of CT scan.
  - *Tumors*: For evaluation of newly diagnosed tumors or staging of pre-existing tumors, MRI may be required during pregnancy as in nonpregnant state.
- *Gynecological causes*: Various gynecological causes such as ovarian cyst, ovarian torsion, uterine leiomyomas, and congenital abnormalities of genital tract may necessitate doing an MRI during pregnancy. If a primary pelvic mass is suspected to be malignant, to ascertain the exact nature of the mass, to look for solid/cystic components, invasion, ascites, peritoneal implants, and lymphadenopathy, MRI may be necessary.
- *Obstetric causes*:
  - *Ectopic pregnancy*: Ectopic pregnancy at extrauterine sites, especially in unusual implantation sites, may necessitate doing MRI to confirm the diagnosis and plan further line of management. Cesarean scar pregnancy and pregnancy in rudimentary horn of uterus in advanced condition may mimic a normal intrauterine pregnancy. MRI due to its large field of view and orthogonal imaging can help in diagnosing ectopic pregnancy in advanced 1st trimester or in 2nd trimester where USG is less useful.
  - *Morbidly adherent placenta*: Diagnostic sensitivity of USG has been reported to be 91% with a specificity of

97%.[1] Features that are used include placenta previa, placental lacunae, abnormal color Doppler imaging patterns, loss of retroplacental clear space, reduced myometrial thickness, and irregular bladder wall. MRI is found to be equally sensitive in diagnosis of morbidly adherent placenta. There is placenta percreta index to help in diagnosing the condition.[2]

Typical MRI findings in morbidly adherent placenta include uterine bulging, thick irregular intraplacental bands, and heterogeneous parenchymal signal intensity. These findings are increased with severity of placental invasion. In placenta percreta, there is full-thickness gap of myometrial signal along with loss of fat planes between adjacent pelvic organs and placenta.

MRI is indicated when USG diagnosis is equivocal or in patients with high clinical risk factor for placenta accreta. MRI is also done to plan cesarean section delivery and peripartum hysterectomy in otherwise diagnosed case of morbidly adherent placenta.

- *Degenerating leiomyoma*: Leiomyoma may increase in size during pregnancy. They can degenerate if they outgrow their blood supply. It is seen more commonly when they are submucosal or retroplacental in location. Though USG is the primary modality of diagnosis, MRI can aid in diagnosis of location, size, and degree of degeneration. On MRI, increased T2 signal is seen in internal necrosis and increased signal in T1-weighted image is suggestive of internal hemorrhage.
- *Placental abruption*: Placental abruption in initial stages may be missed by USG. If clinically suspected, MRI can diagnose the condition with 100% sensitivity and specificity and also the extent of placental detachment. Hyperintense blood products or hematoma between the myometrium and chorionic membrane can be seen on T1-weighted imaging.[3]
- *Uterine rupture*: MRI can help in diagnosing silent uterine rupture by documenting full-thickness tear in myometrium and serosa and presence of hemoperitoneum.

SAFETY OF MRI IN PREGNANCY

Safety concern for mother remains the same as that in the nonpregnant stage during MRI. Concerns were raised for fetus because of rapidly switching gradient fields of noise during the investigation and the heating effect of the electromagnetic field. Increasing evidence is accumulating that MRI is not associated with fetal teratogenicity. Large retrospective study of 1,737 children exposed to MRI in intrauterine life failed to demonstrate an increased risk of stillbirth, neonatal death, congenital anomaly, neoplasm, vision loss, or hearing loss.[4] MRI also does not lead to difference in fetal heart rate pattern during the study. However, safety of MRI during 1st trimester is not yet established and it is a good practice to avoid doing the investigation during this gestation unless the benefits outweigh the risk. Contrast agent used in MRI is gadolinium based and it has been shown to be associated with increased risk of fetal teratogenicity. Hence, a contrast agent should never be used during MRI in pregnancy unless mandatory.

ADVANTAGES

Advantages of MRI over USG include being nonoperator dependent, nonionizing in nature, having better soft-tissue differentiation, and acquiring images in multiple orthogonal planes, but it has its own limitations. In second half of pregnancy, mothers may find it uncomfortable to lie in supine position for MRI due to pain or risk of supine hypotension and may be claustrophobic. Fetal movement in amniotic fluid hampers with image acquisition in MRI and prior to 18 weeks, it is less advantageous due to small size of fetus.

CONCLUSION

While USG remains the modality of choice for imaging the mother and fetus, sometimes MRI may be necessary to confirm the diagnosis or to supplement the USG findings.

REFERENCES

1. D'Antonio F, Lacovella C, Bhide A. Prenatal identification of invasive placentation using ultrasound: systematic review and meta-analysis. Ultrasound Obstet Gynecol. 2013;42: 509-17.
2. Rac MW, Dashe JS, Wells CE, et al. Ultrasound predictors of placental invasion: the Placenta Accreta Index. Am J Obstet Gynecol. 2015;212:343.e1-7.
3. Masselli G, Derchi L, McHugo J, et al. Acute abdominal and pelvic pain in pregnancy: ESUR recommendations. Eur Radiol. 2013;23:3485-500.
4. Ray JG, Vermeulen MJ, Bharatha A, et al. Association between MRI exposure during pregnancy and fetal and childhood outcomes. JAMA. 2016;316:952-61.

21
Genetic Markers in Aneuploidies
Ashok Khurana

INTRODUCTION

The genetic sonogram is an ultrasound examination done on second trimester fetuses that not only evaluates the fetus for structural malformations, but also searches for the sonographic markers of fetal Down syndrome.[1] Most workers have extended the definition to the second trimester fetal anatomic survey targeted at identifying features associated with any aneuploidy.[2-5] It has evolved as an adjunctive screening tool capable of further refining the individualized risk-calculation for trisomy that is based on maternal age or serum screening markers.[6]

The common aneuploidies include trisomy 21 (Down syndrome), trisomy 13 (Patau syndrome) and trisomy 18 (Edwards syndrome), Turner syndrome (XO) and triploidy. Other trisomies are rarer and are encountered most frequently in abortus karyotypes. Trisomy 21 is associated with potential long-term morbidity and has an estimated prevalence of 1.21 per 1,000 live births.[7] Trisomies 13 and 18 usually abort spontaneously or result in intrauterine demise, and, if born alive, rarely survive beyond the neonatal period. The greatest emphasis in the genetic sonogram, therefore, is to screen the population and then follow-up with an appropriate definitive diagnostic procedure for Down syndrome.

Screening procedures refer to tests that define an at-risk population and diagnostic tests refer to an actual demonstration of fetal karyotype. Screening tests for aneuploidies include maternal age, serum markers and ultrasound markers. The chromosomes themselves can be demonstrated by a microarray or conventional karyotyping of cells from amniotic fluid, chorionic villi or fetal cord blood or by identifying an abnormal karyotype by fluorescent in situ hybridization (FISH) or quantitative fluorescent polymerase chain reaction (QF-PCR) studies.

Although, the incidence of Down syndrome increases with increasing maternal age, particularly beyond 35 years, 70–80% of Down syndrome babies are born to women younger than 35 years.[1] The prevalence of trisomy 21 decreases with increasing gestational age and is about 30% higher at 16–20 weeks' gestation compared with term[8] and about 48–50% higher at 9–14 weeks compared with term.[9]

Soon after the finding of an association between low maternal serum alpha-fetoprotein (MSAFP) and Down syndrome, it was discovered that the addition of an assessment of maternal serum unconjugated estriol (E3) and beta-human chorionic gonadotropin (βhCG) in the form of the "triple test" was an effective screening test in women less than 35 years of age with a sensitivity of 57% and a false positive rate of 3.25%.[10]

In recent years, improved resolution of ultrasound and its consequent ability to demonstrate abnormal morphology, have placed the sonographic examination in a more sensitive and specific position than maternal age and maternal serum screening. This is very significant in the perspective of the observation that amniocentesis for prenatal detection of chromosomal aneuploidy, a diagnostic tool offered at one time arbitrarily to all pregnant women aged 35 years or over, has in recent years lost favor as a first-line investigation.[6] This shift in practice stems from a recognition that selection of candidates for amniocentesis on the basis of maternal age alone is an ineffective screening method for aneuploidy.[11] Furthermore, the well-established iatrogenic fetal loss rate associated with amniocentesis[6] or chorionic villus sampling (CVS) in inexperienced hands, although low (<1%), is increasingly being regarded by patients as unacceptable, particularly when the vast majority of apparently at-risk pregnancies are chromosomally normal.

It is reassuring to note that recent evidence puts the miscarriage risk of invasive testing as no higher than the risk of spontaneous miscarriage in a particular individual.[12] In experienced hands, therefore, every patient should be offered invasive fetal testing.

Patient access to information from professional medical counseling, the internet, and, guide-books, has put forth a demand for combining maternal age, maternal serum screening and sonographic findings in order to provide individualized patient-specific risk estimates and refine selection criteria for amniocentesis.[13-15] The manner in which ultrasound information can be utilized to optimize obstetric decision-making in clinical practice is presented here.

SONOGRAPHIC MARKERS FOR DOWN SYNDROME (TRISOMY 21)

Neonatologists have for many years used morphological features to identity Down syndrome. These include a flat facial profile, epicanthal folds, short stature, a mongoloid eye slant, muscle hypotonia, a single palmar crease, excess skin over the back of the neck, hypoplastic middle digit of the fifth phalanx, sandal gap foot deformity, flat iliac wings, duodenal atresia and heart defects. Sonologists have extended morphological feature recognition to identify those fetuses at high risk for trisomy 21 using a combination of major anomalies, major markers and minor markers.

Overview of Markers

Major anomalies are seen in about one-third of affected fetuses and include heart defects particularly ventricular septal defects and atrioventricular septal defects, ventriculomegaly, cystic hygromas, omphalocele and hydrops. Major markers include a thickened nuchal skin fold, short femur, short humerus, echogenic intracardiac focus, echogenic bowel and renal pyelectasis. Minor markers include flat iliac wings, brachycephaly and frontal lobe shortening, clinodactyly, sandal gap great toe deformity, short ear length, cerebellar hypoplasia and a single palmar crease.

A few of these features represent actual structural abnormalities that have clinical consequences regardless of karyotype. Most, however, are considered traits or markers that often have no serious clinical importance with the exception of their relationship with aneuploidy. To make matters more complicated, these features may be transient, resolving by the second trimester of gestation.[16-18]

Major Markers

A thickened nuchal skin fold was the first major marker identified for trisomy 21.[19] This remains the most useful marker to date. This is measured in an axial plane through the posterior cranial fossa and calipers are placed corresponding to the outer surface of the occipital bone and the outer surface of the skin. A thickness of more than 5 mm is significant before 18 weeks of gestational age and a thickness exceeding 6 mm beyond 18 weeks.[20-22]

Although echogenic bowel is often a normal variant in the second trimester, one in eight fetuses with Down syndrome show this feature.[23-25] Bowel should be labeled echogenic only if it is brighter than adjacent bone. It also needs to be remembered that high frequency transducers and equipment with real time enhanced contrast resolution and speckle reduction software options accentuate brightness of bowel. Bowel may also be echogenic in fetuses with cystic fibrosis, mesenteric ischemia and cytomegalovirus infections. Fetuses that swallow blood from a placental bleed also show increased bowel echogenicity consequent to ingested heme pigments.

The echogenic intracardiac focus (EIF) refers to calcified papillary muscle that is seen as a bright dot on ultrasound. This is usually in the left ventricle but occasionally in the right ventricle or both ventricles. It should be as bright as bone. About 16% of fetuses with trisomy 21 and 395 of fetuses with trisomy 13 demonstrate this feature.[18,26,27] The risk for trisomy is higher if the echogenic focus is in the right ventricle or both ventricles. The prevalence of this marker in normal fetuses is as high as 30% in normal fetuses of Asian ethnic origin.[28] As an isolated marker, therefore, it does not warrant further investigation. An EIF is not associated with cardiac anomalies in low-risk patients.[17]

Pyelectasis refers to an increase in the anteroposterior diameter of the renal pelvis beyond 4 mm at 15–20 weeks of gestation. Around 20–25% of fetuses with Down syndrome demonstrate this feature.[29,30] In isolation, this marker is not an indicator for amniocentesis. It should be used in conjunction with other markers.

Short humerus and short femur are defined as an observed-to-expected length of <0.9.[26,31] The expected bone length is based on a biparietal diameter (BPD) measurement. *Expected femur length* = $-9.3105 + 0.9028 \times$ BPD. These have been identified as markers for trisomy 21 and are useful when combined with other markers.[32] A short humerus is more sensitive as a marker than a short femur.[33] Both these markers are limited by the requirement of data specific to the population being studied and by ethnic diversity. Femur/foot length ratio, although useful in assessing skeletal dysplasias are not useful in assessing for Down syndrome.[32]

Minor Markers

A widened iliac angle has been observed in children with Down syndrome and this has been extended to assessing the iliac angle in the fetuses.[34,35] The increase in angle represents an increased distance between the iliac crests and should be measured in a transverse view of the spine. The mean iliac angle is 80 ± 19.7° in fetuses with trisomy 21 and 63.1 ± 20.3° in normal fetuses. The technique of measurement is cumbersome and limits routine use of this marker. Clinodactyly refers to hypoplasia of the middle phalanx of the fifth digit and is a morphological feature of children with trisomy 21 and can be seen in the fetus as well.[3] Although initially regarded with skepticism, this marker has performed well and shows a sensitivity of 17.1% and a false positive rate of 3%.[36] A wide space between the first and second toes is seen more frequently in trisomy 21 fetuses and is called a sandal gap toe deformity. The reliability in various studies is variable.[37-39] Nasal bone hypoplasia[40] is a highly sensitive and specific marker for trisomy 21. It is a feature of 62% of trisomy 21 fetuses and approximately 1% of chromosomally normal fetuses. The nasal bone was initially considered to be hypoplastic if it was either absent or "strikingly small" (<2.5 mm). Later data[41] has described the nasal bone length increasing with gestation from a mean of 4.7 mm at 15 weeks to 8.2 mm at 22 weeks and such normative data is likely to be more specific in assessing this marker. The efficiency of using various nasal bone criteria for the detection of aneuploidy has been studied further[42] and it has been observed that the optimal nasal bone threshold associated with trisomy 21 was a BPD/nasal bone length ratio of 11 or greater. An important prerequisite to consider when using this marker is the angle of insonation of the fetal nose, which should be between 45° and 135° to avoid false shortening. Brachycephaly in fetuses with trisomy 21 reflects a frontal lobe shortening and has been assessed in several studies.[16,43,44] The frontothalamic distance was less than the 10th centile in 52% of fetuses with trisomy 21.[45] Short ear length, cerebellar hypoplasia and amniodecidual separation have been described in literature but their reliability is questionable.

SENSITIVITY OF MARKER DETECTION

There is a wide variation in the detection rates of sonographic markers of trisomy 21.[46] Strict standardization of definitions, operator experience and dedication can largely overcome this.[47]

Other variables that influence detection rates include gestational age and maternal body habitus. The detection rate rises from 1 in 8 at 15 weeks of gestation to greater than 60% after 18 weeks.[48] Serial reviews are, therefore, to be considered if the maternal abdomen is fat and hirsute and if the genetic sonogram is performed prior to 18 weeks of gestation. Pelviectasis is more frequently picked up in male fetuses.

SIGNIFICANCE OF INDIVIDUAL MARKERS

The accuracy of the genetic sonogram and the significance of each marker has been evaluated in several studies.[2,3,15,16,25,36,37,44,49-55] The Agathokleous[15] meta-analysis is currently in wide use as a reliable calculation. All studies refer to the presence of major structural anomaly, soft markers or both. Identification of at least one marker conferred an overall sensitivity of 72-77% with a false positive rate of about 13%.

Significantly, about half of all fetuses had a nuchal-fold thickness of 5 mm or more rendering this as the most sensitive individual marker. The risk of trisomy 21 increases with the number of markers detected.[25,39,49] The prevalence of isolated and multiple markers has been evaluated[14] and is simple to calculate. The absence of a marker is important as well in risk calculation.

The greatest challenge in risk assignment is where a marker is identified in isolation. If isolated soft markers are used as a basis for deciding to offer invasive testing, the resultant fetal loss rate would exceed the number of cases of trisomy 21 detected and indeed, that detection rates would fall. This assertion has been challenged by others[30] who argue that while this may confirm the poor contribution that isolated soft markers make to risk assignment for aneuploidy, the performance of combined markers has been well validated in screening paradigms and furthermore that dismissal of the role of soft markers in screening ignores the pivotal role their absence plays in providing patient reassurance and avoiding invasive testing. The unacceptably high false-positive rate associated with identification of isolated soft markers in low-risk women presents a challenge insofar as there will always be a group of low-risk women undergoing "routine" mid-trimester sonography, in whom soft markers for aneuploidy may not be actively sought but may be incidentally noted. For this, several scoring systems have been devised which correlate maternal age, serum biochemistry and sonographic markers.

A simple sonographic scoring index for the detection of chromosomal aneuploidy was devised by Benacerraf et al.[27,49] Major structural anomalies and a thickened nuchal fold were each given a score of 2, as these are sufficiently strong even when detected in isolation. Soft

Table 1: Meta-analysis of second trimester markers for trisomy 21.[15] (Agathokleous M, et al.; Ultrasound Obstet Gynecol; 2013)

Marker	DR	FPR	LR (+ve)	LR (−ve)	Isolated marker
Cardiac echogenic focus	24.4	3.9	5.8	0.80	0.95
Ventriculomegaly	7.5	0.2	27.5	0.94	3.81
Increased nuchal fold	26.0	1.0	23.3	0.80	3.79
Echogenic bowel	16.7	1.1	11.4	0.90	1.65
Mild hydronephrosis	13.9	1.7	7.6	0.92	1.08
Short humerus	30.3	4.6	4.8	0.74	0.78
Short femur	27.7	6.4	3.7	0.80	0.61
ARSA	30.7	1.5	21.5	0.71	3.94
Absent or hypoplastic NB	59.8	2.8	23.3	0.46	6.58
No markers LR 0.13 = 7.7 fold reduction					

(ARSA: aberrant right subclavian artery; DR: detection rate; FPR: false-positive rate; LR: likelihood ratio; NB: nasal bone)

markers were each allocated a score of 1. The panel of soft markers included short femur, short humerus, pyelectasis, echogenic intracardiac focus (EICF), echogenic bowel, and choroid plexus cysts. The authors demonstrated that, where amniocentesis was reserved for fetuses scoring ≥2, 73% of fetuses with trisomy 21 and 85% of fetuses with trisomy 18 could be identified with a false positive rate of 4%. Using likelihood ratios, two approaches have been proposed by Nyberg and Nicolaides to calculate a revised risk.[6] The Nyberg method involves multiplication of a priori risk by the likelihood ratio (LR) associated with any identified marker or markers. The latter calculation, proposed by Nicolaides, further takes into account the negative likelihood ratios associated with absent markers. The practical application of these two approaches in fact yields similar results. The likelihood ratios applicable in current practice are based on the Agathokleous meta-analysis and are outlined in Table 1. It is worth noting the consistently wide confidence intervals surrounding the point estimates of these likelihood ratios, inferring that while the identification of one or more markers is an effective screening tool, the actual computed risk is only an approximation.

TRISOMY 18 (EDWARDS' SYNDROME)

Ninety percent of fetuses with trisomy 18 have an abnormal early second trimester morphology and up to 100% have an abnormal third trimester morphology.

Common stigmata include choroid plexus cysts, ventriculomegaly, strawberry-shaped skull, a large cisterna magna, agenesis of the corpus callosum, meningomyeloceles, microphthalmos, hypertelorism, low-set ears, cystic hygromas, thickened nuchal skin fold, cardiac defects, diaphragmatic hernia, renal anomalies, omphalocele, short radial ray, clenched hand with overlapping fingers, rocker bottom foot, club foot, polyhydramnios, intrauterine growth restriction (IUGR) and a single umbilical artery, umbilical cord cysts and absent end diastolic umbilical artery flow velocity waveforms.

Ultrasound is often used to detect trisomy 18 when the quadruple screen shows a low alpha-fetoprotein (AFP), low βhCG and low free estriol. In addition, when choroid plexus cysts are present the search for other stigmata should be intensified. Isolated choroid plexus cysts do not warrant an amniocentesis for karyotyping.

TRISOMY 13 (PATAU SYNDROME)

Morphologic abnormalities are evident from 10 weeks onwards and the sensitivity is 90–100%. It is very unusual for an affected fetus not to have a morphological stigma.

Features include holoprosencephaly, agenesis of the corpus callosum, ventriculomegaly, enlarged cisterna magna, microcephaly, microphthalmia, hypotelorism, cyclopia, proboscis, cleft lip and palate, midline facial hypoplasia, nuchal thickening, cystic hygroma, cardiac defects, neural tube defects, echogenic enlarged kidneys, echogenic bowel, echogenic intracardiac focus, omphalocele, cystic kidneys, radial ray aplasia, polydactyly and a single umbilical artery.

TURNER SYNDROME (XO)

This is a syndrome consequent to the loss of an X chromosome, usually paternal. Most fetuses are spontaneously aborted. Ongoing pregnancies are characterized by extensive, often whole body, septated cystic hygromas, which may regress over time and persist as only a webbing of the neck in an adult. Long-term survival is associated with a short stature, ovarian dysgenesis and occasionally mental retardation. It is also associated with left heart defects especially coarctation of the aorta and aortic valvar defects, horseshoe kidney and a short femur. There may be evidence of hydrops consequence to a high output cardiac failure. Mosaicism is common, often resulting in delayed menarche.

TRIPLOIDY

This occurs as a result of a complete extra set of chromosomes. Survival beyond 20 weeks of gestation is rare.

Features include severe early onset asymmetric IUGR, microphthalmia and hypertelorism, micrognathia, ventriculomegaly, midline brain defects, cystic hygromas, omphaloceles, renal anomalies, an enlarged placenta, oligoamnios, and abnormal umbilical artery flow velocity waveforms.

GENETIC SONOGRAPHY AFTER FIRST TRIMESTER SCREENING

First trimester genetic screening is now widely available and involves assessing maternal serum biochemistry and sonographic markers in order to identify patients who should undergo invasive testing. This is carried out between 11 weeks and 13 weeks 6 days of pregnancy and has the advantage of an easier and safer termination of pregnancy and less parental psychological trauma. The combination of maternal serum pregnancy-associated plasma protein-A (PAPP-A) and free hCG along with fetal crown-rump length (CRL) to assess fetal size, and a group of ultrasound markers allows detection of 88–90% of fetuses with Down syndrome[56] (Table 2). The ultrasound markers include nuchal translucency (NT) thickness, nasal bone delineation, fetal ductus venosus studies and fetal tricuspid regurgitation. In this group of patients, sequential screening with a second trimester genetic sonogram enhances the detection rate for Down syndrome to 94–96%.

Currently, a first trimester approach with its high detection rates is the preferred method of Down syndrome screening. A screening method that detects less than 75% of affected fetuses is regarded as inappropriate[57] (Table 3). The triple test is, therefore, inadequate and should not be used.

A summary of the detection rates of various combinations of maternal characteristics, ultrasound findings and biochemical markers in the first trimester is shown here. This list includes newer methods of screening such noninvasive prenatal testing (NIPT), and additional first trimester biochemical markers such as placental growth factor (PlGF), AFP and dimeric inhibin A (DIA).

- Age (not recommended)
- CRL and NIPT (ideal for T1, misses other advantages of a T1 scan, expensive)
- Age, CRL and NT (skill)
- Age and biochemistry (poor detection rate, not recommend)
- Age + CRL + maternal factors + NT + PAPP-A + hCG (combined test)
- Age + maternal factors + CRL + NT + additional markers + biochemistry [enhanced sensitivity and low false-positive rate (FPR): time and skill]
- T1 combined test + T2 Quad (sequential or integrated)
- *T1 Quad:* Age + historical factors + PAPP-A + βhCG + PlGF + AFP (Risk for PE, NTD)
- *T1 Penta:* combined test + nasal bone + AFP + DIA + PlGF (high detection rate, low FPR).

Table 2: Screening for trisomy 21.

Methods of screening	Detection rate	False-positive rate
Maternal age (MA)	30%	5%
First trimester:		
MA + fetal nuchal translucency (NT)	75–80%	5%
MA + serum free βhCG and PAPP-A	60–70%	5%
MA + NT + free βhCG and PAPP-A (combined test)	85–95%	5%
Combined test + nasal bone or tricuspid flow or ductus venosus flow	93–96%	2.5%
Second trimester:		
MA + serum AFP, hCG, µE3 (triple test)	60–65%	5%
MA + serum AFP, hCG, µE3, inhibin A (quadruple test)	65–70%	5%
MA + NT + PAPP-A (11–13 weeks) + quadruple test	90–94%	5%

(AFP: alpha-fetoprotein; hCG: human chorionic gonadotropin; PAPP-A: pregnancy-associated plasma protein-A)

Table 3: Detection rate in various tests.

Methods of screening	Detection rate
First trimester:	
Maternal Age	30–50%
PAPP-A, hCG, MA	60–63%
NT measurement and MA	74–80%
Combine test (NT, PAPP-A, hCG, MA)	86–90%
Combined test plus nasal bone, tricuspid flow, ductus venosus and facial angle	95%
Second trimester:	
Maternal age	30–50%
2nd trimester double test (AFP, hCG, MA)	60%
Triple test (AFP, hCG, E3, MA)	68%
Quadruple test (AFP, hCG, E3, Inhibin A, MA)	79%
Ultrasound (16–33 weeks) with anomaly screening	75%
Invasive diagnostic testing:	
Chorionic villus sampling	Close to 100%
Amniocentesis	Close to 100%

(AFP: alpha-fetoprotein; E3: estriol; hCG: human chorionic gonadotropin; MA: maternal age; NT: nuchal translucency; PAPP-A: pregnancy-associated plasma protein-A)

CONCLUSION

Screening for aneuploidies has shifted from the second trimester to the 11 weeks to 13 weeks 6 days window. This has the additional advantage of screening for fetal size, number and viability, structural defects and screening for pre-eclampsia and fetal growth restriction. The genetic sonogram refines screening for patients who refuse invasive testing for a positive first trimester screen. Second trimester quadruple screening should be used only for those patients where the first trimester screening was missed or was unreliable.

REFERENCES

1. Benacerraf BR. The role of the second trimester genetic sonogram in screening for fetal Down syndrome. Semin Perinatol. 2005;29(6):386-34.
2. DeVore GR, Alfi O. The use of color Doppler ultrasound to identify fetuses at increased risk for trisomy 21: an alternative for high-risk patients who decline genetic amniocentesis. Obstet Gynecol. 1995;85(3):378-86.
3. Nadel AS, Bromley B, Frigoletto FD Jr, et al. Can the presumed risk of autosomal trisomy be decreased in fetuses of older women following a normal sonogram? J Ultrasound Med. 1995;14(4):297-302.
4. Nyberg DA, Luthy DA, Cheng EY, et al. Role of prenatal ultrasonography in women with positive screen for Down syndrome on the basis of maternal serum markers. Am J Obstet Gynecol. 1995;173(4):1030-5.
5. Vintzileos AM, Egan JF. Adjusting the risk for trisomy 21 on the basis of second-trimester ultrasonography. Am J Obstet Gynecol. 1995;172(3):837-44.
6. Breathnach FM, Fleming A, Malone FD. The second trimester genetic sonogram. Am J Med Genet C Semin Med Genet. 2007;145(1):62-72.
7. Hook EB. Chromosome abnormalities: prevalence, risk and recurrences. In: Brock DJ, Rodeck CH, Ferguson-Smith MA (Eds). Prenatal Diagnosis and Screening. Edinburgh, Scotland: Churchill Livingstone; 1998. pp. 351-92.
8. Ferguson-Smith MA, Yates JR. Maternal age specific rates for chromosome aberrations and factors influencing them: report of a collaborative European study on 52 965 amniocenteses. Prenat Diagn. 1984;4 Spec No:5-44.
9. Snijders RJ, Sebire NJ, Nicolaides KH. Maternal age and gestational age-specific risk for chromosomal defects. Fetal Diagn Ther. 1995;10(6):356-67.
10. DeVore GR. Trisomy 21: 91% detection rate using second-trimester ultrasound markers. Ultrasound Obstet Gynecol. 2000;16(2):133-41.
11. Nicolaides KH. Screening for chromosomal defects. Ultrasound Obstet Gynecol. 2003;21(4):313-21.
12. Salomon LJ, Sotiriadis A, Wulff CB, et al. Risk of miscarriage following amniocentesis or chorionic villus sampling: systematic review of literature and updated meta-analysis. Ultrasound Obstet Gynecol. 2019;54(4):442-51.
13. Nicolaides KH, Snijders RJ, Gosden CM, et al. Ultrasonographically detectable markers of fetal chromosomal abnormalities. Lancet. 1992;340(8821):704-7.
14. Nyberg DA, Souter VL. Sonographic markers of fetal trisomies: second trimester. J Ultrasound Med. 2001;20(6):655-74.
15. Agathokleous M, Chaveeva P, Poon LC, et al. Meta-analysis of second-trimester markers for trisomy 21. Ultrasound Obstet Gynecol. 2013;41(3):247-61.
16. Bromley B, Lieberman E, Shipp TD, et al. The genetic sonogram: a method of risk assessment for Down syndrome in the second trimester. J Ultrasound Med. 2002;21(10):1087-96.
17. Achiron R, Lipitz S, Gabbay U, et al. Prenatal ultrasonographic diagnosis of fetal heart echogenic foci: no correlation with Down syndrome. Obstet Gynecol. 1997;89(6):945-8.
18. Bromley B, Benacerraf BR. The resolving nuchal fold in second trimester fetuses: not necessarily reassuring. J Ultrasound Med. 1995;14(3):253-5.
19. Benacerraf BR, Frigoletto FD Jr, Laboda LA. Sonographic diagnosis of Down syndrome in the second trimester. Am J Obstet Gynecol. 1985;153(1):49-52.
20. Gray DL, Crane JP. Optimal nuchal skin-fold thresholds based on gestational age for prenatal detection of Down syndrome. Am J Obstet Gynecol. 1994;171(5):1282-6.
21. Bahado-Singh RO, Oz UA, Kovanci E, et al. Gestational age standardized nuchal thickness values for estimating mid-trimester Down's syndrome risk. J Matern Fetal Med. 1999;8(2):37-43.
22. Locatelli A, Piccoli MG, Vergani P, et al. Critical appraisal of the use of nuchal fold thickness measurements for the prediction of Down syndrome. Am J Obstet Gynecol. 2000;182(1 Pt 1):192-7.
23. Nyberg DA, Kramer D, Resta RG, et al. Prenatal sonographic findings of trisomy 18: review of 47 cases. J Ultrasound Med. 1993;12(2):103-13.
24. Nicolaides KH, Salvesen DR, Snijders RJ, et al. Strawberry-shaped skull in fetal trisomy 18. Fetal Diagn Ther. 1992;7(2):132-7.
25. Nyberg DA, Luthy DA, Resta RG, et al. Age-adjusted ultrasound risk assessment for fetal Down's syndrome during the second trimester: description of the method and analysis of 142 cases. Ultrasound Obstet Gynecol. 1998;12(1):8-14.
26. Benacerraf BR, Gelman R, Frigoletto FD Jr. Sonographic identification of second-trimester fetuses with Down's syndrome. N Engl J Med. 1987;317(22):1371-6.
27. Benacerraf BR, Neuberg D, Bromley B, et al. Sonographic scoring index for prenatal detection of chromosomal abnormalities. J Ultrasound Med. 1992;11(9):449-58.
28. Shipp TD, Bromley B, Lieberman E, et al. The frequency of the detection of fetal echogenic intracardiac foci with respect to maternal race. Ultrasound Obstet Gynecol. 2000;15(6):460-2.
29. Nyberg DA, Souter VL, El-Bastawissi A, et al. Isolated sonographic markers for detection of fetal Down syndrome in the second trimester of pregnancy. J Ultrasound Med. 2001;20(10):1053-63.
30. Hobbins JC, Bahado-Singh RO, Lezotte DC. The genetic sonogram in screening for Down syndrome: response to the JAMA study. J Ultrasound Med. 2001;20(6):569-72.
31. Lockwood C, Benacerraf B, Krinsky A, et al. A sonographic screening method for Down syndrome. Am J Obstet Gynecol. 1987;157(4 Pt 1):803-8.

32. Grandjean H, Sarramon MF. Femur/foot length ratio for detection of Down syndrome: results of a multicenter prospective study. Am J Obstet Gynecol. 1995;173(1):16-9.
33. FitzSimmons J, Droste S, Shepard TH, et al. Long-bone growth in fetuses with Down syndrome. Am J Obstet Gynecol. 1989;161(5):1174-7.
34. Shipp TD, Bromley B, Lieberman E, et al. The second-trimester fetal iliac angle as a sign of Down's syndrome. Ultrasound Obstet Gynecol. 1998; 12(1):15-8.
35. Bork MD, Egan JF, Cusick W, et al. Iliac wing angle as a marker for trisomy 21 in the second trimester. Obstet Gynecol. 1997; 89(5 Pt 1):734-7.
36. Deren O, Mahoney MJ, Copel JA, et al. Subtle ultrasonographic anomalies: do they improve the Down syndrome detection rate? Am J Obstet Gynecol. 1998;178(3):441-5.
37. Hobbins JC, Lezotte DC, Persutte WH, et al. An 8-center study to evaluate the utility of mid-term genetic sonograms among high-risk pregnancies. J Ultrasound Med. 2003;22(1):33-8.
38. Yeo L, Vintzileos AM. The use of genetic sonography to reduce the need for amniocentesis in women at high-risk for Down syndrome. Semin Perinatol. 2003;27(2):152-9.
39. Vintzileos AM, Campbell WA, Guzman ER, et al. Second-trimester ultrasound markers for detection of trisomy 21: which markers are best? Obstet Gynecol. 1997;89(6):941-4.
40. Cicero S, Sonek JD, McKenna DS, et al. Nasal bone hypoplasia in trisomy 21 at 15-22 weeks' gestation. Ultrasound Obstet Gynecol. 2003;21(1):15-8.
41. Guis F, Ville Y, Vincent Y, et al. Ultrasound evaluation of the length of the fetal nasal bones throughout gestation. Ultrasound Obstet Gynecol. 1995;5(5):304-7.
42. Odibo AO, Sehdev HM, Dunn L, et al. The association between fetal nasal bone hypoplasia and aneuploidy. Obstet Gynecol. 2004;104(6):1229-33.
43. Winter TC, Reichman JA, Luna JA, et al. Frontal lobe shortening in second-trimester fetuses with trisomy 21: usefulness as a US marker. Radiology. 1998;207(1):215-22.
44. Sohl BD, Scioscia AL, Budorick NE, et al. Utility of minor ultrasonographic markers in the prediction of abnormal fetal karyotype at a prenatal diagnostic center. Am J Obstet Gynecol. 1999;181(4):898-903.
45. Bahado-Singh R, Oz U, Kovanci E, et al. A high-sensitivity alternative to "routine" genetic amniocentesis: multiple urinary analytes, nuchal thickness, and age. Am J Obstet Gynecol. 1999;180(1 Pt 1):169-73.
46. Shipp TD, Benacerraf BR. Second trimester ultrasound screening for chromosomal abnormalities. Prenat Diagn. 2002;22(4):296-307.
47. Smith-Bindman R, Hosmer WD, Caponigro M, et al. The variability in the interpretation of prenatal diagnostic ultrasound. Ultrasound Obstet Gynecol. 2001;17(4):326-32.
48. Taslimi MM, Acosta R, Chueh J, et al. Detection of sonographic markers of fetal aneuploidy depends on maternal and fetal characteristics. J Ultrasound Med. 2005;24(6):811-5.
49. Benacerraf BR, Nadel A, Bromley B. Identification of second-trimester fetuses with autosomal trisomy by use of a sonographic scoring index. Radiology. 1994;193(1):135-40.
50. Bahado-Singh RO, Tan A, Deren O, et al. Risk of Down syndrome and any clinically significant chromosome defect in pregnancies with abnormal triple-screen and normal targeted ultrasonographic results. Am J Obstet Gynecol. 1996;175(4 Pt 1):824-9.
51. Bahado-Singh RO, Oz AU, Kovanci E, et al. New Down syndrome screening algorithm: ultrasonographic biometry and multiple serum markers combined with maternal age. Am J Obstet Gynecol. 1998;179(6 Pt 1):1627-31.
52. Verdin SM, Economides DL. The role of ultrasonographic markers for trisomy 21 in women with positive serum biochemistry. Br J Obstet Gynaecol. 1998;105(1):63-7.
53. Vintzileos AM, Guzman ER, Smulian JC, et al. Indication-specific accuracy of second-trimester genetic ultrasonography for the detection of trisomy 21. Am J Obstet Gynecol. 1999;181(5 Pt 1):1045-8.
54. Vergani P, Locatelli A, Piccoli MG, et al. Best second trimester sonographic markers for the detection of trisomy 21. J Ultrasound Med. 1999;18(7):469-73.
55. Smith-Bindman R, Hosmer W, Feldstein VA, et al. Second-trimester ultrasound to detect fetuses with Down syndrome: a meta-analysis. JAMA. 2001;285(8):1044-55.
56. Nicolaides KH. Screening for fetal aneuploidies at 11 to 13 weeks. Prenat Diagn 2011;31:7-15.
57. Benn P, Borrell A, Chiu RW, et al. Position statement from the Chromosome Abnormality Screening Committee on behalf of the Board of the International Society for Prenatal Diagnosis. Prenat Diagn. 2015;35(8):725-34.

22
Fetal Medicine Beyond Ultrasound
Pramod Vasantrao Patil

INTRODUCTION
- More than 95% will deliver a healthy baby
- 4–5% will have problems:
  - Structural
  - Genetic
  - Growth
- Prenatal evaluation—a boon
- Universal screening

ROLE OF FETAL MEDICINE SPECIALIST
- *Understanding natural history and course of fetal disorders*:
  - Best example of this is increased nuchal translucency (NT) can have variable outcomes
  - Increased NT can manifest as Tetralogy of Fallot
  - Increased NT can manifest as chromosomal abnormality like Down syndrome
  - Increased NT can manifest as single gene disorder like mucopolysaccharidosis
  - Increased NT—decision making
  - Terminate pregnancy
  - Immediate prenatal invasive procedure
  - IInd trimester amniocentesis + Structural scan
  - >95% of increased NTs with normal KT and normal heart will result in normal childbirth
- *Early and accurate diagnosis*:
  - High-resolution ultrasonography (USG)
  - The shift of targeted scan to 1st trimester
  - Multisystem anomaly
  - *Solving the puzzle:* For example, imaging specialist-posterior fossa cyst + cleft lip and cleft palate (CLCP)
  - *Fetal medicine specialist + Geneticist*:
    - Pallister-Hall syndrome

We can perform prenatal diagnostic procedures like:
- Chorionic villous sampling
- Amniocentesis
- Cordocentesis
- *Counseling:*
  - Counseling can be pre-pregnancy counseling or during pregnancy.
  - Accurate pedigree drawing helps to arrive at pattern of inheritance.
  - It helps in explaining different modes of inheritance such as:
    - Autosomal dominant
    - Autosomal recessive
    - X-linked dominant
    - X-linked recessive
- *Obstetric decision making*:
  - When and where to deliver?
  - Assessment of fetal well-being
  - *Fetal growth restriction:*
    - Diagnosis and classification
    - When to do Doppler and how to interpret?
    - Decision based on Doppler
- *Index case workup with geneticist*:
  - Term small for gestational age (SGA), history of delayed milestone, and failure to gain weight
  - Karyotype 46,XX,del(4)(q12q13.2)
  - Interstitial deletion of chromosome—rare
  - Parental karyotype done—normal
  - Recurrence low in subsequent pregnancies
  - Low recurrence risk
  - Numerical
  - De novo structural

- *Offer treatment in specific conditions*:
  - Intrauterine transfusion in Rh isoimmunization
  - Intra-amniotic installation of thyroxine in fetal goiter
  - Intra-amniotic installation/IM of digoxin in fetal supraventricular tachycardia
  - Thoracoamniotic shunts in pleural effusions/congenital cystic adenomatoid malformation (CCAM)
  - Urinary shunts for bladder outlet obstruction (BOO), distended bladder
  - Fetoscopic laser ablation of anastomotic vessels in monochorionic diamniotic (MCDA) twins
- Complete diagnosis with the help of perinatal pathologist
- *Message*: The job of fetal medicine specialist:
  - Start screening early 11–12 weeks
  - *Counseling*:
    - Premarital
    - Prepregnancy
  - Judicious use of prenatal invasive procedures
  - "Termination of pregnancy only in cases with dismal outcome".

CONCLUSION

The joy of prenatal care—a fetal medicine specialist is one who:
- Does a clinical examination of fetus
- Understands fetal physiology
- Knows how to counsel the patient
- Knows when "not" to intervene
- Reassures the patient.

23
Pre-conception and Pre-natal Diagnostic Techniques: How to Comply with the Law?

Hitesh J Bhatt

INTRODUCTION

When the Medical Termination of Pregnancy (MTP) got legalized in 1972 by an MTP Act in India, authorities thought that it will help India and solve all the problems related to population and poverty. This was correct to the extent that it made abortions safer than before. Then sonography was added as a diagnostic device in the armamentarium of diagnostic tools for the doctors. It became easy to see fetus in utero as well. The problem started when doctors started looking at the sex of the fetus upon requests by the patients. As such, it is a routine practice in the foreign countries. In India, the social situation is quite different from those countries. In India, female child is looked upon as a burden on the family. Due to customs like dowry and undue importance of the male child, females are considered as a liability rather than an asset.

The combination of sonography and MTP Act along with doctors came to help society in its aim to abolish female child even before her birth. This immoral work was done unopposed as there was high demand and there was no law to prevent it!. This continuous demand and supply changed the sex ratio to the extent that only 800 girls were getting born as against 1,000 males. Suddenly, some NGOs and Government became alert and a case was filed in the Supreme Court and as a result, the Pre-natal Diagnostic Techniques (PNDT) Act was formed and it came into existence in 1994.

This is a presumptive act. Presumption of crime is taken when act or any of its rules are not followed. So, please follow all the sections and rules strictly.

DO'S IN PRE-CONCEPTION AND PRE-NATAL DIAGNOSTIC TECHNIQUES ACT[1]

- Registration of place is must and any change in place, person, employee, address, and equipment installed should be intimated to the appropriate authority at least 30 days in advance of such change and should get such change incorporated in the certificate (Rule 13/2).
- Display a board that "sex determination is a punishable crime and prohibited at our place" at conspicuous place in both in English and local language (board should include name and address of clinic also (Rule 17).
 Also, display form B in original (your registration certificate) in waiting room (Rule 6/2).
- It is must to have nameplate on the dress worn by the employee (Rule 18/8).
- Before doing sonography, first fill up form F with full detail of the patient (Part A) and declaration by patient Rule 10 1A (Part D), then do sonography. For accidently diagnosed pregnancy while doing sonography—or abdomen or pelvis, one should fill form F before patient leaves the clinic.
- Always maintain PNDT register 9(1)—make one register showing serial no, name and address of men and woman given genetic counseling or prenatal diagnostic procedures, name of husband/father, date on which they reported first for counseling, procedure, and test.
- Maintain all records [form F, consent form G (in case of invasive procedures)], sonography plate, slides, and referral notes, for minimum 2 years.
- In case the genetic counseling center or genetic laboratory, genetic clinic, ultrasound clinic, or imaging

center maintains records on computer or other electronic equipment, a printed copy of the record shall be taken and preserved after authentication by a person responsible for such record (Rule 9/7).
- In case of closing or selling the clinic or center, change of ownership, change in management, or cessation of function of center, surrender the PNDT registration certificate to appropriate authority (Rule 6/6).
- Keep at least one copy of (bare act) PNDT act in outpatient department (OPD) (Rule 17).
- If your clinic is under renovation and temporary shifting your all machines and staff in different area and place—no need for separate or new PNDT registration, but appropriate authority (AA) has to be informed 30 days in advance of such a change in address with changes duly incorporated into the certificate. Make all applications in duplicate and keep one copy with you taking signature of AA on it "as received" for acknowledgment (Rule 13).
- Keep information, education and communication (IEC) material from Government such as Female Foeticide is Heinous Crime, Beti Bachao Beti Padhao poster at your OPD (supplied by Government authority).
- Renewal date of registration should always be remembered and make an application for renewal in form A at least before 30 days of expiry to the appropriate authority office in duplicate. Please have acknowledgment of the same from authority (Rule 8/1).
- Always send form F monthly report to Government office before 5th of next month (Rule 9/8) and keep record for 2 years at your clinic (Rule 9/6). In case of litigation, till final disposition of the case or 2 years, whichever is late.
- Always cooperate with the authority whenever they visit for inspection.
- Never panic. Be careful before giving signature on commission of offence on inspection. Take time to consult your medicolegal advisor.
- Never sale your machine without proper advised by the lawyer or medicolegal consultant.
- Always give answer to show cause notice related to violation of the Pre-conception and Pre-natal Diagnostic Techniques (PCPNDT) Act in reasonable time to Government authority as prescribed in the notice.
- If records are maintained on computer or other electronic format, a printed copy of the record shall be taken and preserved after authentication by a person responsible for such record (Rule 9/7).
- In vitro fertilization (IVF) centers, assisted reproductive technologies (ARTs), and magnetic resonance imaging (MRI) machines should also be registered under the PNDT Act.
- Always write name and designation in full under the signature (Rule 18/9).

DON'TS IN PRE-CONCEPTION AND PRE-NATAL DIAGNOSTIC TECHNIQUES ACT

- Never do sonography at unregistered place.
- Rules for portable sonography are strict so never do it at any nearer or far place even on request.
- Do not hesitate to refuse or do not promote sonography at polyclinic run by BHMS, DHMS, or unauthorized person. As such if center is registered by appropriate authority owner could be anybody, but if you are visiting sonologist, do not do or encourage sex determination or preconception sex selection in any situation.
- Do not do sonography at more than two places in one district. One cannot visit more than two centers (Rule 3/3).
- Do not hire unqualified person at your clinic.
- Do not encourage patient or person (agent) for sex determination. Any inquiry should be refused at reception counter, and not allowed to enter in your consulting room.
- Do not forget date of your renewal of PNDT registration.
- Do not make any change in original form F prescribed under Act.
- Do not forget monthly report of form F before 5th (of next month).
- Do not make any change in sonography unit, place, or management without prior intimation to appropriate authority before 30 days of expected change.
- Do not sale sonography machine to unregistered place, agent, or do not buy from unauthorized agent or person or unregistered center.
- Do not do sonography without written declaration of patient in form F.
- Do not publish any advertisement relating to pre-conception sex selection and/or prenatal sex determination.
- Do not ignore any new direction or amendment by government authority in the PCPNDT Act.
- Do not get involved in any argument, hot discussion, or misbehave with authority when they come for inspection at your clinic.
- Do not tamper any records after notice issued by Government authority to you in case of violation of the PCPNDT Act.
- Do not send sample to unregistered laboratory in case of invasive procedures, e.g., chorionic villus sampling, amniocentesis, etc. Laboratory should also be registered under the PCPNDT Act.
- Do not forget to send report of form F—nil or zero (even if you have not done single sonography in month).
- Do not forget to inform Government authority in writing in duplicate in event of temporary closure of your

clinic because of renovation or foreign tour or some other reason and keep the sonography machine in safe custody.
- Never allow your hospital staff to sign in Panchanama as a witness in the event of sealing of your sonography machine. Never confess or admit or sign anywhere which mentions that you have done a mistake (because your first confession makes it difficult in court of law to prove your innocence).

CONCLUSION

Pre-natal Diagnostic Techniques is very strict act, this is made so to prevent sex determination high handedly. To save ourself from the punishment under this law, we must follow all the sections and rules of this act. We also should start giving names of the patients asking for sex determination to appropriate authority so that necessary actions can be taken against them as well. There will not be supply if there is no demand. Lets hope for better society and lets support government in its aim to curb female foeticide.

REFERENCE

1. Wikipedia, Acts of the Parliament of India (1994). The Pre-Conception and Pre-Natal Diagnostic Techniques (Prohibition of Sex Selection) Act (PCPNDT Act) and Rules. [online] Available from https://en.wikipedia.org/wiki/Pre-Conception_and_Pre-Natal_Diagnostic_Techniques_Act,_1994#:~:targetText=Pre%2DConception%20and%20Pre%2DNatal%20Diagnostic%20Techniques%20(PCPNDT),act%20banned%20prenatal%20sex%20determination [Last accessed November, 2019].

24
Writing an Ultrasound Report

Chinmay Umarji

INTRODUCTION

Writing an ultrasound report is an integral part of ultrasound scanning which in itself is a learned skill. The report is the communication between sonographer and the treating doctor and as it usually passes through the hands of the patient, it assumes multidimensional significance.

It conveys imaging, it is interpretation and the clinical relevance, diagnosis or prognosis of the patient or the fetus which helps the treating doctor in counseling and planning the treatment. Clarity of the ultrasound report and counseling of the sonographer increases the continuity of care and thus improves patient satisfaction.

AIDS TO THE REPORT WRITING

- A software has now become an integral part of the report writing. It provides easy recovery, safe storage and back up of the reports; also helps with image transfer and storage. Of the many softwares available, some are accredited by international bodies and provide various calculators, e.g., aneuploidy risks, preterm delivery, fetal growth restriction (FGR), pre-eclampsia, middle cerebral artery-peak systolic velocity (MCA-PSV) multiples of median (MoM), ovarian cancer risks, etc. This makes the reports more clinically relevant and aids in patient management. While choosing a software, it is important to make sure of their service (Fig. 1).
- Statutory compliance as per the Preconception and Prenatal Diagnostic Techniques (Prohibition of Sex Selection) (PCPNDT) act is a must. There are certain softwares which can help with the same (Fig. 2).

ATTRIBUTES OF THE REPORT WRITING

- *Demographic accuracy*: Right patient, right test, right report. It is the first and foremost important step which must be followed by everyone involved in the

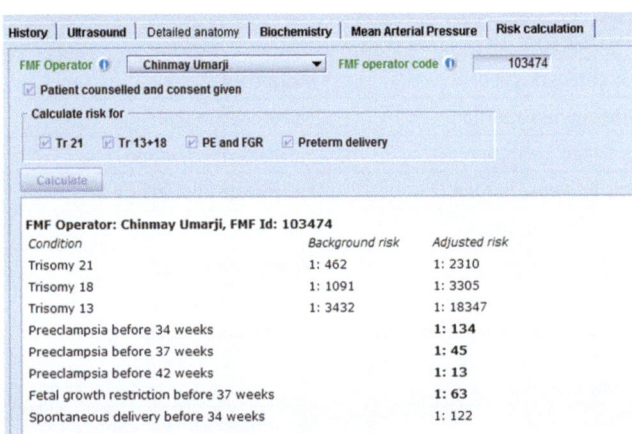

Fig. 1: An example of OBGYN medical software.

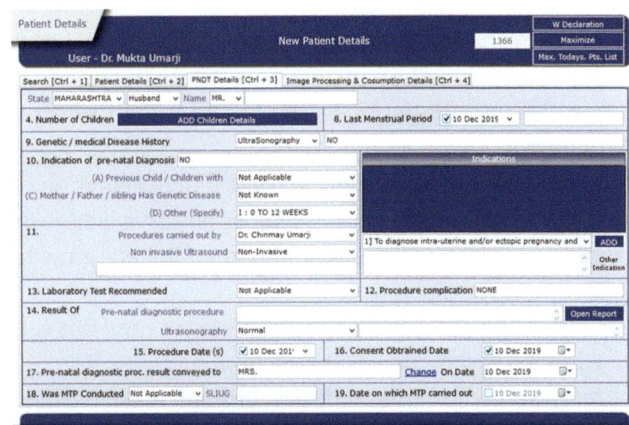

Fig. 2: Sample form of a medical software.

care and an easy way to avoid errors is two parameter confirmation, e.g., name and date of birth.
- *Clinical accuracy*: Patient history, examination findings especially pre-existing diseases, family history, previous obstetric history, etc. may make some ultrasound findings more significant. Thus, it is important to record this accurately, e.g., risk factors for pre-eclampsia, FGR, menopausal status of woman with an ovarian mass, etc.
- *Sonographic parameters in clinical relevance*: It is important to record relevant ultrasound findings in an easy manner which can make the findings clearer to a clinician. One must refrain from using parameters of only academic/research significance and follow the guidelines by the reputed organizations. A standardized examination procedure makes report writing easy, clinically relevant and improves the diagnosis. Also, a note reflecting the actual process that examination was made with a chaperone, two sonographers confirmed a diagnosis, e.g., of an intrauterine fetal death (IUFD) helps with the standardization of the procedure as per the national and international norms.
- *Diagnosis*: It should be clear, unambiguous and phrases used should be in accordance with the current practices/guidelines, e.g., blighted ovum should not be used and replaced by pregnancy of uncertain viability.
- *Prognosis/further management*: As a sonographer has a unique advantage of knowing clinical as well as live ultrasound attributes of a patient, it is important that they give clinician and the patient a feedback about the prognosis of a condition. This helps better continuity of care, more patient satisfaction and aids clinician in counseling. It is important to be on the same page with the clinician to avoid confusion and a clear communication with the clinician aids the same.
- In case if a further test or referral is needed, the same should be clearly mentioned and an offer should be made by the sonologist as well as clinician to make an appointment for the patient. This is especially important for pregnant patients, as they need urgent referral pathways.
- Report should contain the graphical representation of the attributes wherever possible as it makes diagnosis and counseling easier, e.g., nomograms for fetal growth, Doppler (Fig. 5).
- Counseling becomes easier with diagrams and this can go a long way in patient satisfaction.
- *Images and clips*: These help the clinicians in establishing accuracy of the findings, patient counseling and are a must in an examination.
- *Supporting patient information leaflets, websites, guidelines or references*: These further aid in clinical communication and counseling.
- *Statutory requirement*: PCPNDT act mandates a declaration at the end of the report in a prescribed format also a copy of section D of Form F to be carried by the patient and this statutory requirement needs to be followed in every report.

CLINICAL CONTENT OF REPORT WRITING

As discussed earlier, this section of report writing needs to stick to the national and international norms so as to make the diagnosis accurate, clear, concise and aid patient counseling. Following are some examples where the report must follow the standard language and avoid confusion.
- *Early pregnancy*: Using the terms miscarriage and abortions interchangeably causes a lot of patient confusion and should be abandoned. Terminologies like blighted ovum are now obsolete. Adherence to the current terminologies shall reduce confusion[1,2] (Table 1).
- *Multiple pregnancy* report should clearly mention chorionicity, number of pregnancies, there should be a recorded image of lambda or T-sign (Fig. 3).[3,4]
- *Nuchal translucency (NT) scan*: It is important to offer this scan after accurately measuring the crown–rump length (CRL) which should be between 45 and 84 mm. A good software will notify the operator if the CRL is beyond this range, and also help with various calculations, nomograms, etc.[5] (Figs. 4 and 5).
- *Anomaly scan*: It should be preceded by patient counseling clearly mentioning advantages and limitations of the scans[6] (Fig. 6).

Table 1: Terminologies to be used for early pregnancy scanning.

Previous term	New term
Spontaneous abortion	Miscarriage
Threatened abortion	Threatened miscarriage
Inevitable abortion	Inevitable miscarriage
Incomplete abortion	Incomplete miscarriage
Complete abortion	Complete miscarriage
Missed abortion	Missed miscarriage
Anembryonic pregnancy/blighted ovum (these reflect different delayed miscarriage stages in the same process)	• Early fetal demise • Silent miscarriage
Septic abortion	Miscarriage with infection (sepsis)
Recurrent abortion	Recurrent miscarriage

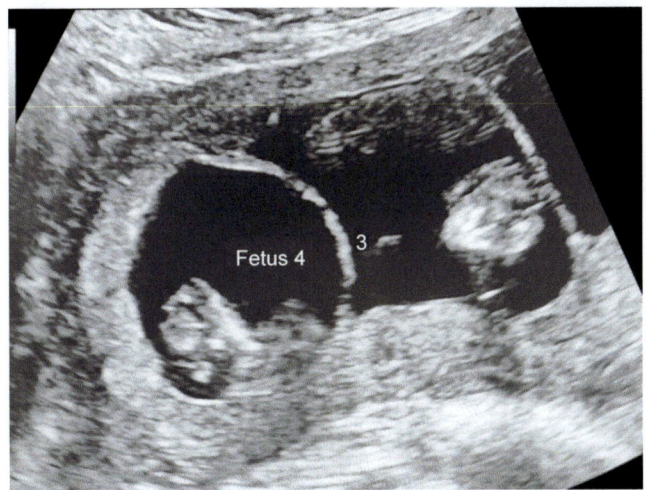

Fig. 3: Documentation of intertwin membrane.

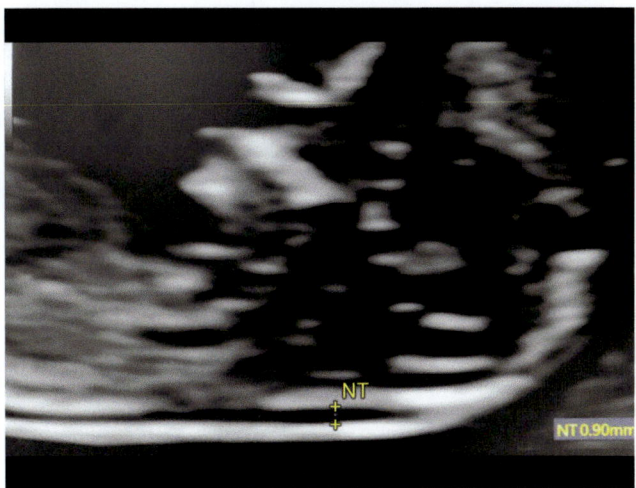

Fig. 4: Sampling of nuchal translucency (NT).

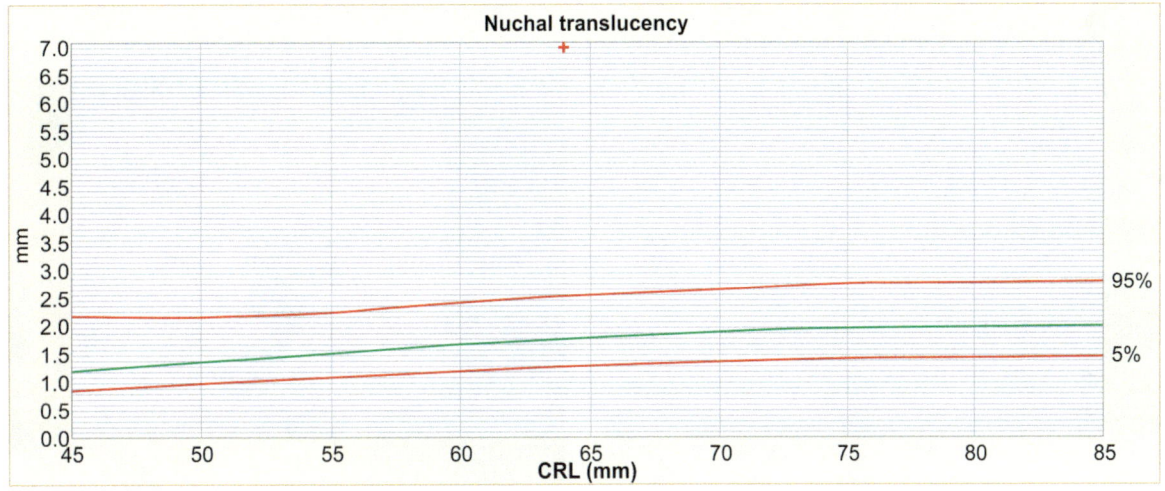

Fig. 5: Nomogram of nuchal translucency (CRL: crown-rump length).
Source: Wright D, Kagan KO, Molina FS, et al. A mixture model of nuchal translucency thickness in screening for chromosomal defects. Ultrasound Obstet Gynecol. 2008;31:376-83.

- *Growth scan*: It should include the parameters with nomograms clearly indicating the growth curve of the fetus. A fetal growth restriction should trigger fetal Doppler assessment[7] (Fig. 7).
- For postmenopausal bleeding, offer transvaginal ultrasound. The pelvic ultrasound report should note—endometrial thickness (ET) (measuring the anteroposterior (AP) 2-layer thickness in the sagittal plane near the fundus), suspected polyps, uterine size, ovarian morphology, presence of fibroids, presence of ascites[8] (Fig. 8).

REPORT STORAGE

It is important to understand that most of the times in Indian settings, patients carry their own reports to the treating consultant and it is suggested that there should be an extra copy for the patient and the consultant in addition to the sonographer's copy. With the advent of three-dimensional (3D) and four-dimensional (4D) ultrasound, obstetric ultrasound examination has started becoming more of an event for the family. They look forward to it as a bonding opportunity with the baby and the partner and getting the souvenirs in the form of images (Fig. 9). This should be supported when possible.

Storage of the report should be in accordance with the existing acts such as PCPNDT for specified duration.

Declaration of interests: Author has not taken any grants or funding from the products displayed in the text.

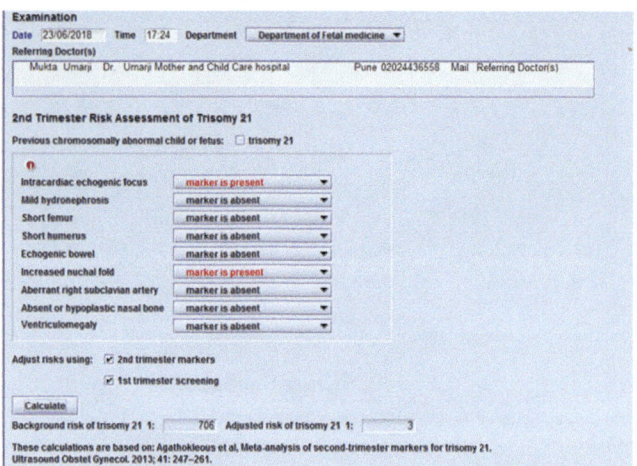

Fig. 6: Documentation of anomaly scan depicting normal variants for aneuploidy risk calculation. *Note:* Findings of more than one variants is associated with increased risk of aneuploidies.
Source: Agathokleous M, Chaveeva P, Poon LCY, et al. Meta-analysis of second-trimester markers for trisomy 21. Ultrasound Obstet Gynecol. 2013;41:247-61.

Fig. 7: Nomogram depicting fetal growth restriction.
Source: Yudkin PL, Aboualfa M, Eyre JA, et al. New birthweight and head circumference centiles for gestational ages 24 to 42 weeks. Early Hum Dev. 1987;15:45-520.

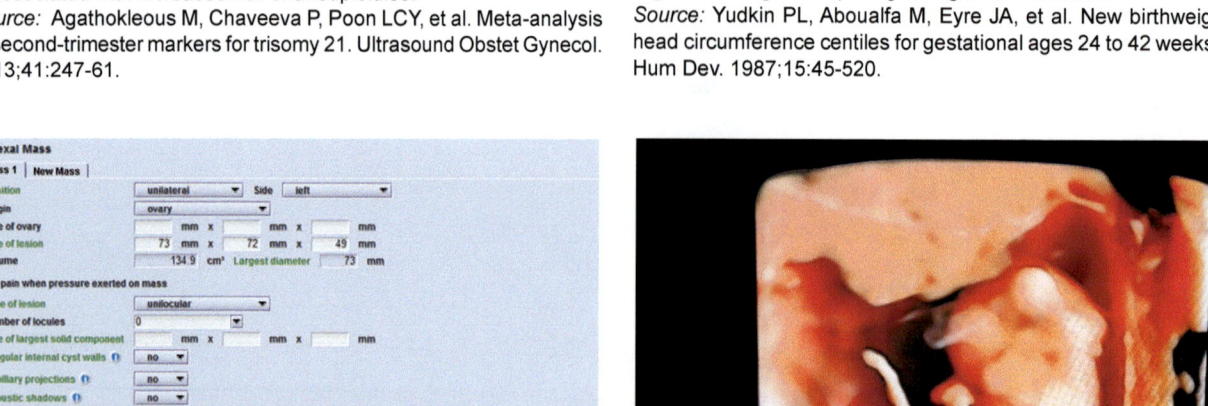

Fig. 8: Software with checklist helps with detailed assessment of adnexal masses.

Fig. 9: Reports can be emotional boosters for the pregnant couple. A 3D image at NT helps with bonding with the baby.

REFERENCES

1. RCOG (2006). Green-top guidelines: Early Pregnancy Loss, Management (Green-top Guideline No. 25). [online] Available from https://www.rcog.org.uk/en/guidelines-research-services/guidelines/gtg25/. [Last Accessed December, 2019].
2. NICE (2019). Ectopic pregnancy and miscarriage: diagnosis and initial management: NICE guideline [NG126]. [online] Available from https://www.nice.org.uk/guidance/ng126. [Last Accessed December, 2019].
3. Images are real life cases drawn from Astraia Obstetrics and Gynaecology database and Diagnoflame ultrasound softwares.
4. RCOG (2016). Green-top guidelines No. 51. Monochorionic twin pregnancy. [online] Available from https://www.rcog.org.uk/en/guidelines-research-services/guidelines/gtg51/. [Last Accessed December, 2019].
5. Fetal medicine foundation: First trimester scan. [online] Available from: https://fetalmedicine.org/fmf.certification/certificates.of.competence/nuchal.translucency.scan#:~:text=Sonographers%20who%20have%20obtained%20the,-hCG%20and%20PAPP-A.
6. ISUOG. Practice guidelines. [online] Available from https://www.isuog.org/clinical-resources/isuog-guidelines/practice-guidelines-english.html. [Last Accessed December, 2019].
7. RCOG Green-top guidelines no. 31. Fetal growth restriction. [online] Available from: https://www.rcog.org.uk/en/guidelines-research-services/guidelines/gtg31/
8. Norfolk and Norwich University Hospitals NHS Foundation Trust (NHS NNUH).

25
Training in Ultrasound in Obstetrics and Gynecology

S Suresh, Indrani Suresh

INTRODUCTION

Over the last few decades, there has been a steady increase in the applications of clinical ultrasound in almost every branch of medicine. Needless to say that ultrasound has become an integral part of women's healthcare and the last two decades has witnessed the integration of ultrasound in obstetric and gynecological practice. Rapid technological advances and increasing availability of equipment at an affordable cost have brought this modality within the reach of the common man and is now available as a "point of care" equipment. Endless debates whether ultrasound should be used in unselected populations have been put to rest and we have truly moved from an era of "obstetric ultrasound" to "ultrasonographic obstetrics" [Professor Yves Ville, Editorial, Ultrasound in Obstetrics and Gynecology (UOG) Journal, January 2006]. The use of ultrasound in obstetrics and gynecology helps in monitoring the pregnancy from conception to delivery and the push toward early screening and diagnosis has resulted in earlier and more accurate dating, diagnosis of birth defects, screening for aneuploidy and pre-eclampsia. Doppler ultrasound has added the ability to manage fetal growth restriction better and time the delivery appropriately thus improving perinatal outcomes. Ultrasound has also become an essential component of gynecological and infertility care.

Technological advances and increasing number of scans being done pose the risk of increasing interpretation errors if adequate training is not imparted. There is no dispute to the fact that ultrasound is a highly "operator dependent modality". The last two decades have also seen the emergence of "fetal medicine" as a subspecialty. Fetal cardiology and fetal therapy are fast becoming subspecialties in their own right! The day is not far off when fetal neurology, urology, and gastroenterology emerge as subspecialties. The fundamental requirement, therefore, is to establish a robust system of training in OBGYN ultrasound and a methodology to assess competence with certification from an authority which will be accepted as a standard. Errors in diagnosis can be minimized by a combination of proper training in understanding the use and limitations of the equipment. We will now consider how this can be achieved.

Who and When should Ultrasound Training be Imparted?

All obstetricians and gynecologists should be able to do basic ultrasound as it is an essential tool for routine clinical decision-making. Hence, there is an urgent need for incorporating ultrasound training as part of the postgraduate training in a structured manner with experienced personnel. The training should result in assessment and certification of competence and should be ideally achieved during the second year of postgraduate training.

What Constitutes "Basic Level Training"?

The basic level training in obstetric ultrasound should aim to impart theoretical knowledge of normal anatomy of the developing fetus at each gestational age, dating and growth assessment using biometry, the placenta, liquor assessment and the fundamentals of assessment of fetal and uteroplacental blood flow. The training should also include knowledge of the most common abnormalities and ability to know when to refer the patient to the next higher center.

In gynecological ultrasound, the trainee should possess the theoretical knowledge of normal ultrasound anatomy of the pelvis, appearances of common gynecological conditions and invasive procedures.

Theoretical training should be accompanied by a logbook of cases and the candidate should log in a minimum number of cases at least 200 obstetric and 100 gynecological cases, according to the standard prescribed by the European Board and College of Obstetrics and Gynecology. In India, the standard requirement can be drawn up by a national body such as Federation of Obstetric and Gynaecological Societies of India (FOGSI).

The bigger challenge is in providing "hands on" training as the "learning curve" of each trainee is different. Most training programs across the world have an unstructured hands-on training due to the paucity of trainers and difficulties of patient acceptance and time availability.

The Educational Committee of the International Society of Ultrasound in Obstetrics and Gynecology (ISUOG) has brought out revised recommendations for basic training for trainees in the year 2003. These recommendations can be considered as a consensus-based approach in formulating a structured training program for residents in India.

What Constitutes Training Basic in Obstetric and Gynecology Ultrasound?

International Society of Ultrasound in Obstetrics and Gynecology recommends considering basic training under three headings:

Step 1: Theoretical which includes didactic lectures and online learning modules complemented by reading textbooks and journal articles. They also suggest that the guidelines issued by ISUOG should also form part of the training. The ISUOG basic training task force has drawn up a curriculum (BT curriculum) which constitutes 30 lectures which are available online or can be run as a 4 day theoretical course. The author of this chapter is a member of this task force and we have piloted this program in his own institution and also at the Sri Ramachandra Medical College. At the time of writing this chapter, the program has been planned for two more rural areas in the coming months. The program can be administered easily and ISUOG provides support for the same. Further details can be seen at www.isuog.org under the heading training.

Theoretical training and certification modules are also available from the Fetal Medicine Foundation, the United Kingdom and a number of private centers in India. The FOGSI training program needs to be restructured, in accordance with international recommendations fine-tuned for Indian conditions.

Step 2: Practical should happen under formal supervision. The trainees should be taught how to perform ultrasound examinations and how to document and report findings and this step must include a logbook of cases done with a standardized reporting format. This is the most challenging part of training and requires a large number of skilled personnel with time for supervision.

It is time to leverage the availability of simulators and artificial intelligence to impart basic hands on skills. Though at present, these are expensive, with increasing demand, the costs are likely to come down.

Step 3: Examination—the trainee should undergo an examination to assess their theoretical knowledge and it is recommended that they undertake a practical assessment of the technical skills learnt in Steps 1 and 2.

Practical training: The practical training should aim to impart a standardized and systematic examination technique.

For obstetric ultrasound, the following checklist is recommended:
- Fetal presentation and lie.
- Fetal viability and fetal movements
- Demonstration of presence of a singleton or multiple pregnancy
- Assessment of gestational age and comparison of biometric values with gestational age
- Assessment of fetal size by recording biometric measurements
- Descriptive evaluation of amount of amniotic fluid
- Evaluation of placental appearance and location

For gynecological examination, the recommended checklist is:
- Visualization of uterus in longitudinal and transverse planes
- Measurement of endometrial thickness
- Assessment of size and morphology of ovaries
- Evaluation of presence or absence of fluid in the pelvis
- Description of any abnormality.

CERTIFICATION

This is the biggest challenge in any training program since the learning curve is highly variable. ISUOG recommends—A minimum of 100 hours of supervised scanning, to include:
- A minimum of 100 obstetric scans covering a wide spectrum of obstetric conditions
- A minimum of 100 gynecological examinations, some of which involving early pregnancy complications.

LOGBOOK

The logbook recommended by ISUOG should include a set of standard ultrasound images obtained from scans they themselves have performed, and that also documents patient history, indication and findings, and includes a formal ultrasound scan report.

TRAINING FOR RURAL INDIA

In a first experiment of its kind, MediScan in association with National Rural Health Mission conducted a basic training program for 352 rural medical officers in 176 primary health centers across 11 districts of Tamil Nadu in 2013. A 12-day program was conducted at the primary health center for each district and for the next 1 year, all images were audited online by experts. The skill sets of the medical officers were assessed by the quality of images. In 1 year, 65,000 scans were done and 1980 abnormal ultrasound were reported. This was a unique experiment which established the fact that basic training was feasible and could be done on a scale.

TRAINING OF PRACTITIONERS

In addition to residents being trained, it is important to address the need for training of current practitioners. The same curriculum can be adopted with mechanisms of certification to be addressed by the national body. There are several training centers across the country and a uniform curriculum would go a long way in standardizing performance and reporting and planning higher level training. This will also improve the confidence and trust of patients in the system.

CONCLUSION

It is time to include a structured quality controlled basic training program in basic obstetric ultrasound in India. This is feasible and the urgent need is to form a national task force to evolve a strategy for implementing basic training in accordance with international recommendations adapted to India. This will go a long way in improving quality of ultrasound and significantly improve women's healthcare in India. The debate must move from "who can do and who cannot do ultrasound" to "How to improve the quality and standards of ultrasound". This alone will make an impact on society.

Index

Page numbers followed by *b* refer to box, *f* refer to figure, and *t* refer to table

A

Abdomen 107
    axial view of 157*f*-159*f*
Abdominal circumference 70, 104, 105, 133, 134*f*
Abdominal distension 70
Abnormal ductus venosus waveforms 85*f*
Abortion 46
    complete 75
    incomplete 75
    missed 75, 76*f*
    threatened 74
Abruptio placentae 80, 80*f*
Absent end-diastolic flow 135, 137*f*
Acardiac twin 98
Acardius acephalus 99
Acardius amorphous 99
Acardius myelacephalus 99
Adenomyoma 29*t*, 32
Adenomyosis 29, 29*f*, 59, 61*f*
    color flow pattern of 29*f*
    ultrasound features of 61*t*
Adherent placenta 167
Adhesions 51
Adnexa 17, 52, 82
    assessment of 68
    solid masses of 72
    ultrasound of 70
Adnexal mass 87*f*
    classification of 28
    near ovary 67*f*
Adnexal ovarian torsion 30
Adnexal pregnancy 68*f*
Adnexal torsion 70, 72
Allister-Hall syndrome 184
Alpha-fetoprotein 180, 181
American College of Obstetricians and Gynecologists 132, 136, 147
American College of Radiology 132
American Institute of Ultrasound in Medicine 132
Amniocentesis 146, 146*f*, 177, 184
    indications for 145
Amniotic cavities 95*f*
Amniotic fluid 23, 124, 124*f*, 157*f*
    assessment 124
    dynamics 125*f*
    index 126, 132, 173
        percentile values 127*t*
        technique for 126*f*
    old blood-stained 146*f*
    volume 124, 125*f*, 131, 136
        assessment 129
        measurement of 125
        normal 125
Amniotic membrane 84*f*
Anal atresia 158, 161
Andometrioma, complex 51
Anembryonic pregnancy 75
Anencephaly 107
Aneuploidy
    risks 189
    screening for 94
Angiogenesis around follicle 35*f*
Angiotensin-converting enzyme inhibitors 127
Anorectal malformations 161
    surgical repair of 162
Antenatal care 131
Antepartum fetal surveillance 135
Anteroposterior abdominal diameter 104, 105
Anti-Müllerian hormone 42
Antral follicle 36
    count 42, 42*f*, 43, 62
Aortic isthmus Doppler 138
Arcuate uterus 59
Asherman's syndrome 60
Assisted reproductive technology 67, 187
Asynchronous color flow imaging 26
Atrial septal defect 95
Atrioventricular septal defect 108*f*
Atypical endometriotic cyst 50*f*
Axial diffusion-weighted imaging 51

B

Backache 70
Benign adnexal masses, causes of 70
Beta-human chorionic gonadotropin 74, 82, 177
Biophysical profile 135
    score 135
Biopsy 52
Biparietal diameter 104, 105, 133, 134*f*
Bladder
    outlet obstruction 185
    wall-serosa interface 116*f*
Bleeding
    causes of 74
    in late pregnancy 78
    in obstetrics, ultrasonography for 74
    per vaginum 153
    subacute 51
Blighted ovum 75*f*, 86, 86*f*
Blood velocity 25
Body mass index 42, 43
Bowel
    atresia 158, 165
    lumen 17*f*
    muscularis 17*f*
Brain 22, 23, 107
Bronchopulmonary sequestration 140

C

Cancer antigen 125 50
Cardiac anomalies 141, 158
Cardiac defects 158
Cardiotocography 135
    computerized 96
Cardiovascular system 129
Caudal regression syndrome 161
Cell-free deoxyribonucleic acid 94
Central cord insertion, normal 120*f*
Central nervous system 95, 129, 139
Cephalopagus conjoined twins 98*f*
Cerebral ventriculomegaly, bilateral 107*f*
Cerebroplacental ratio 135, 137
Cervical
    canal 16*f*, 77*f*
    glands 16*f*
    insufficiency 80, 80*f*
    length assessment 104, 109
    pregnancy 77*f*
Cervix 16, 55, 66
    assessment of 110*f*
    carcinoma of 35
Chocolate cysts 32
Choledochal cyst 164
Chorioamnionitis 153

Chorioangioma
    gross specimen of 119f
    placental 119f
    vascularity of 119f
Chorionic plate 167
Chorionic villus sampling 94, 145, 147, 147f, 177, 184
Chorionicity, ultrasound signs of 92t
Chronic endometriotic deposits 51
Chylothorax 153
Circle of Willis, HD-live flow of 21f
Circummarginate placenta 113f
Circumvallate placenta 113f
Clear cell carcinoma 28
Cleft lip 107, 108f, 184
Cleft palate 129, 184
Cobweb pattern 63f, 71
Cogwheel appearance 72
Coiling abnormalities 120
Color Doppler 3, 25
    in infertility, role of 35
    settings 6
Color flow, role of 25
Complex extra-adnexal cyst 78
Computed tomography scan 49, 51
Congenital anomalies, absence of 135t
Congenital cystic adenomatoid malformation 152
Congenital diaphragmatic hernia 141, 141f, 144, 152
    repair of 152
    treatment of 153
Congenital pulmonary airway malformation 140, 141
    thoracoamniotic shunt for 152
Congenital pulmonary airway obstruction 154
Conjoined twins 97
    classification of 97t
Continuous wave Doppler 26
Cord cyst 121, 121f
Cordocentesis 184
Corpus callosum agenesis 139f
Corpus luteal flow, normal 47f
Corpus luteum 34f, 63, 63f
    color Doppler of 38f
Crescent sign 55, 56f
Crown-rump length 74, 82, 84f, 92, 133, 191f
Cul-de-sac 67f
Cyst adenoma 64
Cystic fibrosis 165
Cystic hygroma 129
Cytomegalovirus 146
    infection, diagnosis of 112f

D

Decidual cyst 78
Deep infiltrating endometriosis 52, 65
Deep peritoneal implants 52
Deepest vertical pocket 101
Degenerating leiomyoma 176
Delivery, timing of 96, 102
Deoxyribonucleic acid 147
Dermoid cyst 64, 70, 71, 71f
Diaphragmatic hernia 107
Dichorionic diamniotic
    pregnancy 95f
    twins 125
Dichorionic pregnancy 94-96
Dichorionic twins 126
Didelphys uterus 59
Dizygotic twins 90
Doppler 3, 56
    angle 9
    bold spectrum of 9f
    calculations in 26
    frequency 3
    in gynecology, use of 27
    safety of 11
    types of 26
    velocity waveform 25
Double bubble sign 140
Down syndrome 144, 158, 177, 178, 184
Ductus venosus 100, 105, 138f
    agenesis 162
        extrahepatic type of 162f
        types of 162
    Doppler 137
Duodenal atresia 158, 158t, 159f
    differential diagnosis of 158b
Dysgerminoma 28

E

Early pregnancy 92, 190
    failure 85
    scan 85
Echogenic bowel 164, 165f
    grading of 165t
Ectopic endometrial glands 51
Ectopic pregnancy 33, 34f, 67, 67f, 68f, 69, 87, 175
    types of 68
    ultrasound of 67
Edwards' syndrome 177, 180
Electrical interferences 11
Electronic fetal monitoring 173f
Embryo 83
    transfer 39
Endometrial blood flow 39
Endometrial carcinoma 34, 35f, 63f
    ultrasound in 62
Endometrial cavity 37f
    fluid in 60, 62f
Endometrial flow 6f, 18f
Endometrial motion 39
Endometrial polyp 29, 60, 62f
Endometrial thickness 39, 63f
Endometrial vascularity 45, 46t
Endometrioma 28, 32, 32f, 51, 63, 63f, 70, 71

Endometrio-myometrial junctional zone 116f
Endometriosis 31, 32, 49, 53, 65
    imaging 49
        techniques for 52
    sites of 52, 52t
Endometriotic cyst 50f, 64
Endometriotic nodules 32f
Endometritis 34
Endometrium 15, 37f, 42, 47, 47f, 55, 66
    changes in 37
    Doppler features of 45
    hypoechoic inner layer of 37f
    like glands 32
    measurement of 59
Endomyometrial junction 56, 57f
Enteric duplication cyst 163
Enterolithiasis 161
Epithelial carcinoma 28
Esophageal atresia 156, 157f, 157t
Estimated fetal weight 132, 135
Estriol 181
European Board and College of Obstetrics and Gynecology 194
European Society of Urogenital Radiology 51
Exomphalos 107
Extrachorial placentation 113
Extrauterine fetal cardiac activity 78
Extrauterine pregnancies 76, 78f
Extremities 22, 23

F

Face 23, 107
Fallot's tetralogy 141f
Federation of Obstetric and Gynaecological Societies of India 194
Female pelvis, ultrasound examination of 13
Femur length 104, 105
Fetal abdomen 156
Fetal activity 167
Fetal anomalies 107t
    scan, targeted imaging for 104, 106
Fetal arrhythmias 150
Fetal biometry 104
Fetal blood
    flow, disruption of 117
    sampling 148
Fetal bradycardia 74
Fetal cardiac activity 132
Fetal central nervous system abnormalities 139
Fetal cord blood sampling 148f
Fetal disorders, prenatal diagnosis of 144
Fetal Doppler 136
Fetal face 22
    HD-live mode for 21f
    multiplanar view of 20f
    surface rendering of 20f
Fetal gastrointestinal anomalies 140
Fetal genitourinary anomalies 140

Fetal growth 131
    restriction 95, 96, 105, 127, 133, 135, 135t, 167, 184, 189
        early-onset growth charts 134f
        late-onset growth charts 134f
    surveillance 133
Fetal head
    attitude 170
    descent 170
    tomographic ultrasound imaging of 20f
Fetal heart
    color spatiotemporal image correlation of 20f
    inversion mode for 21f
    rate 136
    sound 173
Fetal infection 146
Fetal intervention 144
Fetal medical therapy 149
Fetal medicine 144, 184
Fetal middle cerebral artery 135
Fetal musculoskeletal abnormalities 142
Fetal occiput, position of 170, 171t
Fetal spinal column, omniview of 21f
Fetal structural abnormalities 129b
Fetal surgery 149, 152
    prerequisites for 152
    principles of 152
Fetal therapy 144, 149
Fetal tracheal occlusion 152
Fetal tumors 129
Fetal weight estimation 133
Fetal well-being, assessment of 168
Fetoscopic fetal surgery 153
Fetoscopic surgery 149
    limitations of 153
Fetoscopic tracheal occlusion 153
Fetus papyraceus 96
Fibroids 29t, 59, 61f
    ultrasound features of 61t
Fibroma 28
Fibrotic endometriotic deposits 51
First trimester
    placenta, normal 112f
    ultrasound in 82
Fission theory 97
Flow index 58f
Fluorescent in situ hybridization 177
Follicle 63
    B-mode image of 4f
    pulse Doppler image of 44f
    stimulating hormone 42
Follicular ring sign 66
Fraternal twins 90
Free beta-human chorionic gonadotropin 94
Functional cysts 28
Fusion
    defects 59
    theory 97

G

Gastrointestinal system 129
Gastrointestinal tract 156
    anomalies 156
    malformations 156t
Gastroschisis 107
Genetic counseling 144
Genitourinary system 129
Germ cell tumor 28
Gestation sac 75f-77f
Gestational age 134f, 135
    appropriate for 105f
    fetus growth charts, appropriate for 134f
    function of 125f
    growth charts, large for 135f
    large for 133
Gestational sac 46, 82, 83, 83f, 84f, 86f, 88f
Gestational trophoblastic
    disease 32, 65, 76
    neoplasia 33
    tumors 33
Goitre 129
Gonadotropin-releasing hormone 29
Granulosa cell tumor 28
Graves' disease 150
Ground-glass appearance 63, 63f
Growth scan 191
Gynecology, ultrasound in 55

H

Head and neck 129
Head circumference 104, 105, 133
Head-perineum distance 171
    measurement of 172f
Head-symphysis distance 171
    measurement of 172f
Heart 22, 23, 107
    block, complete 150
Hematoma 115f, 117
    collection of 80f
Hematometra 61
Hemoglobin 100
Hemorrhage, subchorionic 74
Hemorrhagic cyst 32, 34f, 64, 70, 71
Hepatic calcification 161
Hepatic cyst 164
Heterogeneous myometrium 29f
Heterotopic pregnancy 78f
High pulse repetition frequency 10f
High-definition flow Doppler 18f
High-resistance
    umbilical artery Doppler 137f
    uterine artery flow waveform 46f
High-resolution ultrasonography 184
Human chorionic gonadotropin 32, 44, 67, 181
Hydrosalpinx 70, 72
Hydrothorax, primary 152

Hyperplasia
    congenital adrenal 149
    endometrial 60
Hyperthyroidism 150
Hypoplastic uterus 59
Hypothyroid fetus 150
Hysterectomy 116f

I

Iliac flow 28
In vitro fertilization 37, 43, 187
Inferior vena cava 162f
Infertility 63, 67
    monitories 25
    ultrasound in 42
Injury, mechanism of 96
Insonation, angle of 25, 56
International Endometrial Tumor Analysis Group 59
International Ovarian Tumor Analysis 28, 64, 72
    Classification 28
    Collaboration 64
    Guidelines 72t
    Terminologies 28
International Society of Ultrasound in Obstetrics and Gynecology 104, 133, 148, 194
Intertwin membrane, documentation of 191f
Intra-amniotic hemorrhage 165
Intracranial lesions 175
Intrapartum ultrasonography 142
Intrauterine adhesion 60
    ultrasonography features of 60
Intrauterine contraceptive device 67
Intrauterine device 91
Intrauterine growth restriction 25, 105, 133, 157, 165
Intrauterine insemination 16, 39, 42
Intrauterine pregnancy 78, 78f
Intrauterine transfusion 150
Intravenous immunoglobulin, maternal administration of 149
Invasive diagnostic tests 49
Invasive mole 77f
Irregular gestational sac 74
Irregular periods 70

J

Jejunal atresia 159f
Jejunoileal atresia 159f

L

Labor, assessment of progress of 170
Lace-like pattern 71
Lambda sign 92
Laparoscopy 52
Large subchorionic hematoma 86f

Length abnormalities 120
Light-emitting diode 12
Limbs 107
    abnormalities 158
Low spiral artery resistance index 35*f*
Lower segment uterine contraction 115*f*
Low-resistance tortuous vessels 32*f*
Lung
    malformations, congenital 140
    maturity, steroids for 149
Luteal phase scan 37
Luteinized unruptured follicle 36
Luteinizing hormone 44

M

Magnesium sulfate, maternal administration of 149
Magnetic resonance imaging 49, 51, 175
    machines 187
Malignant adnexal masses 72
Malignant teratoma 28
Malignant uterine tumors 34
Marginal hematoma 167
Mass
    ground-glass appearance of 32*f*
    lesions 15
Maternal blood flow, disruption of 116
Maternal human immunodeficiency virus 150
Maternal serum alpha-fetoprotein 177
Maternal transmissible infectious disease 146
Mature cystic teratoma 71
Mature follicle
    B-mode features of 43
    B-mode ultrasound image of 44*f*
Mature teratoma 28
Mean sac diameter 74, 83
Meconium ileus 160, 160*f*
Meconium peritonitis 161
Meconium pseudocyst 164, 164*f*
Medical software, sample form of 189*f*
Meigs syndrome 28
Membranes
    funneling of 110*f*
    premature rupture of 127, 153, 167
Meningocele 139*f*
Meningomyelocele 144, 152
    fetal surgery for 152
    surgery for 152
Menstrual cycle 27, 28*t*
    study of 35
Mesenteric cyst 164
Middle cerebral artery 138*f*, 189
    Doppler 136
    peak systolic velocity 100, 150
Midtrimester scan 106*f*
Miscarriage 88*f*
    incomplete 85
    missed 86, 86*f*
    threatened 74

Modified biophysical profile 136
Molar pregnancy 86
Molar tissue, penetration of 77*f*
Monochorionic diamniotic twins 99*f*, 101*f*, 126, 185
Monochorionic fetuses, reduction in 152
Monochorionic monoamniotic twins 90, 102
Monochorionic pregnancy 94-97
Monochorionic twin 90*f*, 95*f*, 100*f*, 126
    pregnancy 94, 96, 97
    classification of 96
Monozygotic twins 90, 90*f*
    genesis of 91
Morbidly adherent placenta 79, 167, 175
Morphological uterus sonographic assessment 59
Mucinous cystadenocarcinoma 28
Mucinous cystadenoma 28
Mucopolysaccharidosis 184
Müllerian duct abnormalities 15
Multicystic dysplastic kidneys 108*f*
Multifetal gestation 91, 94, 95
    invasive prenatal diagnosis in 94
    mechanism of 90
Multifetal pregnancy
    monitoring of 93
    reduction 151
Multilocular cyst 64
Multiple gestation, diagnosis of 92
Multiple pregnancy 87, 90, 102, 149, 190
Multiplex ligation-dependent probe amplification 147
Myometrial blood flow 38*f*, 39
Myometrial contraction 39
Myometrial cysts 29*f*
Myometrial echogenicity 39
Myometrial lesions 61*f*
Myometrium 15, 16*f*, 55, 66, 116*f*
    homogeneous 38*f*
    homogenicity of 15

N

National Cancer Institute 35
Neck 107
Negative predictive values 92
Neonatal intensive care unit 127, 141
Next generation sequencing 147
Nodule, subcutaneous 53*f*
Nonassisted reproductive technology 39
Noninvasive diagnostic tests 49
Noninvasive prenatal testing 181
Noninvasive transplacental route 149
Nonsteroidal anti-inflammatory drugs 127
Nonstress test 135, 173
Nuchal translucency 82, 85*f*, 181, 184
    nomogram of 191*f*
    sampling of 191*f*
    scan 190
    thickness 94

O

Obgyn medical software 189*f*
Obstetrics
    and gynecology, training in ultrasound in 193
    four-dimensional ultrasound in 19
    three-dimensional ultrasound in 19
Obstructive uropathy 152, 153
Occipitofrontal diameter 104, 105
OEIS syndrome 161
Oligohydramnios 101*f*, 112*f*, 127, 165
Open fetal surgery 149, 152
Open spina bifida 107
Ovarian cyst aspiration 152
Ovarian fibroma 72
Ovarian fossae, peritoneum of 52
Ovarian hyperstimulation syndrome 25, 42
Ovarian masses 28, 63
Ovarian polycystic sonomorphology 64*f*
Ovarian stimulation 25
Ovarian stromal
    flow 18*f*, 43*f*
    resistance index 42
Ovarian torsion 30*f*
Ovarian vessels 28
    resistance index for 28*t*
Ovarian volume 36, 42, 43*f*
Ovary 51, 62, 66
    changes in 35
    corpus luteum in 65*f*
    power Doppler in 58*f*
    three-dimensional ultrasound image of 42*f*

P

Pain, acute abdominal 175
Painful umbilical swelling 54*f*
Parasitic twin 97
Paratubal cyst 70, 72
Partial hydatidiform mole 76
Partial vesicular mole 76*f*
Patau syndrome 177, 180
Peak systolic velocity 42, 43, 47, 136, 189
Pedicle artery sign 30, 30*f*
Pelvic
    congestion syndrome 34
    inflammatory disease 32, 72
    mass 70
    organs, sonography of 13
    pain 70
    wall scars 52
Percutaneous ultrasound-guided fetal shunts 153
Perifollicular flow 18*f*
Peritoneal cavity 78
Peritoneal endometriosis 32
Peritoneal inclusion cysts 70, 72
Persistent right umbilical vein 163

Placenta 109f
    accreta 79, 116f
        spectrum 114, 116f
    anatomy of 112f
    normal 111
    percreta 79f
    previa 78, 108f, 113, 114f
        complete 79f
        transvaginal ultrasound of 168f, 169f
    separation of 80f
    succenturiate lobe of 79f
    thickening of 80
Placental abnormalities 111
Placental abruption 80, 113, 167, 176
Placental calcification 118
Placental cord insertion site 133
Placental growth factor 181
Placental hematoma, types of 117f
Placental lacuna 168f
Placental localization 104, 108
Placental location 133
Placental tumors 118
Plasma protein-A, pregnancy-associated 94, 181
Pleuroamniotic shunt 152
Polycystic ovary 28, 71
    disease 70
    syndrome 60, 63, 64f
Polyhydramnios 101f, 113f, 128, 129b
    causes of 128b
Poor decidual reaction 75
Positive predictive value 30, 92
Positive urine pregnancy test 87f
Positron emission tomography scan 52
Postovulation corpus luteum 63
Potassium chloride 151f
Pouch of Douglas 32, 52
Power Doppler 5
    settings 6
Pre-conception and Pre-natal Diagnostic Techniques 186
    (Prohibition of Sex Selection) Act 189
    Act 186, 187
    Registered Center in India 145
Pre-eclampsia 189
Pregnancy 65, 111
    first trimester of 22
    loss, recurrent 60
    medical termination of 186
    poor prognostication of 88f
    prognostication of 87
Preterm delivery 113, 189
Preterm labor, high chances of 153
Pretrigger endometrium, B-mode features of 45
Previous cesarean scar 87f
    endometriosis 53f
Prostaglandin synthetase inhibitors 129
Pseudocysts 72
Pseudogestational sac 78

Pseudomyxoma peritonei 28
Pulsatility index 28, 39, 47, 135
Pulse
    Doppler 47
    repetition frequency 7, 9, 44
Pulsed wave Doppler 8, 26, 26f
Pyometra 61

Q

Quantitative fluorescent 147
    polymerase chain reaction studies 177
Quintero classification 101t

R

Reactive nonstress test 174f
Renal anomalies 158
Reporting pelvic ultrasound 66, 66b
Reproduction, uterine scoring system for 39
Resistance index 28, 43
Resorption defects 59
Respiratory system 129
Reticular pattern 71
Retrochorionic hematoma 86f
Retroplacental collection 167
Retroplacental hematoma, two-dimensional ultrasound image of 117f
Retroplacental hypervascularity 168f
Retroplacental myometrium, thickening of 80
Ring of fire sign 78
Rubella 146

S

Sacrococcygeal teratoma 144
    ligation of 152
    surgery for 153
Saline infusion sonography 30, 30f
Scanning angle 1
Scanning depth 2
Scar
    dehiscence 81
    ectopic pregnancy 34
        diagnostic criteria for 34
    pregnancy 87f
    tissues 15
Second trimester
    biometry 105f
    placenta, normal 112f
    scan, scope of 104
    ultrasound in 104
    uterine artery Doppler studies in 108
Selective fetal
    growth restriction 95, 96
    reduction 151
Septate uterus 59
Serious cardiac abnormalities 107
Serious cystadenocarcinoma 28
Serosa 55
Serous cystadenoma 28

Sex cord tumor 28
Simple adnexal cyst 78
Simple cyst 70, 71f
Single gene disorder 184
Single umbilical artery 118, 120f
Sirenomelia 161
Skeletal system 129
Skills training 23
Skull 107
Sliding sign 51, 55
Small arteriovenous anastomoses 100f
Small bowel atresia 140f, 159
Small for gestational age 113, 133
    age fetus growth charts 134f
Small gestational sac 74
Small stomach 157
Sonography-based automated volume count 19, 20, 64f
Sonography-based volume computer-aided display 19, 21
Spatiotemporal image correlation 19, 20
    fetal heart 21f
Spectral Doppler 5
Spider web appearance 72
Spinal column, skeletal mode for 22f
Spine 107
Splenic cyst 164
Splitting sign 56
Standard fetal biometric measurements 105t
Stomach
    absence of 157, 157f
    nonvisualization of 157
String appearance, beads of 72
Stroma outside uterus 32
Subchorionic hematoma 75f, 167
    two-dimensional ultrasound image of 117f
Subdiaphragmatic vestibulum 162f
Submucous myoma 62f
Succenturiate lobe 112f
Synchronous color flow imaging 26

T

Tachycardia, supraventricular 150
Telemedicine 19
Tetralogy of Fallot 95, 184
Thecoma 72
Third trimester ultrasound 131, 132
Thorax 107
    axial view of 156
    sagittal view of 156
Thrombosis 175
Thyroid
    disorders 150
    stimulating hormone 150
Tomographic ultrasound imaging 19, 20
Torsion 66
Toxoplasma 146
Tracheoesophageal fistula 158
Transabdominal diameter 104

Transabdominal route 13
Transabdominal scan 13f, 14f, 55, 56
Transabdominal sonography 82, 114
Transabdominal ultrasonography 113
    scan 51
Transabdominal ultrasound 114f
    imaging 171f
Transplacental route 149
Transrectal route 13
Transrectal ultrasonography 49
Transvaginal color Doppler 32
Transvaginal probe 14f
Transvaginal route 13
Transvaginal scan 42, 55, 56, 115f
Transvaginal sonography 45, 68, 70, 75, 82,
    110, 114
Transvaginal ultrasonography 49, 50, 50f,
    51, 53f
Transverse abdominal diameter 105
Triamniotic trichorionic triplet pregnancy 87f
Triploidy 177, 180
Trisomy 13 177, 180
Trisomy 18 177, 180
Trisomy 21 177, 178
    screening for 181t
Trophoblastic diseases 76
T-sign 92
Tubal ectopic gestation 78f
Tubal ring sign 78
Tubo-ovarian abscess 70, 72
Turner syndrome 177, 180
Twin anemia polycythemia sequence 92,
    99, 99f, 100
    management of 92
Twin pregnancy
    incidence of 92t
    management of 94, 96
Twin reversed arterial perfusion sequence
    98, 152
    management of 92
Twin-to-twin transfusion syndrome 92, 100,
    101, 101f, 144, 152
    management of 92
Typical Doppler waveform 25f
Typical ovarian endometriomas 52

U

Ultrasonography 38, 50, 55, 70, 175
    limitations of 51
Ultrasound 1, 42, 48, 90, 104
    appearance 157
    frequency 25
    guided interventions 149, 150
    machine, basic principles of 1
    modalities of 56
    practice, empowerment of 22
    scan 50
    screening 94
Umbilical artery 100, 135
    Doppler 136
        normal 137f
Umbilical coiling index 120
Umbilical cord 119f
    abnormalities of 118
    knot 122f
Umbilical endometriosis
    primary 52
    secondary 52
Umbilical vein 100, 162f
Unicornuate uterus 59
Unilocular cyst 64
Upper gastrointestinal obstruction 128
Ureteropelvic junction 95
Urinary bladder endometriosis 52
Urinary tract dilatation 140f
Uterine anomalies, congenital 58, 60f
Uterine artery 18f, 109f, 135
    Doppler
        flow 39
            studies 104, 108
    flows, normal 109f
    high-resistance flows in 109f
    pulsatility index 46
Uterine biophysical profile 38
Uterine cavity 87f
Uterine fundus 87f
Uterine masses 28
Uterine perfusion 36
Uterine rupture 81
Uterine scoring system for reproduction
    scores 39, 40t
Uterine wall 75f
Uterocervical gland 16f
Uterosacral ligament 53f
Uterus 52, 66, 78, 82
    B-mode image of 3f, 4f, 16f
    endometrium of 61f
    high-definition flow of 58f
    power Doppler in 58f
    transverse
        diameter measurement of 17f
        section of 17f
    ultrasound 57f
    ultrasound color Doppler flow in 58f

V

Vaginal bleeding during pregnancy 74
Vasa previa 79, 79f, 111, 120
Vascular tissue, penetration of 79f
Vascularization-flow index 58
Velamentous cord insertion 120f
Ventriculoamniotic shunts 154
Vertebral anomalies 158
Vertebral defects 158
Vesicoamniotic shunt 152
Vesicouterine fold 52
Vesicular mole
    complete 76f
    snowstorm appearance of 87f

W

Waist sign 72
Wall motion filter 6, 7, 9
Weight loss 70
Whirlpool sign 31f
World Health Organization 131
Writing ultrasound report 189

Y

Yolk sac 75f, 77f, 83, 84f, 88f

Z

Z-score 133